Leadership for

EVIDENCE-BASED INNOVATION

in Nursing and Health Professions

Edited by

Daniel Weberg, PhD, MHI, BSN, RN
Director, Nursing Innovation
Kaiser Permanente
Oakland, California
Auxiliary Faculty
College of Nursing
Ohio State University
Columbus, Ohio

Sandra Davidson, PhD, MSN, RN
Dean and Professor
Faculty of Nursing
University of Calgary
Calgary, Alberta, Canada

JONES & BARTLETT
LEARNING

World Headquarters
Jones & Bartlett Learning
5 Wall Street
Burlington, MA 01803
978-443-5000
info@jblearning.com
www.jblearning.com

Jones & Bartlett Learning books and products are available through most bookstores and online booksellers. To contact Jones & Bartlett Learning directly, call 800-832-0034, fax 978-443-8000, or visit our website, www.jblearning.com.

Substantial discounts on bulk quantities of Jones & Bartlett Learning publications are available to corporations, professional associations, and other qualified organizations. For details and specific discount information, contact the special sales department at Jones & Bartlett Learning via the above contact information or send an email to specialsales@jblearning.com.

Production Credits
VP, Product Management: Amanda Martin
Director of Product Management: Matthew Kane
Product Manager: Tina Chen
Product Assistant: Anna-Maria Forger, Melina Leon
Senior Project Specialist: Vanessa Richards
Digital Project Specialist: Angela Dooley
Senior Marketing Manager: Jennifer Scherzay
Product Fulfillment Manager: Wendy Kilborn
Composition and Project Management:
  S4Carlisle Publishing Services

Cover Design: Michael O'Donnell
Media Development Editor: Troy Liston
Rights Specialist: John Rusk
Cover Image (Part Opener, Chapter Opener):
  © Everything Possible/Shutterstock
Printing and Binding: McNaughton & Gunn
Cover Printing: McNaughton & Gunn

Library of Congress Cataloging-in-Publication Data
Names: Weberg, Daniel Robert, author. | Davidson, Sandra, 1973- author.
Title: Leadership for evidence-based innovation in nursing and health
  professions / Daniel Weberg & Sandra Davidson.
Description: 2nd edition. | Burlington, MA : Jones & Bartlett Learning,
  [2020] | Includes bibliographical references and index.
Identifiers: LCCN 2019019347 | ISBN 9781284171365 (paperback)
Subjects: MESH: Nurse Administrators--organization & administration |
  Evidence-Based Nursing | Organizational Innovation
Classification: LCC RT89 | NLM WY 105 | DDC 610.73068--dc23
LC record available at https://lccn.loc.gov/2019019347

6048

Printed in the United States of America
24 23 22 21   10 9 8 7 6 5 4 3

Contents

Chapter 4 From Organization as Machine to Organization as Conversation: Making Sense of Complexity in Health Care 77

Sandra Davidson

SECTION 2 Organizations/ Systems   103

Chapter 5 Evidence-Based Practice and the Dynamic of Innovation: A Model for the Advancing Practice Excellence . . . 105

Tim Porter-O'Grady and Kathy Malloch

Chapter 6 Assessing Your Innovation and Evidence Capacity: Essentials for Organizational Infrastructures 141

Kathy Malloch and Tim Porter-O'Grady

Chapter 7 Shifting Workforce Paradigms: From Quantity to Value-Driven Staffing Using Evidence and Innovation 179

Kathy Malloch and Tim Porter-O'Grady

Chapter 8 Failure and Resilience: Driving Sustainable Innovation 207

Tim Porter-O'Grady

Chapter 9 Leading Innovation and Performance Improvement for High-Performing Systems 235

Daniel Weberg, Jung G. Kim, and John Myovich

SECTION 3 Trends and Issues   259

Chapter 10 The Best Way to Predict the Future Is to [Co]Create It: A Technology Primer for Healthcare Leaders 261

Richard Booth, Gillian Strudwick, Josephine McMurray, Adam Morse, Ryan Chan, and Timothy Zhang

Chapter 11   Incorporating New Evidence from Big Data, Emerging Technology, and Disruptive Practices into Your Innovation Ecosystem 289

Rayne Soriano and Daniel Weberg

Chapter 12   From Patient- to Person-Centered Care: Re-Forming Relationships in Health Care 317

Daniel Weberg and Sandra Davidson

Chapter 13   Toxic Leadership: Leadership Behaviors That Kill Innovation and How to Avoid Them. 345

Daniel Weberg and Courtnay Caufield

SECTION 4   Exemplars   371

Chapter 14   Organizing Systems for Successful Innovation: Examples from the Field 373

Cheryl Hoying

Contributors

Richard Booth, RN, PhD
Assistant Professor
Arthur Labatt Family School of
 Nursing
Western University
London, Ontario, Canada

**Courtnay Caufield, RN, DNP, CENP, CNML,
NE-BC, RN-BC, CPN**
Cedars-Sinai Medical Center
Los Angeles, California

Ryan Chan, MScN, RN
PhD Student
Arthur Labatt Family School of
 Nursing
Western University
London, Ontario, Canada

Kevin Clouthier, MSc, MBA, PhD
Executive Director
Open Doors for Lanark Children and
 Youth
Carleton Place, Ontario, Canada

Denise Duncan, RN
Executive Vice President
United Nurses Association
Union Health Care Professionals
San Dimas, California

Cheryl Hoying, PhD, RN, NEA-BC, FACHE, FAAN
Senior Consultant
Values Coach
Cincinnati, Ohio

Jung G. Kim, MPH, CPH
UC Berkeley School of Public Health
Berkeley, California
University of Washington School of
 Medicine
Seattle, Washington

Cathy Lalley, PhD, RN, MHI
Clinical Assistant Professor
Arizona State University
Phoenix, Arizona

Kathy Malloch, PhD, MBA, RN, FAAN
President, KMLS, LLC
Glendale, Arizona
Clinical Professor
College of Nursing
Ohio State University
Columbus, Ohio

Josephine McMurray, MRT, MBA, PhD, FBTM
Associate Professor
Lazaridis School of Business &
 Economics
Wilfrid Laurier University
Waterloo, Ontario, Canada

Adam Morse, BSc, BScN, RN
PhD Student
Arthur Labatt Family School of
 Nursing
Western University
London, Ontario, Canada

John Myovich, BA, MBA
Healthcare Financial Management
 Association
UC Berkeley School of Public Health
Berkeley, California

**Tim Porter-O'Grady, DM, EdD, ScD, APRN,
FAAN**
Senior Partner, Tim Porter-O'Grady
 Associates, Inc.
Atlanta, Georgia

Joshua Rutkoff, BS
Senior Staff Analyst
Los Angeles Department of Health
   Services
Los Angeles, California

Rayne Soriano, PhD, RN
Regional Administrator
Resource Stewardship
Kaiser Permanente
Oakland, California

Jerry E. Spicer, DNP, RN, NEA-BC, FACHE
Vice President, Patient Care Services
Kaiser Permanente Foundation
   Hospitals, Southern California
   Region
Pasadena, California

Gillian Strudwick, RN, PhD
Independent Scientist, Centre for
   Addiction and Mental Health
Assistant Professor, Institute of Health
   Policy, Management and Evaluation,
   University of Toronto
Toronto, Ontario, Canada

Timothy Zhang, BSc (c)
Undergraduate Student
Faculty of Applied Health Sciences
University of Waterloo
Waterloo, Ontario, Canada

Reviewers

Becca Billings, MLIS
Assistant Professor, Reference
  Librarian
UAB Libraries
Birmingham, Alabama

Nicolette Fiore-Lopez, PhD, RN, CNEP
Adjunct Faculty, Stony Brook
  University
Stony Brook, New York
Chief Nursing Officer, St. Charles
  Hospital
Port Jefferson, New York

Kimberly A. Hires, PhD, RN
Clinical Assistant Professor, DNP
  Program Director at Georgia State
  University
CEO at The Nightingale Firm, LLC
Atlanta, Georgia

Nancy Hoffart, PhD, RN
Forsyth Medical Center Distinguished
  Professor
School of Nursing, University of North
  Carolina Greensboro
Greensboro, North Carolina

Cathy Lalley, PhD, MHI, RN
Professor
College of Nursing and Health
  Innovation
Arizona State University
Phoenix, Arizona

Michele A. Schultz, MPAS, PA-C
Assistant Professor
IUPUI PA Program
Indianapolis, Indiana

Introduction

We are excited to share our second edition of *Leadership for Evidence-Based Innovation in Nursing and Health Professions*. Since the publishing of the first edition, we have been hard at work studying trends, teaching leadership, and pushing the boundaries of healthcare leadership. We are even more certain that this text is needed in our industry.

Health care is the next major industry to be fundamentally disrupted. Sectors such as taxi companies, hotels, retail, and media have already been reshaped by technology. Health care has thus far resisted disruption, relying on the clunky systems of the industrial era, complicated payment mechanisms, and clinical traditions. However, outcomes are lacking, consumers are frustrated, and clinicians are exhausted. We are overdue for a new operating system!

Leaders, all of us, need to develop our ability to lead fundamental change, drive innovation, and improve performance. This new edition provides perspectives that have not been widely acknowledged—let alone published.

We examined high-performing organizations and learned how they combine both innovation and performance improvement. These very different but interdependent processes provide the framework for creating the new and optimizing the known.

The often unspoken phenomena of toxic leadership and toxic teams are infecting our systems and are leading to burnout, waste, and even death. In this edition, we examine the underlying systems issues, the leadership behaviors, and specific strategies to address and avoid toxicity in organizations.

Finally, to round out the new content, we added chapters on the disruptive changes health care faces, including new entrants, technology changes, and ways leaders can learn and adapt no matter what role they have.

These new additions build on the solid evidence base of updated chapters that include contemporary topics that any healthcare professional can apply tomorrow. The text is also rearranged in a more logical grouping to help facilitate curriculum design and conceptual frameworks in innovation.

▶ Section 1—Leaders

This section is focused on developing leaders' innovation skills. We moved the conceptual framework chapters to the front to provide context, invitation, and provocation for individuals to adopt new leadership practices. From framing one's systems view of leadership to specific team behaviors to sense making in complex organizations, this section contains essential foundations for the leaders of the future.

▶ Section 2—Organizations/Systems

Leading systems requires a different way of thinking and interacting. Leaders hoping for system change must understand the foundations of culture, systems thinking, failure, and performance improvement. These areas of focus are rarely seen in leadership texts but are essential to success. Section 2 highlights essential shifts in perspective that leaders need to building organizations where failure is formative, change is viewed as a continuum, and workforce development is essential to innovation.

▶ Section 3—Trends and Issues

As leaders develop their capacity for transformation, they must become increasingly aware of the context that is influencing the healthcare environment. The most influential changes are coming from technology developments, new entrants like Amazon, and consumer demand for a more person-centric health care. In this section we have added several chapters that provide insights into the changes health care is experiencing and the struggles leaders are facing. From toxic organizations and person-centered care to blockchain and machine learning, this section presents leaders with novel perspectives that help make sense of the patterns and chaos that will ultimately disrupt the industry.

▶ Section 4—Exemplars

Every leader needs a proverbial north star to follow, to know that there are others on this journey of transformation and what success might look like. In Section 4, we have provided exemplars of innovation leadership from the real world. Based in theory, we show you how high-performing organizations have worked through major issues like labor relations, building business cases for innovation, and changing education to meet the future needs of the healthcare industry. These examples provide tangible foundations for how the evidence of innovation can be applied and measured.

▶ Summary

It is time we be bold, call out the unspoken, and change the way we lead in organizations. This text is a compendium for leaders to change the conversation, curate the evidence, and foster the skills and strategies to disrupt a system. We hope to encourage positive deviance. Positive deviants are those who thrive in systems that are failing; leaders of evidence-based innovation are those who thrive in the failing healthcare system and find ways to challenge the status quo to deliver value-based patient care. This is for the innovators, the disruptors, and the positive deviants, and the leaders that expect better from their teams and systems.

We hope this inspires you to do something different and make *AND* your new *OR*.

SECTION 1

Leaders

Future of Evidence, Innovation, and Leadership in Health Care: A Model for Leading Change

Daniel Weberg and Sandra Davidson

"The dogmas of the quiet past, are inadequate to the stormy present ..."

— **Abraham Lincoln**

CHAPTER OBJECTIVES

Upon completion of this chapter, the reader will be able to:

1. Describe key leadership elements for building innovative organizations in health care.
2. Synthesize core aspects of evidence and innovation in relation to the changing healthcare system.
3. Discuss a new framework for innovation in health care.

Now more than ever, the need for innovation in health care is clear. A shift from volume to value has disrupted the status quo and demonstrated that the models of the past are no longer relevant or sustainable ways to improve the quality, cost, affordability, and experience for the greater population. Healthcare organizations are struggling to combine, align, merge, adapt, reinvent, and even innovate new ways to provide superior quality while reducing the cost to the consumer and the overall system.

▶ Are We Moving Too Slowly?

Many healthcare start-up entrepreneurs think so! In recent years, venture funding to healthcare-focused start-up companies was the highest in history (Gandhi & Wang, 2015). Innovators, many with little formal healthcare experience, are developing software, devices, systems, and solutions to fill the gaps left by the shifting healthcare system or to capitalize on emerging opportunities. Universities, venture capital firms, and large organizations are creating incubators for healthcare start-up companies to spin out solutions focused on digital health, pharmaceuticals, medical devices, and diagnostics.

Consumers are also demanding and purchasing services outside the traditional medical model. MeMD, Teladoc, and HealthTap are technology companies that decentralize care and allow patients to see a clinician from their computer or mobile device in seconds for a low one-time charge. Robots are enabling specialists around the world to examine, operate, and follow up with patients with solutions from InTouch Health and other companies. Sensor devices are allowing healthcare professionals to amass petabytes of data on patients that could not have been collected previously. These petabytes are expanding the sources of data that can be analyzed and translated into evidence automatically and instantly. There is so much data produced on a continuous basis that practitioners can easily access that we do not know what to do with it all. Traditional health professions education has not yet caught up with the available technology or mounds of data. Healthcare providers today have not been taught how to assess, diagnose, treat, and monitor patients based on this data captured millions of times per second. The episodic basis of care-related data (vital signs, activity, diet, medication absorption, etc.) is quickly becoming irrelevant. Technology is challenging old models of care, enabling new ones, and providing the evidence of what works and what does not work.

It seems obvious that the needs of clinicians, healthcare consumers, and populations are rapidly changing due to technology, health policy changes, and innovations. Equally as important is the changing focus and scope of leaders in the healthcare industry. The call for outside-the-box thinking, leading, and organizing is loud and clear. However, there are few frameworks of leadership, innovation, and evidence that help new and experienced leaders understand the complexities of the new world of health care. This text has provided the content and evidence needed to inform a new framework, and this chapter will present a synthesis and starting point on which we might build and refine such a framework. We argue that by thinking more intentionally about the interdependence and connectedness of leadership, innovation, and evidence, and by utilizing the skills, attitudes, and ideas presented in this text, leaders in health care can create a greater impact on the outcomes across the system. Without a paradigm revolution, entire organizations, professions, and systems may fail and disappear.

▶ The Paradox of the Box: Moving to an Interconnected Framework

What is the box? The phrase *thinking outside the box* has been used to describe anything from innovation to visionary thinkers to disruptive ideas. In many organizational applications, the phrase has been used to describe anything that challenges the normal operating thinking and status quo of the organization. The conceptualization of a status quo box (**FIGURE 1-1**) that requires people to break their normal routine to disrupt creates a culture of episodic change that may not be responsive enough to adjust to the continuous changes that are impacting health care.

The idea that innovation occurs outside a hypothetical status quo or normal operating procedures box presents conceptual problems that undermine the ability of organizations to implement innovation. By thinking about innovation as something external to the day-to-day workings of an organization, we actually build another silo: the silo of the innovation team. To lead organizations and the health system to new ways of work, it is important to design a system that breaks down silos and reduces fragmentation (Berwick & Hackbarth, 2012). Furthermore, innovation needs to be integrated into the learning experiences and preparation for all healthcare disciplines. This text provides evidence that high-performing organizations will not just be competent in performance improvement but innovation as well. These skills are essential to exploring future needs and optimizing current processes. The faster leaders can adapt and adopt, the more likely they are to be flexible about the pressures of a changing system. Innovation cannot continue to stand alone, or separate

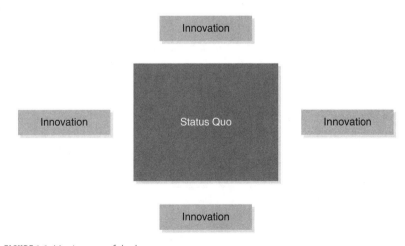

FIGURE 1-1 Moving out of the box.

and apart, from other dimensions of organization and leader learning. Innovation needs to take its place among the other core competencies for healthcare practice in the 21st century.

This text will present content, research, and examples of a three-pronged framework that will help organizations move to a new future of care: evidence-based practice, innovation, and leadership. It is important that we discuss each component, its current status quo, and how the concepts in this text will help disrupt our fragmented system and create more interdependent and relational ways of linking evidence, innovation, and leadership across organizations.

▶ Evidence

Evidence has evolved over time to create rigor, validity, and a rational hierarchy for assessing and appraising research and turning it into insights to improve care outcomes (Melnyk, Gallagher-Ford, & Fineout-Overholt, 2016). This evolution serves as an excellent and needed foundation on which practitioners can build and incorporate new data into the system and turn it into evidence. Current evidence-based practice hierarchies limit sources of valid evidence to systematic reviews, randomized control trials, and so forth. However, by viewing evidence as generated only from the few sources within the box, we fail to integrate the new emerging sources and insights of evidence, like technology and powerful analytics.

Emerging sources of data that are disrupting existing evidence frameworks include big data technologies, wearable monitors, analytics, continuous patient monitoring, and electronic medical records (EMRs) (**FIGURE 1-2**). These outside-the-box disruptions are signposts for leaders and practitioners to innovate new possibilities for the evidence hierarchy and dynamic. In addition to the technologic possibilities for generating and aggregating evidence, we must also consider the relational and contextual aspects of evidence-based practice. How do we engage patients, communities, and providers in collaborative decision making about the evidence?

FIGURE 1-2 Evidence beyond the box.

FIGURE 1-3 Emerging sources that further inform evidence-based practice.

Leaders in health care must be able to identify disruptions, challenge current thinking, and begin to facilitate the integration of these new sources of evidence into new ways of clinical decision making.

As leaders read the signposts, gather learnings, and test ideas, they will begin to break down the rigid walls of the status quo that organizations build. By connecting evidence to innovation and leadership, a new paradigm of evidence begins to emerge that is fluid, permeable, and able to incorporate out-of-the-box thinking to inform proven methods—in essence, getting rid of the box altogether and creating a more networked and complex approach to linking, trying, and implementing evidence-based practice (**FIGURE 1-3**). In a networked complex system, the practices informed by evidence begin to connect and incorporate newer sources and insights, thus strengthening the practice and evolving our thinking. This allows us to stay relevant and nimble in how we respond to shifting information and needs. Some practices, such as big data analytics, may have stronger ties to the new sources, such as continuous monitoring. Thus, the fluidity of the new evidence bubble allows practices to shift based on continuous assessment and learnings from innovative testing of linkages among the elements. For example, the ubiquitous adoption of EMRs may signal a need to link the evidence hierarchy to EMR insights and data sources to build new practices, but the use of continuous monitoring may still be in the early stages and have fewer linkages that inform new care practices.

It is important to also note that evidence is not a silo. The discussion of evidence presented here is intended to help leaders conceptualize one part of the larger framework discussed throughout this chapter. Accepting new forms of evidence informs expansion and connection building, and it helps us anticipate the future directions of care. It allows us to begin to recognize new patterns. Evidence provides the foundations of innovation and leadership, and innovation and leadership are required to build more evidence. It is an iterative and dynamic system with complex linkages. It is essential that leaders have competence in linking a body of evidence to their innovation facilitation and stop thinking innovation results from an "aha" moment or from spending a day putting sticky notes on a wall. Innovation arises when the participants in the innovation work are informed in the body of evidence and build upon it rather than disregard it.

▶ Innovation

From a traditional perspective, innovation as a whole is considered outside the box, but from the perspective of an innovator, there are always radical ideas that continue to inform practice and aid in the evolution of new ways of thinking. New and radical technological disruptions are often considered innovation, but other practices, such as process redesign, failure, and patient-generated innovations, are not. Even innovation has a cutting edge that continually challenges and moves the practice of innovation forward (**FIGURE 1-4**).

Disruptive practices that are changing how innovation is practiced include conceptualizing failure as necessary, incorporating and relying on patient-generated innovations, the use of social labs, and building innovation from a foundation of evidence-based practice. These trends in innovation practice rely on the connections among multiple parts of the organization and cannot be accomplished in isolation. Innovation requires a network of people who can collaborate, envision the future, overcome barriers, and generate a new vision and direction for the healthcare system to evolve.

The practice of innovation (in health care particularly) is maturing from the notion of idea generation and radical product creation to a practice that fundamentally derives value and content from the front lines of the organization. Healthcare leaders should be competent in innovation practice, accept failure as part of the journey, and develop their own competencies to support innovators in their organizations by building partnerships across silos and teams. Leaders must continually evolve the innovation practice, looking for new sources of ideas, implementation techniques, and ways to keep change relevant to the organization. Therefore, the innovation practice should continually test and trial new processes of change. Evidence-based innovation will require more leadership energy because many people conceptualize it as a separate process. Innovation is often viewed as new, exciting, and future oriented, and evidence-based practice is perceived as steadfast, slow, and present focused. Yet

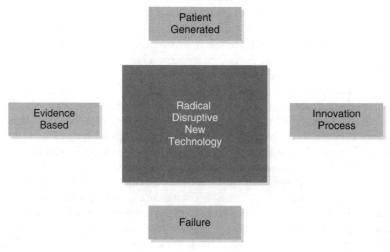

FIGURE 1-4 Innovation as its own box?

if you combine the two practices in new ways, such as using evidence as the foundation from which to inform innovation (new practices and processes), they actually inform each other and synergize the system change. Gone are the days in which we show up unprepared and uninformed to brainstorming sessions. Instead, we should be intimately aware of the evidence around the problem we are trying to solve and make an informed decision to innovate and/or improve. It is also important to know that innovation is not always the process that is needed. Leaders should be adept in assessing the need for innovation or the need for improvement.

The concept of failure can provide a similar example. If failure is viewed through the traditional lens, in which it is punitive, negative, and avoided at all costs, it actually limits the ability of organizations to innovate. By combining the notion of failure and linking it to evidence (knowing what does not work), there emerges another source of innovation rather than a roadblock to it. The failure of practice, process, trials, change, and tests provide a rich source of evidence that can be used as a foundation to improve innovation in the future. Failure should be celebrated for providing insight into all the ways things do not work and providing clues to what is not yet possible. The role of the leader is to document, revisit, and incorporate failures into the conversation regularly in order to ensure movement forward. Failure becomes a body of evidence that can inform future innovation and improvement efforts. It should not be kept secret. Leaders should strive to fail early and often to rapidly move innovation forward because failure is the process from which the new replaces the old.

Innovation is the force that propels evidence creation and provides a practice for leaders to use to evolve the organization, and it infuses energy into the system to catalyze change. Innovation is not a separate team or event but rather the life force that keeps individuals, teams, and organizations relevant (**FIGURE 1-5**). Innovation occurs all the time, at various impact levels, and informs how evidence is created and leadership is practiced. If innovation is absent, so is the ability for the organization to grow, learn, and adapt. Building a competency in basic innovation concepts and practices is a prerequisite for leaders, regardless of your role in the organization or system.

FIGURE 1-5 The edge of innovation: New sources and practices.

▶ Leadership

It is possible that the notion of leadership carries with it the most history, misconception, and biggest lack of evidence of all the elements in the innovation, evidence, and leadership framework (**FIGURE 1-6**). Twentieth-century leadership practices built on the ideas of individualistic power dynamics, followership, command and control, and hierarchy still dominate organizations in health care. Popular media books suggest hundreds of simplistic and overgeneralized tips that leaders should follow to become great but minimize or are completely devoid of research on effective leadership. The disruption of the tradition of leadership thinking and practices is a challenging endeavor that will require evidence, innovation, and significant energy. However, it is an essential element to transform health care. Throughout this text the argument has been made, and supported by evidence, that leadership needs to move toward a distributed, networked, team-based, and relational approach that is supported with the latest evidence and fueled by innovation.

Leadership relies on partnerships, and partnerships are built through networks. To build a network, and thus a partnership, leaders should focus on relationships among colleagues and teams (Porter-O'Grady & Malloch, 2014). The stronger the leader's network, the better the chance that diverse thought and sources of evidence will emerge to inform innovation and change (Weberg, 2013; White, Pillay, & Huang (2016). As the network strengthens, the distribution of decision making can be improved as well. Placing problem-solving and decision-making power at the point closest to the problem allows those with the best connections to relevant evidence to create and sustain solutions (Porter-O'Grady & Malloch, 2014). Distributed leadership requires partnership and team-based models of collaboration to leverage the diverse skill sets of organizations. Partnerships and teams allow groups to leverage their collective expertise and evidence to cocreate innovative changes and move the organization forward.

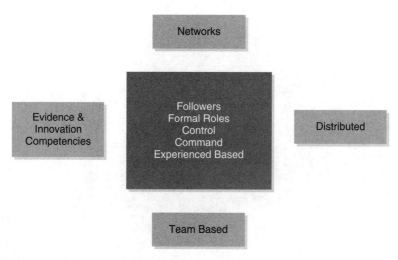

FIGURE 1-6 Traditional in-the-box leadership.

The most important shift in our understanding of leadership is that it is a set of behaviors that helps the organization focus and align time, resources, and energy through relationships and networks. It is not about controlling but rather facilitating, connecting, and emancipating. Leaders may accomplish this by building relationship-centered cultures and translating information in ways that are meaningful and relevant in local contexts. In essence, leaders can help create the organizational norms that value shared decision making, innovation, and evidence integration. These norms will give rise to a culture that supports evidence-based innovation.

Depending on the current practices of the organization, leaders will need to test and try new leadership behaviors in different patterns and ways. For example, if the organization has a strong relational and network culture, the leader may be able to more easily try different practices in distributed leadership. If the organization is steeped in hierarchy, the practice of building evidence-based leadership behaviors may be a good use of energy. There is no plug-and-play methodology to change culture and leadership practice other than to innovate, fail, and support decision making with the best data and evidence available. This is the challenge of 21st-century leadership. Unlike leadership models of the past that rely on neatly listed steps or recipes for change, transformational and relational leadership embraces the messiness rather than seeking to control and confine it. **FIGURE 1-7** represents how leadership might look as more collaborative and networked approaches are incorporated. These new approaches will become the new norm, replacing antiquated practices like command and control tactics. The more networked, distributed, and team-based leadership becomes, the more capacity that is created for evidence-based innovation. As the leadership practice matures, the capacity to incorporate more innovative practices will increase.

This is the challenge of 21st-century leadership. Unlike leadership models of the past that rely on neatly listed steps or recipes for change, transformational and relational leadership embraces the messiness rather than seeking to control and confine it.

FIGURE 1-7 Leadership beyond silos and hierarchy.

▶ The Evidence–Innovation–Leadership Framework

The evidence–innovation–leadership framework proposed in this text is an interdependent dynamic that helps leaders frame behaviors, evidence, and change in a way to further organizational evolution in health care (**FIGURE 1-8**). Often, evidence, innovation, and leadership are seen as disconnected and different, yet this framework

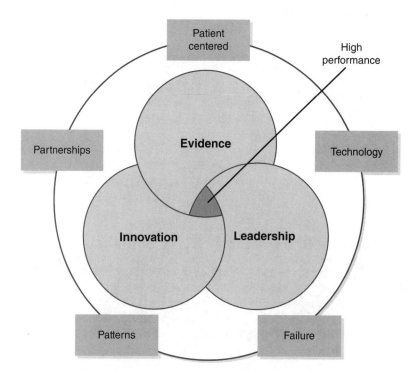

FIGURE 1-8 The evidence–innovation–leadership framework.

describes ways they are synergistic and interdependent. Each concept has been detailed with a description of how organizations have boxed in the notions and created silos around each practice. For example, evidence has been boxed by the rigid use of evidence hierarchy, innovation has been boxed by the expectation for radical change, and leadership has been boxed by the notion that total control is necessary. It is important for leaders to understand the roots and assumptions of these boxes to create new ways of working and integrating concepts that may be more effective.

Building on the boxed assumptions, each concept of the framework has been described in a way that links it to the others and demonstrates their interdependence. This reconceptualization is meant to provide guidance for leaders to build upon and navigate within, to drive evidence-based practice, innovation efforts, and leadership development. Surrounding each of the concepts are the drivers presented throughout this text, including patient-centered care, technology, failure, pattern recognition, and partnerships that keep the framework fluid, informed, and relevant.

Patient-centered care provides relevancy to the framework by grounding it with the viewpoint that patient care is the focus of most healthcare change. Even business model innovations, evidence-based leadership, and technology changes should be done to improve the care experience, health, and safety for the end user of the system: the patient. Relationship-centered care is a framework for thinking about how we engage with patients, providers, and stakeholder communities in the service of patients. Without the perspective of the patient, there is a risk of focusing energy on evidence, innovation, and leadership efforts that are not aligned with the mission of the organization. Removing the patient-centered care driver from the framework changes the balance of the three core concepts of evidence, innovation, and leadership, and it begins to fragment the system. Patient-centered care and relationship-centered care is discussed in Chapter 12.

The technology driver helps accelerate the framework's rate of change and the ability to gather, interpret, and act on data and evidence. Technology is a cultural norm and expectation that can move a process forward by simplifying complex data for interpretation or providing easy access to information to develop new practices. Technology can also speed up failure in a suboptimal system. Implementing technology on top of a broken process only serves to break the process faster. For example, providing clinicians with mobile devices that can access Google and other data sources without ensuring competency in understanding evidence validity and quality may lead to faster access to inaccurate information. Due to the integration of technology into our everyday lives, technology is quickly becoming the interface that drives care decisions and even patient-centered interactions. We can understand all of the various data points about a patient and at the same time instantly connect them with care team members. Leaders should have an understanding of the impact technology has and the speed at which it changes processes within the evidence–innovation–leadership framework. The technology driver is discussed in Chapters 10 and 11.

The failure driver provides the framework with continuous learning feedback loops and a safe environment to test new ways of work. Continuous learning emerges from tried and failed attempts at change, yet failure is continually avoided in healthcare organizations (Porter-O'Grady & Malloch, 2016). By acknowledging failure and diving deep into the insights that can be gleaned from less-than-successful attempts at change or practice, we can avoid making the same mistakes repeatedly. Moreover, we get better at failure, and this means we are able to learn more quickly. Celebrating failure can build learning that then cycles back into the organizational knowledge base and continues the iteration and movement forward to novel solutions. Failure is essential in evidence generation (building on research, learning what does not work), innovation work (quickly iterating to create novel solutions), and leadership (understanding the networks and increasing the span of impact). Without the failure driver, leaders condemn organizations to avoid or ignore failure at their own peril, which limits the creation of innovation and the use of novel evidence. Acceptance (even celebration) of failures requires leaders and organization-wide cultures to transcend ego, blame, and punishment to gain insights and grow stronger. The failure driver is discussed in Chapters 3, 6, and 8.

The pattern driver provides a different lens through which to conceptualize evidence, innovation learnings, and leadership signposts. In complex systems, individuals, teams, organizations, and technologies interact in a multitude of ways to accomplish tasks, work, and achieve outcomes (Uhl-Bien & Marion, 2008). The complexity of the system is so high that the impact of individual actions and interactions are nearly impossible to predict by any one leader. Therefore, leaders should look for emergent patterns in the organization to better understand how evidence, innovation, and leadership actions are changing the system. For example, a care practice based on one expert's opinion would be haphazard compared to looking across multiple sources of evidence, such as systematic reviews, patient preferences, and local best practices, for patterns that support a practice change. In innovation, patterns in technological change, consumer needs, and clinician practices provide the context on which to build novel solutions that add value. Patterns in failure also provide evidence that leaders can use to focus innovation efforts, understand what does not work, and search for more evidence to build stronger solutions. Without pattern recognition as a driver in the evidence framework, innovation and leadership become linear endeavors that rely on predictable processes rather than embracing the inherent complexity of relationships and systems. Linear leadership, prescriptive solutions, and a cookbook approach to evidence implementation may result in simpler solutions that lack relevancy and impact in complex environments. Patterns provide the signposts by which leaders can frame evidence and innovation within complex relational systems. The pattern driver is discussed in Chapters 3, 4, and 13.

The partnership driver provides the energy to create and strengthen connections and relationships among the core concepts. A core belief within this framework is the impact that groups of people, teams, and organizations can have in changing a large system. The partnership dynamic provides the tools, energy, and linkages to strengthen these networks and better link evidence to innovation and leadership practices. Without partnership as a driver, leadership can become an individual endeavor, innovation becomes slower and less relevant, and evidence that emerges tends to be less trustworthy or valid and reliable. Partnership improves diversity of thought, evidence sources, and leadership resources so that more diverse solutions are generated and more impactful outcomes can be achieved. One example of this is the use of unit-based teams. Facilitating local teams to source and implement evidence and innovation at the point of care results in greater fidelity and effectiveness of processes and solutions. The practice of engaging unit-based teams to solve problems instead of relying on individual leader solutions has provided sustainable and highly effective changes in some healthcare organizations. The partnership driver is discussed in Chapters 12, 13, and 15.

The evidence–innovation–leadership framework proposed here is focused by the lens of patient-centered care, accelerated by technology, fueled by failure, guided by patterns, and strengthened by partnerships. The framework provides a way for leaders to think about the interdependencies necessary to change the healthcare system and lead evidence-based innovation. The framework is a foundation and a call for a new healthcare system.

▶ Using the Evidence–Innovation–Leadership Framework to Create Change

For an evidence–innovation–leadership framework to exist as a way of doing business and building new systems, certain organizational and role capacities must be established. Leaders in organizations will need to be intentional about the design, development, and focus to create the context that will ultimately support new ways of care, practice, and health care.

The following components must be incorporated in the design of this new system to create an environment in which evidence, innovation, and leadership intertwine and thrive (Malloch & Porter-O'Grady, 2010):

- A commitment to data and information-driven decision making must be made at the very senior levels of the organization in a way that ensures the decisions will be generated in alignment with the evidentiary dynamic.
- An investment must be made in the resources needed to build the data and information infrastructure. This includes the appropriation of sufficient hardware and software to ensure the utility and effectiveness of information-driven decision making and determination of fixed-process approaches to operational and clinical decision making.
- Meaningful engagement must occur with point-of-service knowledge workers and patients at the outset of the design of management and clinical information infrastructure, software, and processes. This includes using an effectiveness evaluation as a way of ensuring a goodness of fit between the proposed data tools and the utility of their application.
- A commitment must be made to ongoing professional development of managers and leaders in the concepts of complex adaptive and responsive systems, role agency, networks, and emergent leadership. Leaders at every level must develop the competencies necessary to ensure that innovation and creativity are embraced as the way of being in the organization.
- Ongoing engagement must occur with health professions education programs to continually strengthen the practice–education connection. Leadership needs to support connection and integration at every level of the organization. This includes supporting individual practitioners and teams to participate in mentoring and teaching students align leadership activities at the highest levels.
- Reconceptualize healthcare organizations and hospitals as complex systems composed of networked relationships. Multifocal interactions, interdependence, and relational processes become the organizing framework, replacing vertical decision models, operating silos, and nonaligned departmental configurations.

- Eliminate discipline-specific locus of control in favor of interdisciplinary processes, teams, and collaborative decision making, resulting in an integrated model of evidence-driven decision making, practice, and impact evaluation. This includes the acknowledgment that sustainable outcome-oriented, evidence-driven practice represents the synthesis and coordination of the effort of all stakeholders, as opposed to focusing only on unilateral measures of incremental impact (isolated, nonaligned, discipline-specific outcomes).
- Embrace and leverage the organization as conversation perspective to strengthen relationships, communication, alignment, and transparency across the organization.
- Invest leaders' time and energy into building quality relationships, resilience, and capacity in all three domains: innovation, evidence, and leadership.
- Construct and develop a strategic plan and targets for transforming the system environment from a fixed operational model to a fluid, data-driven organizational framework supporting evidentiary systems, structures, processes, applications, and evaluation. This includes consonance among evidence-driven strategic trajectories, resource capitalization, management and operational reconfiguration for leading, and clinical facilities for execution.

These considerations provide starting points or levers that leaders can use to influence their teams, organizations, and broader networks to support movement toward a value-focused healthcare system. The application of these concepts and the evidence–innovation–leadership framework will require risk taking, adaptation, vision, opportunity, facilitation, information, and technology (Weberg, 2013). This means that at an individual level, the leader's own capacity for apprehending these various aspects will determine his or her effectiveness and reach. There are specific competencies leaders can develop that will increase their capacity for changing the system.

▶ Competency 1: Understand the Foundations of the Innovation, Evidence, and Leadership Dynamic

Leaders who wish to change the system must first have an understanding of the complexities and history that are driving current behaviors and the barriers and benefits that allow that behavior to continue (Porter-O'Grady & Malloch, 2016). Specifically, understanding the foundations of evidence, innovation, and leadership in the context of health care is very important.

The foundations of evidence consist of the evidence framework, critical evidence appraisal models, and evidence-based practice models. Understanding these core concepts and practices allows the leader to quickly and accurately gather evidence to inform decision making, leadership, and innovation. Evidence can inform the change in practices and the beginnings of innovation processes, and provide context for the healthcare system as a whole.

The foundations of innovation consist of innovation methodologies like design thinking, innovation frameworks that include failure as normative, and innovation leadership behaviors that support the practice. Understanding basic innovation methodologies allows the leader to view change as normative and develop behaviors that support teams in problem solving. An innovation mind-set also provides a lens for leaders to view new sources of evidence, test new ideas and practices, and develop new models of care to change the entire system. Innovation competence is often overlooked by organizations, but it is an essential skill in remaining relevant and driving improved outcomes in health care. Chapter 9 has a discussion of innovation and performance improvements processes with a focus on how leaders can incorporate both processes in order to create change.

The foundations of leadership are rooted in leadership theories such as trait, style, transformational, relational, and complexity. By understanding the sources of decision making, power, accountability, and the variety of lenses available through which leaders across the system may make sense of their work, the available solutions and directions become more generative rather than prescriptive. The evidence-based and innovative leader can then develop strategies to overcome resistance, build networks, and create teams that are wired for system change. Understanding that leadership is a complex set of interactions and information that is grounded in relationships, evidence, and innovation is key to building the future of health care.

Each of these foundations provides the starting point for research, learning, and the growth of leaders in health care. The beginnings of each of these concepts are presented in this text with specific examples and tools for change. Additionally, leaders should read seminal texts and articles and search for new evidence to continually build their knowledge and skill. The point is to not silo one's competency in one discipline but to see the patterns and connections among all the disciplines of change. Additional topics that should be studied include culture, communication, health policy and law, business operations, and basic technical and informatics knowledge.

▶ Competency 2: Leading Yourself

Leadership, especially in health care, requires significant energy, reflection, and networking. It can be easy for leaders to focus energy on others, the organization, or the work without regard to their own health and family. Leading yourself includes the concepts of creating your own context for action and balance. Energy management, nutrition, wellness, reflection, and renewal are concepts that professional athletes use for peak performance, and similar concepts can be translated to leadership peak performance. Leaders should make time to build energy through physical fitness and proper nutrition and snacking routines. Wellness and renewal activities, like vacations, deep breathing between meetings, and making time for friends and family, allow leaders to stay grounded in all aspects of their lives and maintain energy throughout the day. Additionally, leaders are visible role models to others in the organization. By modeling self-leadership and encouraging self-care in others, leaders can have a secondary positive effect on the health and resilience of the wider organization. Leaders can also build mental and emotional capacities through emotional intelligence work, mindfulness, and reflection. All these skills help you as an individual engage fully in leadership behaviors. It is necessary to build your own endurance and capacity to weather the stress of challenges that are an inevitable aspect of change and innovation. It is also important for leaders to recognize and intervene in their own burnout and toxicity. If self-care, team-care, and organizational values are not aligned there becomes a real risk for individual leaders to experience negative emotional, physical, and psychological impacts. Toxicity in teams and organizations is real and under-reported in systems. We discuss this in depth in Chapter 13.

DISCUSSION

What self-leadership practices do you currently engage in? What do you think are the biggest barriers to self-leadership? Are there self-leadership behaviors and practices that you want to start? How can you set yourself up for success? Are there peers and/or mentors that you could invite to join the journey toward self-care with you?

▶ Competency 3: Building an Advanced Innovation Skill Set

After leaders have a good foundation in evidence, innovation, and leadership and have begun to reflect on their leadership journey, more advanced innovation competencies can be introduced. These include advances in design thinking, risk taking, strategic alignment, and culture-building skills that can further develop an ecosystem of innovation across departments, organizations, and systems. Concepts such as systems thinking, complexity leadership, and network interaction theory are examples of advanced innovation perspectives that leaders can use to shape change and create lasting innovation structures.

Innovation competency for leaders is not the ability to generate significant numbers of ideas but rather the ability for leaders to create safe conditions for risk taking and leverage resources to support teams to create novel ideas. Rather than the leader acting as an innovator (which may be the case at a basic competency level), this advanced innovation competency for leaders is about creating the conditions for innovation to happen through the actions of others. Leaders with advanced innovation skills can view complex systems as interconnected wholes and recognize emergent patterns that guide evidentiary and innovation dynamics. Complex adaptive and complex relational perspective taking can result in the creative emergence of new ideas and information. Leaders must be aware of the emerging edge of the healthcare industry and respond accordingly. The advanced innovation leader has multiple streams of information, learning, and insight that help inform decision making. These can be informal sources, such as friends, coworkers, and perspectives outside health care social media and popular culture; or they can be formal, such as journals, research, or organization-specific channels of knowledge dissemination like clinical practice guidelines, intranet resources, and special interest groups. Advanced leaders should have competency in developing and accessing both formal and informal networks.

Viewing the system in novel ways is important, but equally important is measuring the impact of innovation and evidence. Leaders of innovation need to understand and look for ways to assess, measure, and otherwise illuminate how new evidence and innovations are changing and influencing the system. This requires an understanding of metrics. For example, failed innovations may be unsuccessful from an individual project standpoint, but the ripples of failed projects or patterns of innovation activity can open new opportunities, break down previous barriers, or inform others to change efforts in the organization. These impacts are complex and at times difficult to see, but advanced innovation leaders can utilize their networks and pattern recognition to gather diverse sources of information and translate this information into meaningful measures of evidence and innovation.

Building relationships across networks requires leaders to create connections beyond the span of their everyday work and to develop the capability to communicate with diverse groups for information and knowledge sharing. Building your network occurs on two levels: informational and relational. First, the leader should create ways for information to be shared with their team members and with members of other teams. Connections enable sharing information through e-mails, conversation, technology, and interaction. For example, moving from data sharing at a physical location, like a whiteboard, and digitizing it into a secure web-based platform that allows for real-time viewing and manipulation of the information, and is accessible by multiple teams who may be working at a physical distance would be a connection for sharing information. The second level of building a network is to develop relationships. The leader's relationships determine the quality, strength, and longevity of connections that are made. By building strong relationships, the leader increases the likelihood that the information exchanged between the teams will be of better quality, accuracy, and relevance. It also increases the likelihood that team members will develop relationships with counterparts of other teams. Mutual respect, trust, and valuing the expertise of others are foundations of relationship building. Creating connections, building relationships, and knowing how and when to mobilize them is a key advanced innovation skill.

Finally, advanced innovation leaders foster high-performing cultures, and this enables innovation. Cultures are the accumulation of behaviors and interactions that occur among people in an organization. Behaviors turn into norms, and these norms turn into subconscious (unspoken) rules that govern future behavior (Schein, 2004). Leaders have the ability to influence behavior by creating the conditions and structures that foster, for example, open communication and acknowledging and learning from mistakes.

The complex relational perspective is also useful in fostering high-performing cultures. Leaders can begin to transform patterns of meaning and patterns of relating in ways that will support and align with the innovation–evidence–leadership framework. Patterns of meaning within organizations can be influenced by paying attention to what people are talking about, what is rewarded, or what energy and resources are focused on. If leaders discern that patterns of meaning are not in alignment with the framework, they can begin to change the patterns of meaning by shifting the attention, rewards, and language in ways that are more generative and aligned with the importance and value of innovation and evidence. Patterns of relating are equally as powerful. Leaders should be aware of the reasons, issues, and events that people organize their interactions around. For instance, if there is a monthly full-day meeting that brings stakeholders together to discuss a certain topic (e.g., risk management), leaders should evaluate if that topic and the intended purpose of the meeting are time and energy well spent. If the organization wants to foster innovation and empower providers at the point of care to engage in tinkering and process improvement, a full-day meeting spent scrutinizing deviations from the status quo and consistency might be sending the wrong message. Leaders should seek to align patterns of meaning and relating with the organization's highest aspirations and priorities (Suchman, 2011). **TABLE 1-1** summarizes the requisite skills associated with advanced innovation competency.

TABLE 1-1 Advanced Innovation Competency

	Skills
Complex adaptive systems view	▪ Pattern recognition ▪ View complex interrelationships among teams and systems ▪ Establish strong feedback loops with formal and informal sources
Measure system-level outcomes	▪ Recognize impacts of innovation and evidence across the system ▪ Determine appropriate metrics to understand impacts
Relationships across the network	▪ Span boundaries across organizations ▪ Influence the network ▪ Model effective network development
Create high-performing cultures	▪ Align energy and resources to match organizational goals ▪ Model and facilitate open communication ▪ Notice and leverage patterns of meaning and patterns of relating

▶ Competency 4: Communicating and Connecting

Leaders who wish to transform systems must be masters at communicating and connecting across networks, teams, and organizations. Communication competencies include the ability to build relationships and networks, as discussed previously, and also the ability to communicate vision and information in a way that influences others to change. The term *influences* is intentional in this context. Leadership is the influencing of others to adapt and change in the face of complex and unpredictable situations (Weberg, 2013). To influence teams of people, leaders must be able to articulate rationale, evidence, data, meaning, and impact clearly, linking those elements to the broader mission of the team or organization. This act is different from motivation. Leaders are influencers more often than they are motivators.

Another important competency related to connecting and communicating is the notion of transparency. In organizations, information is interpreted, analyzed, and acted upon at each level. For example, uninformed rumors of an organizational change can lead people to quit preemptively, look for other opportunities, or launch negative campaigns before official announcements are made. Leaders who value transparency and can communicate effectively are able to anticipate or gain insight about these rumors and work with their teams to communicate and connect concepts in a more focused and meaningful way. For example, the leader may learn of the rumor from his or her professional network and hold a staff meeting to answer questions openly and honestly, providing information proactively. A noninnovative leader would shy away from such conflict and allow team energy to be spent on anxiety-generating activities, thus pushing productivity down and chaos up.

Relationship-centered care comes to bear in our discussion of communicating and connecting, which are an elemental aspect of effective relationships.

Relationship-centered care is supported by what Suchman (2011) described as relationship-centered *administration*. In essence, if we as leaders want care providers to engage patients and families in respectful, honest, and deeply engaged relationships, we must communicate and connect with care providers and patients in ways that resonate with those very same qualities. It is the epitome of walking our talk. But communicating and connecting is not only about talking. Leaders must also be astute listeners. The skills of deep listening (empathically and emergently) are essential for fostering high-quality relationships that ensure connections (Scharmer, 2007). The concept of relationship-centered care is discussed in Chapter 12.

Communicating and connecting is a competency that innovation leaders must hone and continually demonstrate. Deep listening, influencing, transparency, and relationship building are critical to fostering a culture where evidence and innovation are valued and seen as resources for creating high-quality patient care experiences.

▶ Competency 5: Building Momentum and Initiating Change

The fifth competency for healthcare leaders is the ability build momentum that results in system change. This requires a skillful synthesis of the previous four competencies. The important part of this competency is not the magnitude of change or innovativeness of the change but rather that the leader builds confidence and comfort in trying new things. This also extends to fostering self-efficacy for change and innovation among your team and the larger organization. From a complex relational perspective, even the largest of changes begins with a single step (so to speak). Often, there are also missteps and steps backward in this process toward change. Perseverance, learning from (celebrating) mistakes, and failing forward are all important elements of building momentum for change. Leaders who are new to this way of being may be frustrated because they expect that change needs to happen on a grand scale to be meaningful, or they might be anxious because change may not be a controlled process. The following are some points to ponder for leaders seeking to build momentum:

- Any movement in the right direction is worthy of celebration. Celebrating small wins creates energy and visibility, which in turn creates momentum for change.
- Think of a flywheel, where accumulated small incremental movements can eventually lead to the release of tremendous momentum that reinforces itself, and the pace of change accelerates when a critical mass is reached.
- Small steps that occur over a longer period of time may be more sustainable than taking larger steps too quickly (go slow to go fast).
- Leverage the organization as conversation perspective to gain momentum. How can you use rhetoric and patterns of relating and meaning to move change along?
- Fail often to succeed sooner. Reframe failures into learning. Do not pass up an opportunity to learn from something that did not work.
- Do the work of translation. Listen to your stakeholders to understand what the change means for them. Align your messages about change with their needs and interests (help them see what is in it for them).

- Leverage high-quality relationships and robust networks to communicate about the true nature of change. Replace rumors with transparent, open communication about change.
- Change requires endurance and optimism. Good self-leadership helps leaders to maintain focus and energy and remain committed to the change.
- Continued practice at change and successful implementations of smaller change projects can build momentum for further innovation and change on a larger scale.
- Over 2,500 studies of the diffusion of innovation have been conducted and support the idea that roughly 16% of any group will resist change. Leaders should focus not on that 16% but on the 84% that will move forward.

▶ Summary

The complexity of transforming health care is daunting to even the most seasoned executives and clinicians. The traditions, culture, and knowledge base of the existing system are deeply rooted in the symbols, language, and behaviors of mechanistic, linear, and hierarchy-based organizational ways of being. Leaders of innovation and change must become habituated to new ways of being and doing (**FIGURE 1-9**).

FIGURE 1-9 Leadership competencies that enable healthcare transformation.

Leaders will need to develop specific skill sets, behaviors, and competencies to work effectively within the innovation–evidence–leadership framework. Understanding and leveraging the drivers that enable this framework will be integral to moving health care from its siloed and mechanistic structures to more dynamic, integrated, relational, and value-driven structures that can meet the needs of patients and providers today and into the future.

References

Berwick, D. M., & Hackbarth, A. D. (2012). Eliminating waste in US health care. *JAMA, 307*(14), 1513–1516. http://dx.doi.org/10.1001/jama.2012.362

Gandhi, M., & Wang, T. (2015). Digital health funding: 2014 year in review. Retrieved from http://rockhealth.com/2015/01/digital-health-funding-tops-4-1b-2014-year-review/

Malloch, K., & Porter-O'Grady, T. (2010). *Introduction to evidence-based practice in nursing and health care*. Sudbury, MA: Jones & Bartlett Learning.

Melnyk, B. M., Gallagher-Ford, L., & Fineout-Overholt, E. (2016). *Implementing the evidence-based practice (EBP) competencies in healthcare: A practical guide for improving quality, safety, and outcomes*. Indianapolis, IN: Sigma Theta Tau.

Porter-O'Grady, T., & Malloch, K. (Eds.). (2014). *Creating and sustaining a culture and an environment for evidence-based practice* (3rd ed., Vol. 3). New York, NY: Wolters Kluwer.

Porter-O'Grady, T., & Malloch, K. (2016). *Quantum leadership: Building better partnerships for sustainable health* (3rd ed.). Burlington, MA: Jones & Bartlett Learning.

Scharmer, C. O. (2007). *Theory U: Leading from the future as it emerges*. Cambridge, MA: Society for Organizational Learning.

Schein, E. H. (2004). *Organizational culture and leadership*. San Francisco, CA: Wiley & Sons.

Suchman, T. (2011). How we think about organizations: A complexity perspective. In A. L. Suchman, D. J. Sluyter, & P. R. Williamson (Eds.), *Leading change in healthcare: Transforming organizations using complexity, positive psychology and relationship-centered care*. London, UK: Radcliffe.

Uhl-Bien, M., & Marion, R. (2008). *Complexity leadership part 1: Conceptual foundations*. Charlotte, NC: Information Age.

Weberg, D. R. (2013). *Complexity leadership theory and innovation: A new framework for innovation leadership* (Doctoral dissertation). Arizona State University, Tempe, AZ.

White, K. R., Pillay, R., & Huang, X. (2016). Nurse leaders and the innovation competence gap. *Nursing Outlook, 64*(3), 255–261.

CHAPTER 2

Innovation Leadership Behaviors: Starting the Complexity Journey

Daniel Weberg

"…we must think anew and act anew…"

— **Abraham Lincoln**

CHAPTER OBJECTIVES

Upon completion of this chapter, the reader will be able to:

1. Identify three leadership theory classifications and their impact on innovation and evidence-based practice (EBP).
2. Discuss basic theoretical foundations of complexity science and complexity leadership.
3. Describe and recognize seven characteristics of innovation leaders.

This chapter will describe how leadership emerges from the interactions of team members to move innovation forward in an organization. The chapter will also describe organizational pressures impacting innovation and the innovation leadership gap, discuss the inadequacies of antiquated leadership practices in addressing innovation behaviors, and discuss seven behaviors of innovation and how leaders can recognize and apply them to their practice.

The creation, implementation, and measurement of innovation backed by evidence requires organizations to reconceptualize the notion of leadership from being embodied and centralized in a single individual to leadership emerging through the interactions among teams. Technology has also enhanced the complexity of the healthcare system and has created a change in the ability of individuals to understand and move the system while operating in silos. The future of healthcare transformation requires innovation practices steeped in evidence-based principles and implemented across organizational silos to improve health outcomes. Change and leadership in complex environments emerge as the result of team behaviors rather than simply the actions of a single administrator or manager working through the hierarchical organizational structure alone.

▶ Leadership as a Team Dynamic

As information, globalization, and technology continue to grow and impact organizations, the traditional conceptualization of the leader as an individual is no longer adequate. The volume and vastness of evidence available create conditions in which the administrative leaders or healthcare organizations can no longer possess or access enough information to make well-informed decisions (McKelvey, 2008). The same is true not only for administrative leaders but also for frontline clinicians, managers, directors, and physician leaders.

Clinical teams and organizations that rely on a disconnected group of individuals to guide evidence and innovation will, over time, fail to meet the dynamic changes that are present in health care. **TABLE 2-1** demonstrates the dynamic shift

TABLE 2-1 New Models of Care		
	Old Approach	**New Approach**
Care	Episodic care	Continuous relationship
Management	Clinician	Clinical team
Decision making	Training and experience	Evidence
Control	Care system	Patient
Variability	Clinician autonomy	Patients' preferences, needs
Information flow	Restricted	Encouraged
Safety	Responsibility of the clinician	Responsibility of system
Needs	System reacts	System anticipates
Financial goals	Reduce cost	Reduce waste
Process visibility	Secrecy	Transparency

Data from Kohn, L. T., Corrigan, J. M., & Donaldson, M. S. (Eds.). (2000). *To err is human: Building a safer health system*. Washington, DC: National Academy Press.

in expectations and deliverables present in the healthcare system. Only a small percentage of hospitals, health plans, and physician groups have been able to fully embrace these transitions in transparency, evidence generation, patient-centered care, and innovation despite the national shift to embrace new organizational models. The reason only a few organizations have been able to fully adapt is that most of organizational leadership and clinical practice is guided by individuals working in silos rather than leveraging the collective knowledge of the larger system. External and internal pressures are pushing for health care to change its organization, its leadership models, and its embrace of innovation.

▶ Organizational Pressures That Facilitate Adaptation

The implementation of an innovation is not a single planned event but rather the synthesis of multiple interactions and changes that occur as the innovation is introduced into the system (Goldstein, 2008; Hazy, Goldstein, & Lichtenstein, 2007; Uhl-Bien & Marion, 2008). This structure affirms that innovation occurs over time as interconnected individuals in the organization adapt, through small changes, to environmental pressures. These pressures may be financial, social, cultural, or market forces that require adaptive changes to the current operating schema of the organization and its workers. According to Plowman and Duchon (2008), these emerging actions are the essence of change: "Change occurs continuously, as minor adaptations, which can accumulate, amplify and become radical" (p. 145).

Organizations are influenced by both external and internal pressures. External pressures occur among industry competitors, systems, and regulatory environments that an organization operates in. For example, federal policy changes, new competitor services or products, and changes in consumer demand all represent external pressures to the organization that could catalyze changes, innovations, and the need for new evidence to guide practice. Leaders can observe and use external pressures as signposts that are signaling changes that require their organizations or departments to innovate. One specific example of an external pressure that is driving health system change is the consumerism of health care that is sparked by the social-technical revolution of apps, access to data, and focus on user experiences.

DISCUSSION

Health care has traditionally been slow to adopt disruptive technologies compared to other industries, but consumers are demanding that their experience at the physician's office or hospital mimic their experience at a nice hotel or on Amazon.com. Healthcare teams can look at this consumer shift as a signpost to improve care experiences and interactions with the healthcare system and as a litmus test to decide what work in the organization is no longer needed.

Discuss three consumer-driven shifts you have seen in health care and the leadership behaviors that are driving these shifts. Are the shifts based in evidence or simply a response to consumer demand?

Internal pressures arise from the interactions among people and groups within an organization. Some examples of internal pressures include organizational culture, hierarchy restructuring, employee satisfaction, staffing issues, and budget surplus or deficit. Leaders and teams can facilitate, influence, and impact internal pressures to create conditions for innovation, change, and adaptation to occur. For example, leaders can impact staffing concerns through facilitating a culture of unit-based teams to enable complex problem solving rather than attempting to only individually address staff concerns. Healthcare systems are complex and networked organizations, and both internal and external pressures can cause varying shifts requiring adaptation and leadership from the frontline caregivers to the executive team.

CASE EXAMPLE

Consumer demand is driving the massive changes in health care. New entrants from outside the system are creating external pressures that will force incumbents to adapt or die.

We can look at how external market pressures are changing health care as an example. The healthcare system in the United States has been costly and the outcomes are below our peer countries. Companies that buy health care for their workforce are becoming increasingly frustrated with the antiquated model and high costs of the system. Additionally, individual purchasers are finding the system to be a large financial burden. These pressures are pushing new entrants into the system. Amazon, Google, Apple, and others are using their size and influence to disrupt the traditional structures of health care. The system is now being influenced by consumer demand and not the incumbent insurance behemoths of the past. The pressure that these new healthcare entrants will place on the system will require those in established healthcare organizations to shift, adapt, and evolve their companies quickly. The evolution will require new leadership ideas and will create internal pressures to either maintain the status quo or evolve.

▶ Innovation and the Leadership Gap

The integration of innovation into healthcare organizations is a social practice focused on developing new processes, products, and services to improve quality and reduce costs (Drucker, 1985; Gubin et al., 2017). Innovation processes are full of paradoxes and tensions, yet much of the literature reflects innovation as a uniform or linear process. This dichotomy suggests a gap between the current perceptions of how innovation occurs and how innovation is led. The innovation leadership gap originates from a difference between traditional notions of leadership that are grounded in command-and-control and linear assumptions, and the idea of complexity or innovation leadership, which is based on leadership occurring as a result of teams, network effects, and unpredictability. According to Rosing, Frese, and Bausch (2011), innovation requires leadership that can facilitate nonlinear and emergent social process that lead to improved organizational outcomes. This can be translated to mean that leaders must facilitate teams that can work together to create novel changes. Because innovation is a nonlinear social process that requires complex and nonlinear leadership behaviors, individual-based problem solving, silo-based conversations, and misaligned ideation are not behaviors that will lead to successful innovation. Healthcare leaders who hope to drive organizational success must facilitate teams. Innovation requires different leadership behaviors than those that were successful in the past, and leaders and teams must practice differently to facilitate adaptation and change in health care.

Traditional leadership methods, such as command and control (controlling), leader-centric decision making (autocratic), and a one-size-fits-all (standardized) management style, were negatively associated with acceptance of change and the implementation of innovation. Innovation is more successfully implemented when progressive leadership behaviors, such as engaging the organizational network and proactively seeking out innovations, are practiced. Leadership is an influencing factor in how innovation occurs in organizations, and, more specifically, traditional leadership behaviors appear to limit innovation in organizations (Howell & Avolio, 1993; Rosing et al., 2011). Healthcare knowledge workers need to develop competencies for innovation. Leadership theories and subsequent leadership behaviors and tactics that focus on command and control, standardization, and autocratic tactics are incompatible with the emergent, complex, and social characteristics of innovation in organizations. Before innovation leadership characteristics are introduced, it is helpful to understand the theoretical basis of traditional leadership models.

▶ Leadership Research

There are four global conceptual frameworks in the study of leadership theory evolution: trait, style, transformation, and complexity (Bass, 2008; Northouse, 2018). Each evolutionary stage has informed the development of the next phase. The role of the leader grew from focusing on individuals running entire enterprises to a broader role of facilitator of employee transformation and ultimately to the catalyst, regulator, and meaning maker of change and innovation. Leadership theory progressed from describing organizational power as being held in a single individual leader to describing the power as concentrated among the team members. These role and power distribution changes provided insight into the future role of leadership and the leadership of innovation. This section will present the history and description of four important conceptual frameworks in leadership theory, beginning with the three traditional frameworks, and discuss how they inform future leadership practices and evidence-based innovation (**TABLE 2-2**).

▶ Trait Leadership Theories

Early leadership theories that focused on individual leaders were called "great man" theories. The great man theories assumed that a leader was born to lead and held traits that were universally tied to good leadership (Northouse, 2018). The great man concept, which dominated leadership from 1904 until 1970, was developed during a time of industrial revolution in which the goal of organizations was to increase production and quantity. The leaders' actions focused on productivity, motivating employees to work, and contingent rewards (Bass, 2008).

Nursing and healthcare literature continues to reflect traits as a part of leadership definitions. Yoder-Wise (2007) and Kelly (2008) discussed nursing leadership

TABLE 2-2 Description of Leadership Theories Pertaining to Innovation and EBP		
Leadership Theory	**Innovation**	**EBP**
Trait	Initiated by leader, problem focused.	Linear process tied to leader. Leader as source of evidence.
Style	Congruent with team's style, initiated by leader, problem focused.	Leader as champion. Evidence must align with leader opinion.
Transformational	Vision set by leader; leader empowers and motivates followers.	Evidence helps teams transform. Leader focuses team on correct evidence.
Complexity	Responsibility of all agents in the system; leaders create conditions to focus innovation.	All users consume evidence, interpret it, and adapt based on it. All sources of evidence are considered and incorporated.

as one individual using traits and styles to influence others toward goal achievement. These definitions do not account for other factors that may influence goal attainment in organizations, such as collaboration and emergent leadership. Crosby and Shields (2010) attempted to identify effective nurse leader traits and found that behaviors that facilitated collaboration were more prevalent than any innate traits.

The foundations of change and innovation for trait-based leaders were ensconced within the individual leaders, not teams. The goal of organizations during the time of trait theory was to control resources, avoid uncertainty, and control change (Poole & Van de Ven, 2004). Innovation, under trait-based leadership, occurred only when embedded routines were broken and novel solutions were implemented by the leader in a problem-focused approach. However, leaders who made unilateral decisions were much less successful than collaborative leaders in creating innovation within their organizations. This highlights the fact that individual leaders are less likely to create novel solutions to problems if they act alone.

Equally important is the impact of trait leadership ideals on EBP. Trait leadership theories can manifest EBP as a linear process with a single unidirectional answer that originated from the leader with little input from the team. Examples of this type of EBP practice can be found in outdated clinician-centered models of care in which questioning the expert on care interventions was heavily discouraged and could result in a formal reprimand or humiliation. This type of culture does not support evidence- or team-based care and can create organizational cultures that lead to poor quality, uncoordinated care, and cost increases (Wong, Cummings, & Ducharme, 2013).

Trait theories have several limitations. There is a lack of research on women and minority leaders, which created a gap that limits the understanding of the traits of successful leaders (Bass, 2008). Additionally, no universal traits have been linked to a significant number of successful leaders. The lack of cultural discernment creates assumptions and values that center on mechanistic workflow and productivity. Staff motivation is assumed to be driven by the leader and supported by the organizational operational theories of command and control. Current literature and understanding of motivation overwhelmingly refute the idea that individual motivation is extrinsic.

The trait era identified certain aspects the leader needed to achieve success. Anderson, Manno, O'Connor, and Gallagher (2010) linked several traits, such as approachability, conflict management, and honesty, among others, to the improvement of quality measures on nursing units. These studies focused only on the individual leader's actions, and the researchers did not investigate the influence of other nurses and health professionals in the system. The lack of evidence confirming a set of universal leader traits that was independent of cultural context led researchers and theorists to change focus from universal traits to examining individual leadership styles.

▶ Style Leadership Theories

As the industrial revolution gave way to more complex organizational forms, and because trait theories did not adequately explain all the facets of leadership, a new group of leadership theories emerged. The style theories contended that leaders emerge when their style fits that of the group from which they are emerging (Bass, 2008; Northouse, 2018). For example, a leader might have an autocratic or democratic style of leadership rather than universal leadership traits. According to the style theory, leaders were successful when their pattern of behavior had a goodness of fit with the group they were leading (Bass, 2008). To maintain power, leaders select followers that fit best with the leader's personal style.

Leadership style theories did not account for all the factors that impacted innovation. Cummings, Midodzi, Wong, and Estabrooks (2010) found that leadership style alone is not connected to patient mortality. Rather, the researchers found that when the organization had a connected and consistent organizational culture, patient mortality was lower. Cummings and colleagues (2010) found that regardless of style, leaders who used relational and transformational styles have better quality outcomes than those who practice autocracy.

In style leadership, innovation typically occurs in response to an identified issue or problem. The leader's approach to innovation is limited based on the style of leadership he or she displays and will be successfully implemented only as long as the approach and solution is congruent with that of the whole team. Leaders who utilize assumptions of style theories as the predominant base of their leadership practice may limit innovation in organizations. Style leaders may have the tendency to select teams of followers based on similarity to the leader's view. This creates homogeneous teams with less diversity, which thus limits the amount of divergent thinking that is a proven catalyst to innovation. Additionally, certain styles of leadership can lead to poor innovation sustainability. For example, teams led by charismatic leaders may have early innovation success, but when the charismatic leader is not present, an innovation void is created because the followers are reliant on the leader for direction and inspiration.

In similar ways, style leadership theory assumptions can also impact EBP. Much like innovation, the sustainability of the EBP interventions may be reliant on the individual leader supporting the process. For example, a charismatic physician champion may support and manage the organizational dynamics to implement a complex fall intervention, but when that physician is absent, the organization moves back to old practices. Other styles, such as autocratic leadership, can support the leader in demanding certain practices, which may cause resentment, rebellion, and frustration in the followers who must implement a practice in which they were not involved in creating (Aarons & Sommerfeld, 2012; Bass, 2008; Porter-O'Grady & Malloch, 2015).

Leaders who practice only a single leadership style or set of assumptions may not be successful in innovation because there are several styles of leadership that were found to be successful depending on the context of the group goals and organizational structure (Cooper & Brady, 1981). The practice of one leadership style places the leader at risk for stagnation and poor adaptability to the constantly changing organizational environment. The discovery of successful styles led other leadership scholars to shift the focus of leadership research to the idea of contextually based leadership. In contextually based leadership theories, leaders change their style to meet the immediate needs of the followers and the organization (Cooper & Brady, 1981; Northouse, 2018). Leadership theories that grew from the contextual assumption are transformational and charismatic leadership (Bass, 2008).

▶ Transformational Leadership Theories

The third conceptual framework of leadership theory development includes transformational leadership. Transformational leadership elevated the leader from planner and motivator to a role that lay at the boundaries of the organization (Bass, 2008). No longer did the organizational leader work as a planner and productivity manager but rather as a vision setter and boundary manager. This elevation of the leader role left a gap between the leader and the point of production in hierarchy-based organizations. To fill this gap, the role of the manager emerged. The manager was expected to assume the role of motivator, productivity controller, planner, and supervisor, and it perpetuated the industrial idea of productivity management (Bass, 2008). With the creation of the manager role in the organization, the leader was freed from the day-to-day work and could focus attention on the relationships among organizational stakeholders and followers. The leader, as opposed to the manager, now focused on external pressures, while the manager was left to manage internal pressures. Networking among organizations quickly became the source of the competitive advantage and was a valued skill for the individual leader.

Transformational leadership theories conceptualize the locus of control originating from the followers rather than the individual leader. This conceptual shift changed the focus of leadership research to relationships leaders had with their followers and their organization. Networking and building relationships with the team became the main activities of the leader role.

Significant research has been conducted on the impact of transactional (trait and style) and transformational leadership styles on organizational quality, innovation, and cost (Avolio & Bass, 2002; Failla & Stichler, 2008; Nielsen, Yarker, Randall, & Munir, 2009; Stordeur, D'hoore, & Vandernberghe, 2001). Gowan, Henegan, and

McFadden (2009) found that transformational leadership, when combined with quality management, improved knowledge acquisition in healthcare organizations. Saint and colleagues (2010) studied healthcare leaders around the country and discovered that those with more transformational behaviors fostered cultures that had a lower incidence of hospital-acquired infections. Transformational leadership was found to be preferable and generally to have a more positive impact in terms of staff satisfaction, employee retention, innovation implementation, and organizational success (Failla & Stichler, 2008). These studies also conceptualized the leader as an individual and demonstrated that the main responsibility of the transformational leader was to motivate staff, which is a hierarchal approach to leadership.

Transformational leadership theory purports that the individual leader must help his or her followers transcend to become extraordinary organizational teams (Northouse, 2018). The impact of transformational leaders on innovation can be mixed. Although transformational leaders focus on empowering their followers to become more adaptable, the underlying assumption of transformational leadership is that followers are powerless to become intrinsically motivated, initiate change themselves, or lead themselves. These assumptions can cause the leader to reject innovations that originate from the front lines because it might not align or represent the vision of the transformational leader. Additionally, leaders who practice transformational leadership might also spend a disproportionate amount of time on setting an organizational vision where the vision can become restrictive and reflective of the individual leader's vision, not that of the organization or the other members of the organization. As we will discuss later in this chapter, misaligned or individual-focused visions actually restrict innovation in organizations. One thing is clear: transformational leadership will create more innovation opportunities than simply practicing reward and punishment styles, such as transactional leadership behaviors (Weberg, 2013).

Transformational leadership has been linked to positive outcomes for the implementation of EBP frameworks in health care (Aarons & Sommerfeld, 2012). The assumptions that transformational leaders appeal to the higher moral values and ethics of the followers may be one reason why transformational leaders can accomplish EBP more effectively, although studies have also shown that transactional leadership has improved EBP adoption as well. This may suggest that any leadership that focuses on EBP will improve adoption in the short term. Because organizational growth and development are not short-term goals, the focus of innovation and EBP leadership shifts to determine what type of leadership will sustain the practice of EBP and allow the organization to enculturate it rather than treat it as yet another transformational initiative.

▶ Outcomes of Traditional Leadership Models

Traditional leadership theories and models are limited in their description of leadership behaviors. Historically, leadership theory focused on special traits of leaders, situational demands, the interaction of leader traits and situational context, and the dyadic relationship between leader and follower (Bass, 2008). Traditional leadership studies have studied only two outcomes: how leaders are chosen, and how well leaders function. These research traditions have defined a leader only as an individual who can influence followers through motivation, manipulation, action, reward, or punishment. For example, one limitation of transformational leadership research is that the leader is conceptualized as an individual, and the organizational culture and emergence of unpredictable leadership within followers and teams in the organization is ignored. Ignoring organizational culture leads to narrow conclusions regarding why the organizational change occurred.

Leadership in the traditional sense is a role rather than a set of behaviors, and it places power in the position rather than in relationships. Leaders who assume command-and-control behaviors and operate from the traditional paradigm of leadership damage organizations, create dysfunctional teams, and kill innovation by creating inefficient and broken systems. Health care has been directly impacted by these leadership traditions.

Boonstra and Broekhuis (2010) cited risk-averse and innovation-naive leadership and resistance to change as major reasons for the slow adoption of electronic medical records (EMRs) and possibly EBP. Further, traditional models of leadership are associated with high staff burnout, poor patient care outcomes, high turnover of staff, and negative impact on cost and outcomes (Kaiser, 2017). Losada (1999) found teams that focused on personal agendas were lower performing than teams that allowed for emergent leadership. Other research has uncovered that transactional leadership behaviors in healthcare leaders has led to worse patient outcomes as well.

The leader's role from the traditional perspective was developed in an age in which the world was focused on industrialization and production quotas (Bass, 2008). Two of the problems associated with poor quality and traditional leadership assumptions are top-down linear thinking and a focus on individuals.

Traditional Leaders as Top-Down Linear Thinkers

Leadership theories that were developed during the industrial era, on the basis of which many current healthcare leaders were trained, focused on maximizing production through linear processes (Bass, 2008; Porter-O'Grady & Malloch, 2015). Linear models assume that the input to the system will yield a proportional and predictable output. For example, a leader who attempts to reduce budget overruns by simply cutting supplies, staff, or hours is employing linear leadership without taking unpredictable system impacts into account. A focus on linear processes removes the capacity for the system to effectively change and innovate because effective change and innovation take place through relationship building, nonlinear processes, and coevolution. When interaction and connections are removed from the system, the system becomes weaker and less able to translate information into knowledge for change (Delia, 2010). Specifically, if leaders are always the source of solutions, their team will rapidly become incapable of solving problems on their own. This will reduce that ability of the team to adapt to critical situations and place more pressure on the leader, thus isolating the leader even more.

By reducing the number and quality of relationships within the organization, the organization voids its alignment with the complexity level of the environment, making the organization reactive rather than proactive. Leaders can reduce relationships, and consequently the power of the network, by limiting interactions among team members. This may be through leader-focused problem solving, reducing interactions or meetings to discuss department needs, or repeatedly dismissing staff concerns or ideas. The reduction in relationships can take place because of impediments to information flow, poor relationships among team members or departments, lack of diversity in the system, and ineffective communication patterns, among others.

Leaders using linear thinking contribute to the system inefficiencies in health care today. For example, EMR implementation is now a core concern for healthcare organizations and leaders, yet the first EMR was planned back in 1970 and was launched as a free application by the U.S. Department of Veterans Affairs in 1997 (Kumar & Aldrich, 2010). Now, nearly 50 years later, organizations are scrambling to optimize electronic records in massive rollout campaigns that cost millions of dollars and result in years of work. Innovations like EMRs require complex systems leadership and adaptive behaviors to be successful. Leading in top-down and linear methodologies results in missing key complexities in implementation, such as training, adoption, user interfaces, and nuances in practice that can result in major inefficiencies in the system.

Leaders as Individuals

Stacey (2007) suggested that leaders who are disconnected from the organizational culture and create visions and plans without input from the team can push the system away from its desired state and thus increase organizational anxiety. Leaders can become disconnected from the organization if they conceptualize leadership as an individual endeavor. All the leadership theories discussed thus far in this chapter have conceptualized leaders and leadership as originating from individuals instead of from the interactions of groups and teams. Although organizations can be influenced by individuals, leadership that results in organizations adopting new work or adapting to environmental pressures results from many more sources, including the organizational interactions that make up culture.

Schein & Schein (2017) suggested that organizational culture is made up of deep assumptions that drive behavior at the subconscious level, values that influence day-to-day work, and physical rituals or objects that define the work, called artifacts (see **BOX 2-1**). By understanding the impact of leadership behaviors within the organizational culture, the leader can better work with the complex variables of personality, and other people in the system can aid in the development of appropriate solutions and trajectories for the organization.

▶ Summary of Traditional Leadership Theories

The progression of leadership theories demonstrates the evolution of the leader's role from command and control to transforming followers to networking and relationships. This progression of theory also moves from simple to more complex ideas regarding what influences organizational change. According to trait theory, inborn traits alone create good leaders. As the concept of transformational leadership became more widely studied, the idea of leadership as a dynamic relationship among culture, followers, self, and organization became increasingly accepted. Although transformational leadership began to better explain leadership in organizations, there was still a gap between the individual stakeholders and the emergent leadership that was being seen in organizational culture research. Practicing leadership using traditional behaviors also led to specific problems in healthcare organizations.

BOX 2-1 What Are Artifacts, Values, and Deep Assumptions?

Artifacts are physical representations of the organization's culture. Signs, banners, decorations, unit setups, and trinkets in a unit or department can give the leader clues about the values of the organizational culture. For example, at the start of each shift, nurses may place yellow sticky notes with their names on mobile computer workstations to claim them as theirs. If others use the claimed workstation, the associated nurse may reprimand the violator and proceed to discuss the many ways the person had disrupted her workflow. This example provides insights into the values of the unit, including poor adaptability to workflow disruption, individual nurse-centered care practices, and potentially a lack of computer resources to carry out work. Just as leaders can use artifacts to gather information about a culture, leaders can also use artifacts to begin to change culture. For example, leaders can post innovation quotes in the break room to support innovation thinking. A more active intervention would be to set up meeting space in a way that enables discussion and discourse rather than classroom-style seating charts.

Values and deep assumptions also underlie an organization's culture. Unlike artifacts, values and deep assumptions are shared by actions, interactions, and discussions among the members of the culture. For example, a care team that is unwelcoming to new or inexperienced staff may signal a value placed on years of service over competency of care. To explore values and deep assumptions, the leader must walk in the shoes of the culture and spend time reflecting and interpreting actions, clarifying their meaning with the members, and experiencing the behaviors of the culture to understand and intervene.

Discussion

What artifacts, values, or deep assumptions exist in your place of work, and what do they tell you about the culture of the department or organization? How do these artifacts, values, or deep assumptions assist or inhibit innovation leadership behaviors?

A gap also exists between the ways in which leadership scholars and organizational culture scholars conceptualize the creation of innovation and organizational life. Complexity leadership theory provides a lens through which this gap narrows by combining leadership and culture as a dynamic that influences one another rather than being discrete. That having a different lens will lend further insight into the realities of organizational life, something Lord (2008) suggested, was not addressed through existing leadership methodologies.

DISCUSSION

Think about the leadership in your current organization or past organizations. What types of leadership (trait, style, transformational) were practiced? Provide a few examples of behaviors you witnessed to support your answer. How did they impact your practice? How did they impact evidence-based practice?

▶ Complexity Leadership

Leaders are finally realizing that the world is filled with uncertainty, interrelationships, and self-organizing that does not align well with the linear thinking of trait and style leadership assumptions. In contrast, complexity leadership challenges the long-held assumptions of linear thinking, emerging as a new paradigm of organizational leadership. Complexity leadership behaviors have been shown to improve team performance, increase the ability of the organization to adapt and innovate, and promote quality outcomes (Losada 1999; Shipton, Armstrong, West, & Dawson, 2008; Uhl-Bien & Marion, 2008). For example, Losada (1999) found that teams displaying complexity leadership behaviors performed better than teams that demonstrated command-and-control characteristics.

The characteristics of complexity leadership theory (CLT) include leadership recognition of interrelationships, emergence, and fostering innovation (Uhl-Bien & Marion, 2008). CLT recognizes the dynamic interactions that take place within organizations as they change, create innovation, and evolve with a focus on complex relationships and network interaction rather than controlling, standardizing, and autocracy (Uhl-Bien & Marion, 2008) (**FIGURE 2-1**).

For healthcare organizations to accommodate innovations, and EBP to increase quality and shift from volume to value services, leadership must focus on collaboration, self-organization, and the construction of strong networks among agents in the system (Uhl-Bien & Marion, 2008).

CLT was developed to address the shortcomings of traditional leadership theory in explaining the way organizations evolve through leadership in the knowledge era. CLT focuses on leadership rather than the leader. Leaders are individuals who influence others toward an outcome, and leadership is the process by which agents of a system learn their way out of problems toward adaptive outcomes. There are three leadership behaviors within CLT: administrative, adaptive, and enabling.

Administrative leadership is conceptualized as the formal hierarchy of the organization, including the chief executive officer, directors, managers, and other formalized leadership positions. The administrative leadership behavior is closely related to the traditional leadership ideas presented earlier in this chapter. Administrative leadership is conceptualized in CLT because of the underlying assumption

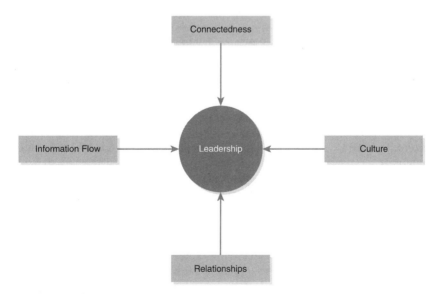

FIGURE 2-1 Elements of complexity leadership.

that organizations cannot exist without some formal structure (Uhl-Bien & Marion, 2008). Although this framework is similar to traditional notions of leadership, CLT describes administrative leadership as being only one piece of leadership rather than the predominant function of leadership within organizations. Administrative leadership in CLT improves applicability to current organizations by acknowledging their existing structures as a relevant part of leadership and innovation.

The second leadership component is the adaptive leader. According to Uhl-Bien and Marion (2008), adaptive leadership is "an emergent, interactive dynamic that produces adaptive outcomes in a social system" (p. 200). Adaptive leadership differs from administrative leadership in that adaptive leadership is the collective action that emerges from interactive exchanges among agents in the system (Delia, 2010). This means that adaptive leadership is not an action of any one individual but the collective influence that occurs as teams of people interact over time. For example, clinical teams that create interactive journal clubs begin to influence practice change over time without a formal leader intervention. The change in practice is influenced by the continual debate and assessment of the latest evidence, which is internalized by the group to inform their daily clinical practice.

The third leadership dynamic is enabling leadership. Enabling leadership is a person or group that brings together diverse agents in a system and creates a catalyst for the self-organization and emergent action of adaptive leadership to take place. In essence, an enabling leader is also an innovation leader. Enabling leaders connect people across the organization in meaningful ways to accomplish adaptive problem solving. All three leadership dynamics are entangled and cannot be separated and studied alone. As the three complexity leadership behaviors arise in an organization, they shape the complex adaptive system, and in return the complex adaptive system shapes the leadership behaviors.

Although a bit dated, Burns (2001) surveyed healthcare leaders on their acceptance of the core underpinnings of complexity leadership in relation to creating successful organizations. The results suggested that leaders had intuitive support for the concepts but were uncomfortable with the concepts that required them to give up some control over processes. Specifically, 41% disagreed with the complexity leadership concept that advised leaders to "build a good-enough vision and provide minimum specifications, rather than trying to plan out every little detail" (p. 480). This result suggests that although leaders intuit that complexity leadership is a good practice, they have trouble accepting a loss of direct control that accompanies complexity leadership behaviors.

A study by Hanson and Ford (2010) that used dynamic network analysis, a quantitative complex system analysis tool, demonstrated that the core leaders in a hospital laboratory setting were not formal directors or administrators but rather customer service representatives—workers on the front line. The study showed through social network analysis methods that the customer service core played an important role in conducting information flow to all others in the lab and had a heavy influence among other lab sections. These findings are contrary to what a traditional leader might expect, but from the complexity perspective, to get work done in the lab, an employee would have to interact with customer service workers due to their high influence and information. Hanson and Ford suggested that the assumption that formal leaders hold the core information for operation of the organization is not accurate. Instead, the department's network was able to accomplish work through distributed power networks rather than strong administrative leadership.

Complexity leadership suggests that the network contains significantly more influence, power to change, and capability to accomplish outcomes than any one individual, regardless of that individual's expertise. Departments in which the reliance of work is on one or two individuals have very weak network strength and are at risk of poor adaptability and ultimately failure. For example, if a department relies on a manager to make all decisions—from staffing to supplies to change management—the capability of the unit to function without that manager is very low. This puts the entire unit at risk for chaos when that leader departs. Complexity leaders should focus energy on building strong networks that are able to nimbly adapt to departures, crises, and environmental pressures.

Rowe and Hogarth (2005) used a complex adaptive systems metaphor intervention to facilitate change in public health nursing. The study examined pilot sites that instituted a complex adaptive system tool that was a vehicle for discussion of the strengths and weaknesses of organizational change. This tool was used to facilitate change in behavior and service among public health nurses. According to the researchers, when the formal leaders, from administrators to the nurses on the front line, embraced the movement of decision making and policy setting, an increase in experimentation and innovation arose that led to new service delivery models and to higher levels of responsibility and decision making for the practitioners. This means that when operating under complexity principles, practitioners are more autonomous, make better decisions, and innovate more.

Sweetman (2010) used surveys and social network analysis and found that the characteristics of leadership, innovation, and creativity in organizations were much more decentralized than previously thought. The sample consisted of a 60-person nonprofit that provided a leadership development program to high school and college students. The participants constituted a diverse group: managers, financial services representatives, engineers, and educators. Sweetman (2010) found that innovation was highly correlated with adaptive function (.59, $p < 0.001$), collective creativity (.67, $p < 0.001$), and shared leadership (.59, $p < 0.001$). All three must be present for innovation to occur. Additionally, Sweetman (2010) concluded that one individual is not primarily involved in all innovations and that numerous actors innovate, with innovation occurring across the organization. This finding supports the complexity leadership concept that leadership and innovation can occur at any level and between any individuals in the organization. Sweetman's work was limited to describing specific behaviors of leaders in the decentralized leadership role, or how these behaviors connected with innovation implementation.

Complexity leadership provides a foundation for conceptualizing leaders and leadership differently to facilitate innovation. Additionally, complexity leadership characteristics are congruent with healthcare leaders' ideas of ideal leadership behaviors (self-organizations, emergence, etc.) and improve creativity, lead to more innovation, and engage care providers. The results of these early studies provide evidence that further understanding of the characteristics of complexity leadership in healthcare organizations may provide a new framework to increase innovation, reduce costs, and improve quality.

Innovation in CLT

Complexity leadership suggests that interactions among all agents shape the organizational context and thus deviant or abnormal agents are the result of deeper assumptions in the organization. For example, agents in the system may test outdated or irrelevant polices through positive deviant behavior. Positive deviance is behavior that challenges organizational norms to find better ways of working (Jaramillo et al., 2008). When faced with positive deviant behavior, the complexity leader reviews organizational incongruence that may signal needed change. Behavior that is not consistent with past assumptions may be a sign that innovation is needed rather than considered negative or a threat to stability. The role of leadership as seen through the complexity lens is to help shape a context by translating information to teams so that they can make informed and relevant decisions to conduct their work and solve problems they face.

EBP in CLT

Data and evidence are part of the organization's information flow and influence how agents in the system act and interact. The leader's role is to ensure that the information flowing through the system is based on the best evidence and not on rumor, past practices, linear sources, or misinterpretations. It is important that information is not shared without regarding its validity, source, or reliability. In the absence of validated information, agents will begin to make assumptions based on the information at hand. Instilling a culture of EBP in the organization will help remove gaps in information and support more informed adaptations.

Complexity provides a different lens to view interactions and leadership in organizations. Innovation is a core behavior as people adapt based on information flow, interactions, relationships, and organizational culture. Evidence is generated, interpreted, and acted upon across all areas of the system. Leaders should work to build cultures that support interactions, build relationships, and improve information flow to all areas of the organization.

▶ Healthcare Quality and a Lack of Innovation

Traditional and less adequate leadership practices in healthcare systems that lead to practice variation and poor innovation implementation include autocratic, standardized, controlled, and profit-driven behaviors as the means to achieve organizational outcomes. Leadership scholars have proposed that the pathway to improving organizational outcomes, and ultimately patient outcomes, may indeed be found in a different leadership model. A leadership practice that is shared among employees, where uncertainty is normative, mutual goals are facilitated, and innovation behaviors are foundational characteristics will support organizations to radically change to meet the challenges of healthcare reform and improved quality. In essence, a model in which teams of nurses, physicians, administrators, and other healthcare workers demonstrate leadership behaviors that facilitate change and innovation supported by data and evidence is essential.

> A leadership practice that is shared among employees, where uncertainty is normative, mutual goals are facilitated, and innovation behaviors are foundational characteristics, will support organizations to radically change to meet the challenges of healthcare reform and improved quality.

Quality issues such as inappropriate variations in care, consumer dissatisfaction, adverse events, medication errors, falls, and surgery mistakes have plagued the U.S. healthcare system for decades. Solutions to many quality issues have been found through innovation in practice supported by evidence, yet implementing, spreading, and sustaining these solutions in practice has been difficult. There is a need to better understand and utilize specific innovation leadership behaviors to improve health care.

DISCUSSION

Lack of innovation leadership is one reason we have a gap in quality health care. Describe one failed implementation you have witnessed and the leadership characteristics that may have hindered the innovation or evidence-based intervention. What would you have changed?

▶ Seven Characteristics of Innovation Leadership

In many cases, the implementation of innovation or EBP is not a single planned event but rather the synthesis of multiple interactions and changes that occur as the innovation is introduced. Innovation occurs over time as interconnected individuals in the organization adapt, through small changes, to pressures internally and externally by displaying leadership behaviors and influencing teams. Plowman and Duchon (2008) described these emerging actions as the essence of change: "Change occurs continuously, as minor adaptations, which can accumulate, amplify and become radical" (p. 145). The innovation in organizations occurs as information flows through the organization, is processed, and disrupts or shifts the normal operating procedures. These disruptions are reflected as team members challenge their assumptions of how to best complete work and interact, and the organization changes its structure to accommodate the innovation. These structural changes can be in culture, the hierarchical organization, or care delivery.

Leadership behaviors are exhibited by all members of the organization and are not solely expressed by individuals acting alone or those with formal leadership roles. Leadership behaviors are displayed when opportunities are presented in the organization's internal and external environment. The seven innovation leadership characteristics described in the following sections have been identified as influencing the movement of the organization toward adaption to the changing conditions: boundary spanning, risk taking, visioning, leveraging opportunity, adaptation, coordination of information flow, and facilitation. Each of these seven characteristics will be summarized and discussed in the context of innovation leadership.

Boundary Spanning

In traditional leadership, boundary spanning is reserved for top levels of the organizational hierarchy (Bass, 2008; Poole & Van de Ven, 2004). Boundary spanning is the process of agents in a system making connections to otherwise unconnected groups. Boundary spanning is usually demonstrated by multiple team members regardless of their formal titles. Boundary spanners look for outside guidance, ideas, and relationships to secure resources and increase knowledge within the organization. Boundary spanning activities increase the information flow into the organization and provide other team members with vital data that influences their leadership behaviors and subsequent actions. Boundary spanning also increases the connections and relationships of the organization, effectively building a larger network through which information could be exchanged and used to continually shift the work of the organization.

Boundary spanning is a behavior demonstrated by multiple individuals in the organization. This characteristic emerges as a team recognizes its deficits in knowledge about an innovation or organizational shift. Team members with connections external to the organization seek out information from these sources and introduce this information to the rest of the team to facilitate decision making and innovation integration.

Recognizing Boundary Spanning

CLT provides a framework to better understand boundary spanning by categorizing the administrative, enabling, and adaptive leadership behaviors (Schreiber, 2006; Uhl-Bien & Marion, 2008). Boundary spanning is demonstrated by multiple agents at different times in the innovation process, which is inconsistent with traditional notions of individual-focused leadership (Schreiber, 2006). Recognizing how boundary spanning occurs in organizations may inform how other teams gather external information to facilitate innovation implementation.

Administrative leadership behaviors include boundary spanning across disciplines and individuals to support funding, planning, and space allocations that help introduce resources needed for innovation to enter the system. Administrative leadership is demonstrated by both formal leaders and informal leaders within the system (Uhl-Bien & Marion, 2008).

Enabling leadership behaviors can occur in both formal and informal leaders as they gather external expertise to consult on ideas or projects in which internal capacity was limited. User design experts, technology experts, and even frontline administrative assistants can provide information to build futuristic innovations and EBP rather than having a single leader plan and design the innovation with his or her individual expertise.

Enabling and administrative behaviors facilitate adaptive leadership behaviors. Adaptive leadership is reflected as team members process the new information gained by the boundary-spanning behaviors and integrate this information into decisions that result in new buildings, new techniques, and shifts in values. For example, team members may process information gathered through boundary spanning and begin to shift their value of their current organizational practices to new, possibly better, practices learned from outside entities. Thus, boundary spanning facilitates allowing team members in the organization to gather enough information to begin challenging assumptions and start taking risks.

Risk Taking

Risk taking is reflected as individuals begin experimenting with untested technologies or practices and gather information about them. Risk taking is dependent on team members actively identifying internal and external pressures and processing the impact and fit with organizational practices and context. A lack of fit creates tension or chaos and provides the needed push to try new ways of work. This process is congruent with the notion that innovation occurs when organizations are near chaos (Porter-O'Grady & Malloch, 2015; Stacey, 2007; Uhl-Bien & Marion, 2008). Fit finding and testing activities reflect risk-taking behaviors because innovation practices that are tested usually have little evidence supporting them, and there is no blueprint for implementing innovation into the organization. Many risk-taking behaviors focus on trial-and-error efforts that test different technologies and implementation strategies to find the goodness of fit with the organization. The trial-and-error activities challenge the assumption that current practices or methods are adequate and introduce complex technologies and practices to individuals who were not previously comfortable with those technologies and practices. Trial-and-error activity generates information about the innovation that allows team members to assess its value, learn about the functionality, and better understand how to integrate it into the day-to-day activity of workers. Leaders must create a safe environment to support risk taking by using course correction rather than punishment as the norm in dealing with failures. Risk taking also increases the visibility, trialability, and usability of the innovation, which allows others to experience the innovation and create their own assessments of it (Rogers, 2003).

Recognizing Risk Taking

The behaviors of risk taking can also be explained using CLT. Administrative leadership behaviors describe how team members experiment with innovation by remaining open to new teaching modalities and feedback from individuals who are internal and external to the system to help create the future movement of the department. Leaders in the organization should remain open and supportive of risk-taking behaviors.

Enabling leadership behaviors reflects experimentation with an innovation after that innovation was introduced into the organization and its practice was supported through feedback and information flow. Adaptive leadership is demonstrated as the individuals evolve over time, testing the innovation and practice against previous operating schemas and remaining open to adaptive outcomes that differ from the traditional methodology. The adaptive function is a result of the agent's ability to process information and make decisions at the point of service and integrate new practices into his or her work.

Risk-taking behaviors reflect a decision by a team to gather more information about the innovation. Individuals challenge current organizational assumptions, which creates opportunity for change in the organization. Risk taking disrupts the context of the organization and provides an opportunity for other team members to observe the innovation and develop their own assessments of its usefulness. This behavior seems to emerge from the risk taker's focus on maintaining quality of care while adapting to the stresses and opportunities presented by the environment. Risk takers seek out opportunities to test innovations to achieve high-level outcomes based on their professional values and their desire to improve work environments and outcomes.

Visioning

Groups of interconnected agents display the characteristic of visioning in organizations. Visioning is not an individual or isolated activity, and if practiced in a silo, it will lead to dysfunctional and fragmented organizational work. One example occurred in a case study in which faculty members adopted a simulation program into their college. The individual faculty members described their leadership roles as informal, but when these same faculty members described the faculty group as a whole, they described a decision-making body with inherent power. Axelrod and Cohen (2000) suggested that the coevolutionary process of organizations is reflected in the combination of the individual strategy decisions made at the agent level. Uhl-Bien and Marion (2008) suggested that networks of agents work together to create the future. Some decisions may be made in cooperation with other agents, while others are made to further an individual agenda. Both types of decision making—group and individual—occur in organizations and influence the outcomes of the team and the larger departments. The innovative leader must recognize this and learn how to facilitate either process to advance practice and innovation. The visioning process is reflective of the coevolutionary process in which individuals collaborate as a group to create the vision for the team, department, or organization. This dynamic contrasts with many traditional leadership theories that suggest the formal leader must create a vision for the future (Bass, 2008). Formal leaders should provide input and suggestions but not create the vision in isolation.

Recognizing Visioning

Visioning reflects the notions of macro-level strategy as described by Dooley and Lichtenstein (2008). Macro leadership behaviors include strategic planning, resource support, gathering funding, and moral support. Leaders who display macro influence and thinking have a disproportionate impact on the organizational trajectory (Dooley & Lichtenstein, 2008; Hazy et al., 2007). For example, agents in a network whose roles are frontline in nature can, through their actions and interactions, create change in the mission of the organization even though leading such change is not within their formal job descriptions. Individuals are able to adjust their behaviors and relationships to translate their day-to-day work to the long-range planning and strategy of the organization as they meet in groups, teams, and cohorts both in formal and informal ways. Collaborative leadership occurs through group interaction and dialogue. Macro-leadership behaviors occur through connections and information flow between agents, not through individual decision making and control (Uhl-Bien & Marion, 2008). Leaders and frontline workers, who individually may not carry out strategic planning, come together as a group and exercise macro-level leadership influences that build strategy and inform the organization's vision.

Many professions describe autonomy of decision making as a core value of the professional practice model. This value allows for the professionals to combine autonomous efforts, and create robust strategy and operational standards that are important to the success of the innovation. The traditional notion of managers and directors as planning, leading, and controlling the change process is challenged by recent evidence and complexity research (Weberg, 2013). Rather, formal leaders should view their role as facilitator and influencer. The absence of command-and-control leadership allows for individuals and teams in the organization to develop strategy by connecting the day-to-day work and resulting innovations to the desired outcomes of professional practice, patient outcomes, and organizational success.

Leveraging Opportunity

Leveraging opportunity is a characteristic that is demonstrated by all individuals in an organization. The behavior of leveraging opportunity is reflected in the actions of individuals who look for creative solutions to opportunities that presented themselves in the organization and in the environment. This may be looking for creative funding for innovations, linking current initiatives to support needed changes, or connecting teams working on similar projects to build stronger efforts. For example, the risk-taking behaviors that are adopted in an effort to find a new way to complete work demonstrates a focus on the opportunity rather than on the problem. More specifically, work-arounds, adaptations to EMR templates, and adopting new EBP in complex situations with unclear answers are ways that healthcare workers demonstrate leveraging opportunity.

Recognizing Leveraging Opportunity

Much of the traditional leadership literature highlights problem solving as a key characteristic of formal leaders (Bass, 2008; Plowman & Duchon, 2008; Poole & Van de Ven, 2004). Complexity literature reflects a different focus of leaders in that formal leaders are not equipped to solve all organizational issues and are more effective leaders when they facilitate the team to tackle these issues. Thus, formal leaders should help create and identify the opportunities that teams can leverage in order to innovate. Plowman and Duchon (2008) proposed that conflict and divergence are the first steps in a change process. Further, leaders must be aware of conflict, look for patterns in the disruption, and see the opportunities these disruptions provide for innovation. Leaders who leveraged opportunity displayed enabling and adaptive leadership behaviors (Uhl-Bien & Marion, 2008). Enabling behaviors are reflected in the way opportunities are presented to the others in the organization. Instead of framing the external pressures as problems requiring cuts and reductions, leaders can frame external pressures as opportunities requiring novel solutions. Adaptive behaviors are reflected in the way teams self-adapt and begin implementing new work strategies in response to opportunity and shifts.

Adaptation

The interconnectedness among agents continually restructures as innovation adoption spreads. This is evident as individuals in the organization adapt their roles depending on the opportunities presented by innovation or EBP implementation. For example, in an EMR implementation, some nurses shifted roles from bedside care to solving technology issues and troubleshooting with their colleagues. The technology support role was not part of the formal job expectations, but it was required by the organization to maintain member buy-in for the EMR implementation. These role changes reflect the ability of agents to adapt based on information and need, without requiring a formal hierarchal change or command decision. Many adaptations are based on the drive to implement innovation and more individual-focused human behaviors. Stacey (2007) suggested that complex systems are not predictable because they are impacted by unpredictable human behavior.

Recognizing Adaptation

Individual team members consistently assess their own value to the organization and the need to adapt behavior. When individuals adapt their behaviors from facilitating connections (nursing care) to more managerial work (solving technology issues), the network strength is impacted, resulting in changes to innovation adoption and success. Teams and leaders must recognize the need for coordination in the system and adapt new roles and leadership behaviors to continue the innovation trajectory of the organization.

Usually innovation work ebbs and flows with the connections of the network over time; reduced network coordination results in fragmented innovation. Schreiber and Carley (2008) stated that the collective action of change agents is a source of learning and adaptive response in the system. Further, they described collective change as being fostered by decentralized decision making and strong learning cultures. Both decentralized decision making, in the form of autonomous practice, and a learning culture may help explain how organizations are able to adopt innovation successfully.

Coordination of Information Flow

Individuals and teams in the innovation process should be able to influence how information is shared and interpreted and how agents in the system relate to each other in order to implement successful innovation through coordination of information flow. This leadership characteristic helps to evolve the organizational context by using connections and relationships to share new information while making it relevant to the organization's work. For example, innovation champions may express the successes of innovation to other departments through meetings, one-on-one conversations, and stories. These leadership actions reflect enabling behaviors (Uhl-Bien & Marion, 2008).

Enabling leadership behaviors are demonstrated as the individual team members influence one another by changing how artifacts and values are communicated and by shifting information flow in the organization to influence how other team members perceive an innovation. Strategy documents may be written, and innovation adopters may praise the use of the technique in open forums. Leaders should challenge their own assumptions about the current work and shift their actions and language to convey more positive outcomes of a change in work if there are possible or perceived benefits. This activity gathers buy-in and adds other agents to the network to begin to adapt to the innovation implementation. The actions of value shifting and adaptation align with the work of scholars who described the coevolution of systems toward adaptive outcomes (Axelrod & Cohen, 2000; Hatch, 2000; Hazy et al., 2007; Uhl-Bien & Marion, 2008; Van de Ven & Hargrave, 2004).

Recognizing Coordination of Information Flow

Leaders can recognize messengers of innovation by looking for evangelists who promote the innovation, examine documents that reflect the underlying response to the innovation, and assess the information that is created about the innovation. For example, innovation champions may promote the use of the innovation and communicate the successes through connections and relationships. Strategy documents can reflect the desire to grow the innovation and to continue to refine and coordinate the efforts when using the innovation. Additionally, formal leaders should continue to assess the organizational context to determine if and when resources or administrative influence is needed to overcome stagnated processes.

Healthcare organizations are complex systems that contain subsystems of a large organization, and leaders must navigate through the bureaucracy by catalyzing change through resource allocation and facilitating a context that values agent autonomy and decentralized decision making. Formal processes such as shared governance, administrative approval processes, and bureaucracy are a normal part of organizational life, but formal leaders can help reduce the restricting impact of these structures on the innovation at the front line of the organization by promoting shared decision making by the end user. As Uhl-Bien and Marion (2008) suggested, leaders can overcome stagnating structures by becoming catalysts and resource gatherers for change. Stacey (2007) described these processes as balancing negative and positive feedback loops in the system to keep it moving at the edge of chaos. Messaging innovation reflects targeted information flow through the organization and results in improving interest in the new techniques.

Facilitation

The role of leaders in influencing information flow centers on helping organizational members to see an innovation as relevant to their work through the characteristic of facilitation. Complexity research shifts the leader's focus from controlling actions of individuals to influencing and facilitating the information those individuals get and use in the process of decision making. These behaviors influence the system to consider new ways of operating by allowing for professional decision making and innovation. The leadership actions should not be aimed at directing the work of nurses, for example; there should be, instead, a high degree of value placed on professional autonomy. Leaders in the system facilitate and coordinate opportunities for the agents to build connections and relationships with one another and experience the innovation firsthand. Facilitation is displayed in gathering information, making sense of it, and allowing the autonomous agents to integrate it through resource allocation and relationships rather than through command-and-control tactics. Many times, formal leaders may feel they have little direct-line authority to force change on the professional. Their only option is to facilitate and influence innovation.

Recognizing Facilitation

By fostering interactions, facilitating information, and understanding that leadership is a system behavior, leaders can look for the points in the system where their influence is most needed and valued. Developing and facilitating these network interactions helps to build the organizational context that sets the rules of engagement that can lead to emergent displays of leadership without requiring or depending on formal leader input to the system. Facilitation is reflected in practice as team members adopting an innovation aid others to use the new technique through trial and error rather than initially creating perfectly working systems. This process creates a context of ownership around the innovation and allows the team members to develop new skills through utilization of the new technology or practice. Additionally, facilitation allows the team members to customize the innovation to their objectives, which allows them to find the fit between the new technique and their own practice philosophies. This customization improves buy-in to using an innovation and reflects enabling leadership behaviors (Uhl-Bien & Marion, 2008).

Summary of Leadership Characteristics

No one individual reflects the risk taker or the boundary spanner, as is suggested in traditional leadership literature (Bass, 2008). Instead, boundary spanning, risk taking, and the other five leadership characteristics are reflected and practiced through the complex interaction of leadership behaviors by multiple individuals in response to emergent opportunities in the internal and the external environments. Boundary spanning and risk taking reflect the ability of the team to recognize knowledge deficits and seek out external information sources and bring them into the system for processing by other members. Visioning and leveraging opportunities reflect the team's ability to process information, look for opportunities to integrate the new technique into the organization's context, and create desired outcomes from the information. Adaptation, coordinating information flow, and facilitating reflect the ability of the team to adapt to changing conditions by creating internal emergent structures such as new roles, strategies, and information sharing that facilitate the adoption of the innovation. These characteristics reflect a new framework from which to understand leadership of an innovation—not through the direction of an individual formal leader but rather as a team focused on achieving the shared outcome of student success.

Leadership of innovation emerges from individual and group interactions. Formal and informal leaders influence information flow by boundary spanning, risk taking, visioning, leveraging opportunity, adaptation, coordination, and facilitation. The system then processes the information through autonomous decision making, collaboration, and formal structures that result in an organizational context that guides the implementation of the innovation. Leaders in health care should work to remove barriers to interaction and collaboration, create opportunities to catalyze innovation, and gather resources to further the innovation agenda. Leadership occurs at all levels and ranks in the organization, and the role of leaders of teams and leaders of innovation is that of building alignment and relationships rather than implementing command-and-control tactics.

▶ Implications

The seven behaviors of innovation leadership provide a new understanding of how leaders in health care can facilitate innovation in their organizations. Groups that will benefit most from these implications include nurses and other healthcare professionals, healthcare organizations, healthcare leaders, and researchers. The data and concepts support a new lens to view leadership, organizations, and innovation.

Implications for Nursing and Health Professionals

The seven behaviors of innovation leadership and the underlying CLT framework have several implications for the nursing profession and provide a new lens through which nurses and nursing leaders can facilitate innovation and EBP. Nurses in all roles of the profession can use this framework to begin to build innovation teams to respond to the changing healthcare landscape and align new care innovations with new and existing organizations. Nurses are uniquely positioned to lead the next revolution in health care because they are the hub of care coordination.

Nursing and healthcare leaders can use boundary spanning, risk taking, and messaging to improve information flow into their organizations. Nursing leaders must span beyond their nursing colleagues and the healthcare industry to find novel approaches and technologies to solve the problems of cost and quality facing today's healthcare organizations and nursing workforce. Healthcare professionals at all levels should use risk-taking characteristics to continually test new workflows, technologies, and patient care interventions using early evidence and clinical judgment. This can be done only if information about the changing healthcare landscape, organizational quality metrics, budget, and mission flows to the frontline nursing staff. Without this information, innovation may be restricted or fragmented.

Professional leaders can take risks by helping to recognize the innovative potential of work-arounds and new practices that are unproven but show promise in improving patient care. Leaders can also provide resources and support; additionally, they can facilitate cross-discipline interactions to build these new innovations. Most importantly, formal healthcare leaders can help coordinate the innovation occurring across the organization and facilitate alignment of these innovations with the trajectory of the organization.

Nurses are traditionally the hub of care for patients in hospitals and other places of care. Nurses connect multiple disciplines and coordinate care with a holistic patient focus. Nurses must leverage these connections to build strong collaborative relationships among team members and to design new models of care that are both patient-centric and cost-effective. They can do so by facilitating learning, exposing the care team to new innovations, and adopting risk-taking behaviors in regard to technology and care innovations.

The proposed leadership behaviors focus on organizational context, which, for nurses, may be of paramount importance. Cultures of nursing, as well as other professions, that are guided by punishment for error, negative attitudes toward young innovators, and the worship of ineffective past practices may lead to stagnated care and worsening quality. This chapter suggests that a culture in which trial and error is welcomed and learning is facilitated leads to new models of work that are more effective than past practices. It is imperative that nursing leaders and frontline nurses take note of the large impact that organizational context has on innovation and change.

Nursing and healthcare professionals have an obligation to the patient to continue to improve care and reduce cost while maintaining the highest ethical principles. Similarly, innovative change can be achieved while maintaining the core values of patient safety and professionalism. This endeavor requires new ways of leading and new definitions of leaders.

Implications for Healthcare Organizations

The described leadership behaviors challenge the traditional hierarchical structures and leadership methodologies present in many healthcare organizations. These traditional structures may be restricting innovation by limiting information flow, restricting connections among agents, and limiting diverse relationships, potentially resulting in fragmented organizational cultures and innovation.

Organizations need to consider restructuring their reporting hierarchy to mimic network relationships and promote information flow to the front line. Additionally, healthcare organizations have to refocus their organizational cultures to promote and support innovation competencies, such as risk taking and boundary spanning, to gain new insights to solve cost and quality problems. Similarly, organizations must focus resources on aligning new ideas with the work of the organization by intentionally crafting innovation messages, facilitating learning about innovations, and creating flexible roles that can adapt to shifting conditions. Proactively seeking innovations to overcome external pressures and working to align the innovation internally with the core mission of the organization are proposed new organizational competencies that are needed to navigate the changing healthcare landscape by facilitating innovation.

Implications for Healthcare Leaders

Healthcare leaders may stand to benefit significantly from the reframing of leadership and leadership behaviors presented in this chapter. The term *leader* refers to all individuals in the organization who administer, enable, and adapt novel solutions to complex situations. Burns (2001) found that healthcare leaders approved of the concepts of complexity leadership and, with the preliminary findings of the proposed framework of this case study, a new leadership framework presents tangible behaviors and characteristics of complexity leadership that healthcare leaders can use to build innovation competency in teams across an organization.

Most importantly, research suggests that formal leaders may be ill equipped to individually promote innovation. Instead, leaders should focus on building teams with the characteristics described in this study to create novel solutions. The focus of leadership should not be on controlling the process but rather on facilitating the optimization of leadership behaviors across the organization.

Information flow allows the group to have access to and gather needed information to make decisions concerning problem solving and innovation alignment with the organization. Formal leaders can facilitate this process by sharing data and explicating its relevance to the organizational mission. Additionally, formal leaders can eliminate traditional structures that dilute or restrict the sharing of information across groups in the organization. They may do so by reducing the focus on hierarchal reporting structures and individual-focused leadership practices. Adopting a focus on facilitating shared leadership structures may be more advantageous in terms of implementing innovations. All members of an organization can practice risk taking, boundary spanning, and visioning behaviors that aid in challenging less adequate organizational norms, build connections and relationships beyond the walls of the group or organization, and create compelling visions of the future. These behaviors are reflective of complexity leadership and facilitate the recognition of opportunities, improve information flow through the organization, and translate that information into a relevant trajectory for the organization.

Connections and relationships allow a group to access information and share it effectively. Connections without strong relationships reduce information flow and reduce innovation capacity and relevancy. These connections must also be easily changeable as internal and external pressures dictate. This chapter demonstrates that if resources are not available to solve management-type problems, such as technical issues, the innovation process may stagnate or stop altogether. Leaders in healthcare organizations can reduce this effect by building diverse connections and relationships among teams to leverage unique skill sets as issues arise. For example, if a team is working to implement a technological innovation, building relationships with information technology and electronic media teams may be necessary. Simply connecting these teams is not enough. The teams working toward innovation implementation need to have strong collaborative relationships as well. This means they must be able to move toward a common goal, freely exchange relevant information, and make coordinated decisions to advance the innovation. These relationships can be influenced by leaders in the organization through facilitating shared leadership, improving information flow, and helping build an organizational context that is supportive of teamwork and collaboration.

Organizational context is another factor that influences innovation implementation. Healthcare leaders need to recognize the role this factor plays in facilitating or limiting innovation in organizations. Cultures in which one group dominates decision making, collaboration is not facilitated, and trial and error is punished may be less likely to innovate. For example, a healthcare organization that values only physician leadership without input from nursing and ancillary care providers may result in a culture that restricts information flow about core business practices. This restriction in information flow limits the possible decision options and makes the implemented decisions less relevant to the nonincluded groups. This result leads to maladaptive behaviors and promotes a context of stagnation rather than innovation. An organization that values autonomy of decision making and has a context focused on organizational outcomes can collaborate across specialties to implement an innovation that meets the needs of several different groups.

Formal and informal leaders must recognize the impact and interrelatedness of information flow, connections, relationships, and culture on the innovation work of an organization. By developing new competencies for leadership, removing restrictive organizational context and structures, and facilitating rather than controlling, leaders can build an innovative organization that is ready to adapt and evolve to meet the cost and quality issues that continue to impact the U.S. healthcare system.

References

Aarons, G. A., & Sommerfeld, D. H. (2012). Leadership, innovation climate, and attitudes toward evidence-based practice during a statewide implementation. *Journal of American Academy of Adolescent Psychiatry, 51*(4), 270–280.

Anderson, B. J., Manno, M., O'Connor, P., & Gallagher, E. (2010). Listening to nursing leaders: Using national database of quality indicators data to study excellence in nursing leadership. *Journal of Nursing Administration, 40*(4), 182–187.

Avolio, B. J., & Bass, B. M. (2002). *Developing potential across a full range of leadership cases on transactional and transformational leadership.* Mahwah, NJ: Lawrence Erlbaum.

Axelrod, R., & Cohen, M. D. (2000). *Harnessing complexity: Implications of a scientific frontier.* New York, NY: Basic Books.

Bass, B. M. (2008). *The Bass handbook of leadership: Theory, research, and managerial applications* (4th ed.). New York, NY: Free Press.

Boonstra, A., & Broekhuis, M. (2010). Barriers to the acceptance of electronic medical records by physicians from systematic review to taxonomy and interventions. *BMC Health Services Research, 10,* 231.

Burns, J. P. (2001). Complexity leadership and leadership in healthcare. *Journal of Nursing Administration, 31*(10), 474–482.

Cooper, J., & Brady, D. W. (1981). Institutional context and leadership style: The house from Cannon to Rayburn. *American Political Science Review, 75*(2), 411–425.

Crosby, F. E., & Shields, C. J. (2010). Preparing the next generation of nurse leaders: An educational needs assessment. *Journal of Continuing Education in Nursing, 41*(8), 363–368.

Cummings, G. G., Midodzi, W. K., Wong, C. A., & Estabrooks, C. A. (2010). The contribution of hospital nursing leadership styles to 30-day patient mortality. *Nursing Research, 59*(5), 331–339.

Delia, E. (2010). *Complexity leadership in industrial innovation teams: A field study of leading, learning, and innovation in heterogeneous teams* (Unpublished doctoral dissertation). Rutgers, Newark, NJ.

Dooley, K., & Lichtenstein, B. (2008). Research methods for studying the dynamics of leadership. In M. Uhl-Bien & R. Marion (Eds.), *Complexity leadership part 1: Conceptual foundations* (pp. 269–290). Charlotte, NC: Information Age.

Drucker, P. (1985). *Innovation and entrepreneurship: Practice and principals.* New York, NY: Harper and Row.

Failla, K., & Stichler, J. (2008). Manager and staff perceptions of the manager's leadership style. *Journal of Nursing Administration, 38*(11), 480–487.

Goldstein, J. (2008). Conceptual foundations of complexity science: Development and main concepts. In M. Uhl-Bien & R. Marion (Eds.), *Complexity leadership part 1: Conceptual foundations* (pp. 17–48). Charlotte, NC: Information Age.

Gowan, C. R., Henegan, S. C., & McFadden, K. L. (2009). Knowledge management as a mediator for the efficacy of transformational leadership and quality management initiatives in U.S. health care. *Health Care Management Review, 34*(2), 129–140.

Gubin, T. A., Iyer, H. P., Liew, S. N., Sarma, A., Revelos, A., Ribas, J. . . . & Lee, C. X. (2017). A systems approach to healthcare innovation using the MIT hacking medicine model. *Cell Systems, 5*(1), 6–10.

Hanson, W. R., & Ford, R. (2010). Complexity leadership in healthcare: Leader network awareness. *Procedia Social and Behavioral Sciences, 2,* 6587–6596.

Hatch, M. J. (2000). Dynamics of organizational culture and identity with implications for the leadership of organizational change. In N. Ashkanasy, C. Wilderom, & M. Peterson (Eds.), *The handbook of organizational culture and climate* (2nd ed., pp. 341–356). Thousand Oaks, CA: Sage.

Hazy, J. K., Goldstein, J. A., & Lichtenstein, B. B. (2007). *Complex systems leadership theory: New perspectives from complexity science on social and organizational effectiveness.* Mansfield, MA: ISCE.

Howell, J. M., & Avolio, B. J. (1993). Transformational leadership, transactional leadership, locus of control, and support for innovation: Key predictors of consolidated-business-unit performance. *Journal of Applied Psychology, 78*(6), 891–902.

Jaramillo, B., Jenkins, C., Kermes, F., Wilson, L. Mazzocco, J., & Longo, T. (2008). Positive deviance: Innovation from the inside out. *Nurse Leader, 6*(2), 30–34.

Kaiser, J. A. (2017). The relationship between leadership style and nurse-to-nurse incivility: Turning the lens inward. *Journal of Nursing Management, 25*(2), 110–118.

Kelly, P. (2008). *Nursing leadership & management* (2nd ed.). Clifton Park, NY: Thomson Delmar Learning.

Kohn, L. T., Corrigan, J. M., & Donaldson, M. S. (Eds.). (2000). *To err is human: Building a safer health system* (Vol. 6). Washington, DC: National Academies Press.

Kumar, S., & Aldrich, K. (2010). Overcoming barriers to electronic medical record (EMR) implementation in the US healthcare system: A comparative study. *Health Informatics Journal, 16*(4), 306–318.

Leykum, L. K., Pugh, J., Lawrence, V., Parchman, M., Noel, P. H., Cornell, J., & McDaniel, R. R. (2007). Organizational interventions employing principles of complexity science have improved outcomes for patients with type 2 diabetes. *Implementation Science, 2*(28).

Lord, R. (2008). Beyond transactional and transformational leadership: Can leaders still lead when they don't know what to do? In M. Uhl-Bien & R. Marion (Eds.), *Complexity leadership part 1: Conceptual foundations* (pp. 155–184). Charlotte, NC: Information Age.

Losada, M. (1999). The complex dynamics of high performance teams. *Mathematical and Computer Modeling, 30,* 179–192.

Lotrecchiano, G. R. (2010). Complexity leadership in transdisciplinary learning environments: A knowledge feedback loop. *International Journal of Transdisciplinary Research, 5*(1), 29–63.

Marion, R. (2008). Complexity theory for organizations and organizational leadership. In M. Uhl-Bien & R. Marion (Eds.), *Complexity leadership part 1: Conceptual foundations* (pp. 225–268). Charlotte, NC: Information Age.

McKelvey, B. (2008). Emergent strategy via complexity leadership: Using complexity science and adaptive tension to build distributed intelligence. In M. Uhl-Bien & R. Marion (Eds.), *Complexity leadership part 1: Conceptual foundations* (pp. 225–268). Charlotte, NC: Information Age.

Nembhard, I. M., Alexander, J. A., Hoff, T. J., & Ramanujam, R. (2009). Why does the quality of healthcare continue to lag? Insights from management research. *Academy of Management Perspectives, 23*(1), 24–42.

Nielsen, K., Yarker, J., Randall, R., & Munir, F. (2009). The mediating effects of team and self-efficacy on the relationship between transformational leadership, and job satisfaction and psychological well-being in healthcare professionals: A cross-sectional questionnaire survey. *International Journal of Nursing Studies, 46*(9), 1236–1244.

Northouse, P. G. (2018). *Leadership: Theory and practice.* Thousand Oaks, CA: Sage Publications.

Plowman, D. A., & Duchon, D. (2008). Dispelling the myths about leadership: From cybernetics to emergence. In M. Uhl-Bien & R. Marion (Eds.), *Complexity leadership part 1: Conceptual foundations* (pp. 129–153). Charlotte, NC: Information Age.

Poole, M. S., & Van de Ven, A. H. (2004). *Handbook of organizational change and innovation.* New York, NY: Oxford University Press.

Porter-O'Grady, T., & Malloch, K. (2015). *Quantum leadership: Building better partnerships for sustainable health.* Burlington, MA: Jones & Bartlett Learning.

Rogers, E. M. (2003). *Diffusion of innovations* (5th ed.). New York, NY: Free Press.

Rosing, K., Frese, M., & Bausch, A. (2011). Explaining the heterogeneity of the leadership-innovation relationship: Ambidextrous leadership. *The Leadership Quarterly, 22*(5), 956–974.

Rowe, A., & Hogarth, A. (2005). Use of complex adaptive systems metaphor to achieve professional and organizational change. *Journal of Advanced Nursing, 51*(4), 396–405.

Saint, S., Kowalski, C. P., Banaszak-Holl, J., Forman, J., Damschroder, L., & Krein, S. L. (2010). The importance of leadership in preventing healthcare-associated infection: Results of a multisite qualitative study. *Infection Control and Hospital Epidemiology, 31*(9), 901–907.

Schein, E. H., & Schein, P. (2017). *Organisational culture and leadership* (5th ed.). Hoboken, NJ: Wiley.

Schreiber, C. (2006). *Human and organizational risk modeling: Critical personnel and leadership in network organizations.* Carnegie Mellon University, School of Computer Science, Institute for Software Research International. Technical Report, CMU-ISRI-06-120.

Schreiber, C., & Carley, K. M. (2008). Dynamic network leadership: Leading for learning and adaptability. In M. Uhl-Bien & R. Marion (Eds.), *Complexity leadership part 1: Conceptual foundations* (pp. 291–332). Charlotte, NC: Information Age.

Schwandt, D. R. (2008). Individual and collective co-evolution: Leadership as emergent social structuring. In M. Uhl-Bien & R. Marion (Eds.), *Complexity leadership part 1: Conceptual foundations* (pp. 101–127). Charlotte, NC: Information Age.

Shipton, H., Armstrong, C., West, M., & Dawson, J. (2008). The impact of leadership and quality climate on hospital performance. *International Journal for Quality in Health Care, 20*(6), 439–445.

Stacey, R. D. (2007). *Strategic management and organizational dynamics* (5th ed.). New York, NY: Prentice Hall.

Stordeur, S., D'hoore, W., & Vandernberghe, C. (2001). Leadership, organizational stress, and emotional exhaustion among hospital nursing staff. *Journal of Advanced Nursing, 35*(4), 544–542.

Sweetman, D. S. (2010). Exploring the adaptive function in complexity leadership theory: An examination of shared leadership and collective creativity in innovation networks. *Dissertations and Theses from the College of Business Administration.* University of Nebraska-Lincoln.

Uhl-Bien, M., & Marion, R. (2008). *Complexity leadership part 1: Conceptual foundations.* Charlotte, NC: Information Age.

Van de Ven, A. H., & Hargrave, T. J. (2004). Social, technical, institutional change: A literature review and synthesis. In M. S. Poole & A. H. Van de Ven (Eds.), *Handbook of organizational change and innovation* (pp. 259–303). New York, NY: Oxford University Press.

Weberg, D. R. (2013). *Complexity leadership theory and innovation: A new framework for innovation leadership* (Doctoral dissertation). Arizona State University, Tempe, AZ.

Wong, C. A., Cummings, G. G., & Ducharme, L. (2013). The relationship between nursing leadership and patient outcomes: A systematic review update. *Journal of Nursing Management, 21,* 709–724.

Wu, K., Yang, L., & Chiang, I. (2011). Leadership and Six Sigma project success: The role of member cohesiveness and resource management. *Production, Planning & Control, 23*(9), 1–11.

Yoder-Wise, P. S. (2007). Key forecasts shaping nursing's perfect storm. *Nursing Administration Quarterly, 31*(2), 115–119.

CHAPTER 3

Emergence and Disruption: Working on the Edge of Evidence

Cathy Lalley and Kevin Clouthier

In the long history of humankind (and animal kind, too) those who learned to collaborate and improvise most effectively have prevailed.

— **Charles Darwin**

CHAPTER OBJECTIVES

Upon completion of this chapter, the reader will be able to:

1. Identify human patterns of interaction with a complexity science lens.
2. Compare and contrast characteristics of complex responsive processes and complex adaptive systems.
3. Describe innovation emerging in real time.
4. Define the practice of reflexivity.
5. Outline the effects of relational leadership to advance evidence and emergence in healthcare practices.

▶ Meaning Making in Organizational Life

Health care is frequently referred to as a system as if this "system" were providing care to people. In this chapter, change will be described as the emergence and disruption in human interaction. Health services will be presented as ongoing interactions among people where norms, values, and power relations influence and are influenced by every interaction. Human interactions occur at the point of care, when creating structures to facilitate care at the point of service, and when designing tools to be used at the point of service.

A significant and broadly acknowledged challenge to advance healthcare innovation is to develop practices that disrupt the healthcare system so solutions can emerge. An often cited desired effect of such innovation would be a personalized healthcare system liberated from the faceless, anonymous system that engages people with resources specifically designed for their unique needs in a form that they prefer (Snowden, Schnarr, & Alessi, 2014; Fredrik, Gunnar, Lars, Annica, & Kerstin, 2016). Yet, individually, how do I, or, collectively, how do we innovate this vast system?

One can only imagine change and innovation will be pursued and ultimately achieved through a process of relating to people in a collective effort to influence others and quite naturally, be influenced in return. Success will be earned through this collaborative and competitive process organized through interactions rather than prescriptions. Adopting a micro, or perhaps more appropriately a local, view provides a perspective of healthcare organizations as continuous interactions between people involved in the action of health care. As opposed to contemplation of the "system," embracing health care as a process of relating together provides opportunities to inform, to influence, and to be informed and influenced by colleagues and patients through the course of responsive processes. As a member of a team, as a healthcare professional engaged with people seeking service as we work within a complex network of other healthcare providers, it is a complex process to innovate. As these practices occur on a daily basis, relational patterns emerge (Homan, 2016). Yet holding a view that health care is a complex process of patterned relationships engaged in complex processes creates potential for new solutions to emerge (Flinn, 2018). When you influence another, who in turn influences you, there is potential for the genesis of new transformative small shifts with latent energy to energize larger change experiences. It all begins with a complex responsive process of relating. Working on the edge of evidence is a disruption to outdated practices allowing improved outcomes to emerge.

▶ Complexity Science for Complex Environments

Complexity science gives us a lens to explore and understand human interactions because it is the study of dynamic behaviors of many complexly interacting, interdependent, and adaptive agents responding to internal and external forces in the environment (Marion, 2008). The practice of health care takes place in the context of human interactions in complex environments. When they are viewed through this lens, healthcare organizations come to life through these human interactions. When a complexity science lens is adopted, it becomes abundantly clear that it is no longer adequate to describe and understand healthcare organizations in terms of linearly organized, control-based, and predictable organizations (Lindberg, Nash, & Lindberg, 2008; Porter-O'Grady & Malloch, 2015; Uhl-Bien & Marion, 2008). What emerges instead is an appreciation that healthcare services are delivered in relationships between clinicians who engage in multidirectional interactions with people who have sought the support and intervention of the healthcare providers. These relational interactions are not predictable and occur through power influencing the interactions as opposed to the presence of an outside force. Thus, emergence and disruption occurs on the edge of evidence, on the edge of what we have previously determined to be the best way of doing our work, when we, in the moment, recognize the work we are doing is no longer relevant to our practice.

When our work and our practice are no longer congruent, our behavior changes slightly. We feel it in our gut, the values we hold as guidance for our interactions with team members and patients have been challenged. It's this feeling, this recognition that something is no longer working that can catapult individuals, teams, and systems into dynamic change efforts. The role of the evidence-based innovation leader is to live in the moment and to recognize the incongruencies that will spark innovative change.

▶ One Umbrella

Fitting within the umbrella of complexity science, two leadership theories have been generated in an attempt to understand and describe organizations: complex adaptive systems (CASs) and complex responsive processes (CRPs). Common elements of theories based in complexity science are the temporal nature of being relationships is constantly changing. Time in complexity theories is described as emergent and irreversible. Leadership theories understood from a complexity science lens recognize that agents are humans who are interdependent, engage in self-organizing nonlinear interactions, require diversity to survive, embrace uncertainty, and are able to respond rapidly and creatively to environmental changes (**BOX 3-1**). Both CAS and CRP leadership theories recognize that change emerges in response to internal and external pressures; change is continuous in living systems (CAS) or in human interactions (CRP). For example, clinicians' responses to evidence in clinical practice occurs continuously. Clinicians respond to practice recommendations based in evidence while continuously seeking to improve quality of care. Within complexity-based theories of leadership there is variation in the unit of analysis and power dynamics.

BOX 3-1 Common Characteristics Among Leadership Theories Based in Complexity Science

- Time is emergent and irreversible.
- Agents are interdependent.
- Agents participate in self-organizing nonlinear interactions.
- Diversity is required to survive.
- Leaders thrive in uncertainty.
- Agents are able to respond rapidly and creatively to environmental changes.

▶ Unit of Analysis

CAS leadership theory describes the evolution of complex systems with multiple, diverse, interconnected elements. When using a CAS model, the investigator must define the system's boundaries, including what is inside the system and what is outside the system (Dooley, 2004), recognizing the primary unit of analysis is the defined CAS itself such that the behaviors of the agents are always understood within the context of the CAS (Uhl-Bien, Marion, & McKelvey, 2008). The boundaries of the CAS are permeable so that agents and other CASs can cross over the boundary (Bennet & Bennet, 2004). When exploring outcomes of a defined system or group, this leadership theory can offer insight. However, when using a CAS perspective, the specific interactions and movement among agents within the CAS are overlooked for the outcome of the whole CAS. Thus, nurses may be diverse interdependent agents participating in self-organizing nonlinear interactions, capable of responding rapidly to environmental changes when evidence is generated to guide their practice, although the specific behaviors of the nurses are not explored within the CAS; only the behaviors and outcomes of the entire CAS are measured. To explore the emergence of evidence, the behavior of diverse interdependent agents participating in self-organizing nonlinear interactions is needed.

An assumption within CRP is that the reason for organization is purposeful joint action required for human living and sustained by individual and group identity with the potential to transform it (Stacey, 2001). CRP provides a view of change where apparently paradoxical perspectives, such as the application of evidence into practice, can be embraced in the living organization, including a healthcare work group, through human interaction. The unit of analysis in CRP is the interaction. Human interactions do not have boundaries around them; they include agents within a work group as well as agents in other work groups. CRP is the lens to observe change occurring in the here and now among diverse interdependent agents participating in self-organizing nonlinear interactions (**FIGURE 3-1**).

Power Dynamics

Power dynamics refers to how change occurs. Traditionally, healthcare leaders have attempted to control change through defined processes, such as planned

CAS

CRP

FIGURE 3-1 Change in CAS compared to CRP.

implementation of evidence-based practice guidelines. Although we have observed change that is both planned and unplanned, there have been successful campaigns for planned change that are consciously conceived of and implemented by knowledgeable actors; it was scripted or controlled and left little opportunity for innovation (Poole & Van de Ven, 2004). In planned change, the potential for local response and modification are limited because a normative cast is applied to improve a situation with a stated reference point (Poole & Van de Ven, 2004). Unplanned change implies that change to some degree is a force in its own right and is not susceptible to control or management (Poole & Van de Ven, 2004). Often with planned change, such as implementation of evidence-based practice guidelines, unplanned domestication occurs at the local level (Poole & Van de Ven, 2004). Poole and Van de Ven cautioned managers and change agents, suggesting that they "should realize how difficult change and innovation are to script and manage, as these processes constantly move in unexpected directions and are driven by dynamics that are either too powerful to control or too subtle to understand" (2004, p. 5). The mechanisms for change among CAS and CRP leadership theories are diverse.

Change in CAS

After the boundaries of a CAS are defined, the agents inside and outside the CAS are defined as well, including the leader of the CAS. The administrative leader of a CAS is an outside objective observer of the CAS who creates the conditions for change and observes movement of the CAS. The outside objective observer role of the leader appears much like the traditional leader role from the industrial age. The leader plans, organizes, leads, implements, controls, and evaluates change programs. When the leader attempts to control change, such as with the implementation of evidence-based guidelines, the leader attempts to hold power over workers by defining steps in the change process and identifying the persons involved in the change. To advance the goals of the system, the leader will implement practice patterns based in evidence, while agents or healthcare clinicians within the CAS participate in self-organizing interactions to respond to environment pressures. In this example, the outcome of the CAS is practice based in evidence according to a predefined metric, and the agents that respond to the environmental pressures are found within the boundaries of the system. From the CAS perspective, change in practice is measured by the outcome of the CAS.

After the boundaries are described in a CAS, change is explored at those boundaries. According to Poole and Van de Ven (2004), change is a difference in state, quality, or form measured at two or more points in time in an organizational entity. Change is the outcome of the system where one looks for new patterns or products. In this approach, the micro interactions within the CAS go ignored and change is not identified in the human-to-human interactions. The leader tries to influence the outcome of the system by standing outside it and directing activities. When the focus is on change of the CAS as a clearly defined system, then the human-to-human interactions are seen as a means to the outcomes but not quantifiable or describable in any outcome metrics. The dynamic power of human interaction can be seen through the lens of CRP.

Change in CRP

CRP is a lens used to explore the conditions for change or the power dynamic within an organization without defined boundaries but with purposeful joint action. With a CRP perspective, power or the force for change occurs in human interactions. It

Is in micro interactions that variation arises from diversity within the organization (Stacey, Griffin, & Shaw, 2000). The power dynamic occurs in the micro interactions where ideology and power relations are negotiated among those in the interaction; power is with the interaction rather than a force over interactions.

According to Stacey and Griffin (2005), the cooperative social process of self-organization is both enabled and constrained by rules of power relations, including norms, values, and accounting to one another. The organizing principles governing fluid human interactions are formed by and form power relations and ideology. Stacey and Griffin (2005) explain that ideology is composed of norms and values and is how choices are evaluated. Norms are "evaluative criteria taking the form of obligatory restrictions which have emerged as generalizations and become habitual in a history of social interaction" (Stacey & Griffin, 2005, p. 6). Values are "individually felt voluntary compulsions to choose one desire, action or norm over another" (Stacey & Griffin, 2005, p. 6); they arise in social acts.

Power relations are ongoing processes clinicians participate in as they negotiate with each other regarding what they do or do not do. In these processes, clinicians may find that by using language that is persuasive, they are in, or accepted, while others may find themselves out, or not accepted. It is in processes of accounting to one another on the basis of ideology and power relations that clinicians' individual and collective identity is formed, and so are differences. The application of evidence to clinical practice is influenced by power relations in such a manner that those who are most persuasive to implement a specific guideline or those who are most persuasive to customize the evidence-based guideline find themselves in the in group that forms the norms and values of the larger group.

▶ Working in Real Time: Sensing the Emergence of Innovation

The ancient Greek philosopher Heraclitus observed that the only constant in our world is change. Improved outcomes, higher profitability, faster production cycles, and higher quality represent a partial list of the drivers of innovation that motivate leadership in the clusters of human interaction that have been stabilized around specific themes that are continually reproduced—what we more commonly refer to as organizations (Fonseca, 2002). In a seemingly contradictory note to Heraclitus's observation, the previous statement (referencing human interactions that are stabilized around themes) suggests that while there is a drive for innovation, there is also a need for stability in human interactions in organizations to sustain an identity as an organization. At the same time, there would be a similar requirement for members of an organization to sustain their identity within an organization. Simultaneously there exists both stability and change. The potential for transformational change emerges as people conduct their business through local interactions.

What has hopefully become apparent in what has been described thus far is that through a lens of CRP, the emphasis or focus of observation is not a presence of a superordinate system that extends control of processes. Rather, attention is directed to the interdependent processes that occur among people—in this case, healthcare professionals and their interactions as they simultaneously influence and are influenced by the evolution of the organization. Due to contemporary interprofessional practices that are inherent in healthcare organizations, there is a fundamental degree of complexity present as the various roles interact with each other and alongside ever-increasing technological innovations. While there are actions that support continuation of the identity of individuals and the organization, so too are novel actions introduced in practice or process (Mereth, Aasen, & Johannessen, 2009). Meanings are continuously negotiated as people go about the tasks in their work (Durrant, 2004). As you can anticipate, there is a dynamic tension that exists between what is and what is aspired to be achieved in a desired future. The dynamic nature of this tension is not played out in a sequential, linear manner. Rather, it is evidenced in the paradoxical occurrence of the desire to sustain identity through stability in combination with the desire to effect change simultaneously.

These desires to advance the work of the organization commonly referred to as innovation practices emerge through the patterning of power relations and novelty that are introduced to the interactions among interdependent people (Fonseca, 2002). As members of a clinical team interact, the power relations that emerge are asymmetrical. Elias (1978) has offered that the nonlinear nature of human interaction has the potential to lead change that is disproportionate to the initial condition from which that change has emanated. The introduction of novelty that emerges as people negotiate meaning through their interactions represents the foundation of difference that is potentially amplified through conversational processes leading to change in practice or innovation (Fonseca, 2002).

Imagine a clinical team that has engaged in a familiar practice over an extended period of time. Their experience and interactions are based on known meanings of words and actions that have become well established. Such norms formed as meanings are established through the responses that are provided to gestures that have been expressed (Mead, 1934). Imagine further that this work process is interrupted through the introduction of a novel interaction that represents a difference in the usual process. In this circumstance, the previously held meaning associated with the interaction no longer holds true. In effect, there emerges various degrees of misunderstanding about what the meaning now entails (Fonseca, 2002). As the team members grapple with this potential transformation through social interactions of gesture and response, the misunderstanding that has been generated through the dissolution of the previously held norm is dissipated and new meanings are negotiated that become associated with the introduction of new practices. As the conversations ensue, additional ideas are introduced as diversity and the process of cocreating meaning of the new process expands. Should there be a successful negotiation of new meaning through conversation and actions among participants, the newly formed norm signals a successful innovation to the previous way of accomplishing the task. The process that has been described may be regarded as a counterintuitive perspective of innovation in that the introduction of novel ways of interacting creates a new pattern of behavior. This is contrasted with a more traditional view of innovation process that proposes people coalesce around a common cultural attribute designed to transform the organization (Fonseca, 2002).

▶ The Iterative Innovation Process

In this CRP way of understanding innovation, what cannot be overlooked is simultaneous potential of both change and stability. A shift in power relations through the introduction of novelty leading to increased levels of diversity can prompt the experience of a risk to identity. This dynamic tension may be experienced when one is excluded through persistent association with a preference to sustain known processes associated with previously held narrative themes and meanings (Stacey, 2001). The dynamic tension can be seen when a clinician is reluctant to implement a new evidence-based practice guideline because the practice is outside his or her comfort level. This person is commonly understood by others as a laggard. These sorts of experiences inherently possess the potential to increase anxiety (Fonseca, 2002). When the level of experienced anxiety is overwhelming, the transformational power of the proposed novelty is likely to be squelched by the desire to reduce anxiety by maintaining the status quo. Unlike the generative conversations that promote transformation, conversations occurring under this kind of threat are dominated by repetitious meaning associated with the usual way of conducting business. The result of this pattern of interaction is the victory of stability over change.

How is it that a proposed diversity of practice can overcome the retreat from anxiety to fulfill its transformational potential? Sproedt (2012) has proposed that innovation is largely achieved through the creation of social interaction grounded in trust and identity that emerges through the process of interactions that encourage and promote common meaning. Stated otherwise, the presence of positive relationships among interdependent members of an organization is a necessary precondition for innovation success.

▶ Using Our Words to Leverage Relational Practices

Before proceeding, allow us to refine some earlier points as we return once again to this notion of relationship. We proposed in the introduction that there were three separate elements involved in sharing our work: you the reader, we the authors, and this chapter as the vehicle for communication. Our hope is that our words have assisted in identifying these three objects that together forge our emerging relationship. We premise this notion on the assumption that the authors and readers have a shared understanding of our chosen words. If the words that we were using to write this story were uniquely our own, it would be likely that you would not recognize them. If this were so, we could hardly expect that the publisher would print them. In actuality, as you are no doubt aware, the words that we have chosen are ones that we have encountered innumerable times, and these words form meaning through our communal understanding. In an effort to be completely transparent, we also acknowledge that many of the words that we have chosen to make up this chapter are words that have come to us from others who, in turn, had borrowed them from still others. In effect, who do these words belong to as you read them? Gergen (2009) raised this very issue and proposed that through these words, we share a relationship.

Yet it is a frequently held view that the sole purpose of words is to identify objects within our reality. If this were the only purpose of words, we would discover that we were living an experience in which we would be separated from the reality that words describe (Shotter, 2012). In truth, the flexibility with which we use words, according to Lock and Strong (2012), accomplishes far more to contribute to our reality other than merely naming objects in the world. Lock and Strong suggest that words accomplish additional achievements, such as performing acts as demonstrated in the statement "I pronounce thee husband and wife." While reading the words "I pronounce thee husband and wife," you may well experience an image of a wedding in a house of worship, at city hall, or perhaps in a meadow or on a seashore. In effect, what you accomplish through such visualization is the creation of a social context in which the words have relevance (Shotter, 2012). Absent a context, words cannot convey a story that is comprehensible. Thus, the context that serves as the backdrop in the service of words offers opportunity for another important capacity of language: to provide meaning.

A shared network that is based in common context is necessary for meaning to emerge. Through these networks, people do not merely utter words to each other but instead engage in a responsive interactional process (Lock & Strong, 2012; Shotter, 2012). Reaching back to Foucault for support, Lock and Strong identify that as we engage each other in this form of social interaction, we find that we are on a journey of sharing ideas, thoughts, beliefs, and ways of understanding that all coalesce into a discourse that constructs our world.

For example, suppose we declare that stealing is a good action. You may be confused and perhaps incredulous that we would utter such a statement. However, when we set the context for this statement to be in reference to the game of baseball, we may be more readily greeted with understanding of our meaning by some readers. In such a situation, the baseball discourse constructs meaning. Others, even with this additional information, may be less inclined to agree and remain confused because they do not share this discourse that permits understanding of the game of baseball. These people might be immersed in a discourse pertaining to social justice that provides a negative evaluation of stealing. These people may remain confused because they would not include themselves in the group that shares in the meaning attributable to this baseball discourse. In effect, these people remain excluded from the meaning system that has emerged and thereby cannot claim to share in this construction of stealing.

What becomes available to us in this example is that there are at least two meanings of the word *stealing*. Neither of these meanings is reflective of an external reality. It is rather the cocreated meaning that is shared. The conceptualization of stealing is made possible through a shared discourse premised upon the presence of a relationship among members. All that remains is for members of the group with knowledge to share their knowledge with those who are excluded so they can be in a relationship with others who are knowledgeable of the nuances of baseball.

This is relevant to the discussion of CRP. Remaining momentarily with our baseball stealing metaphor, those people who did not comprehend the unique meaning of stealing in baseball find themselves excluded from the conversation. The transformation of their membership group occurred through the transfer of knowledge via communication (Stacey, 2001). Through a process of being in a relationship and sharing conversation, knowledge or the meaning of stealing in baseball emerged.

From a more generic frame of reference, what can be claimed through this metaphorical example is that change can and is achieved through a process of shared knowledge that has been organized through relationships and that organizes the relationships. More specifically, change occurs through the process and patterns of communication. The transformational power resides in the interaction that occurs among participants. Gergen (2009), who has proposed that process informs evidence in a similarly counterintuitive perspective, has proposed that individuals do not create relationship. Rather, individuals emerge from relationship.

Such a frame of reference holds huge potential for healthcare organizations and those who work within them. The reductionist metaphor of an organization that is compartmentalized through boundaries that define roles, divisions, and functions recedes as human interaction gains prominence (Wheatley, 2006). By implication, Wheatley highlights that when operating from a framework that honors human interaction, leaders will organize their practices to engage the energy inherent in power that is generated through high-quality relationships. Plowman and colleagues (2007) note that rather than seeking stability through control and planning, leaders might instead become enablers of the emergence of the future by engaging in dialogues that create meaning of events. They continue to encourage leaders to promote dialogical practices, noting that unlike a traditional organization, one that is based in emergent dialogue leads to the realization of work contexts in which workers do not wait for direction from managers. Instead, their experience indicates that workers demonstrate ownership of their performance.

Inherent in the adoption of these practices is a concomitant shift from seeing events as isolated incidents. Pronouncing a couple husband and wife is an experience that will endure through time, although the words are uttered in mere moments. Enabling emergence within the workplace through dialogue similarly occurs through ongoing processes. Splicing these experiences together into a tapestry of continuing processes further expresses the emerging stories of our relationships in the world (Shotter, 2012).

▶ Relationship as the Vehicle for Change

Meanings of words and actions emerge through social interaction. Purposeful change in health care that utilizes evidence-based practice is facilitated through human relationships. The human relationships that influence practice patterns include the researcher or author of the evidence, clinicians, patients or clients for whom the evidence supports improved care, professional practice communities, and other individuals in the organization who also must make sense of the evidence to create implementation methods.

As described in the discussion of CRP, organizations are understood as processes of conversations through which power relations and ideology emerge in the living present. One of these power relations that has the potential to be overlooked is the relationship between evidence-based practice and practice-based evidence. Swisher (2010) pointed to the inseparability of the two forms of research. They are in relationship with each other. Swisher, who is a practitioner, observed the necessity to decipher the findings of empirical research in combination with evidence based in practice. For a practitioner to fully participate in an individual relational practice with another, it is necessary for the practitioner to engage in the reflexive practice with both forms of evidence. How does a clinician engage in such a reflexive practice? To develop a relationally grounded practice with individual clients that is based in evidence, the practice of reflexivity is needed.

▶ Reflexivity

Reflexivity is the activity of paying attention to one's experience. These experiences are simultaneously individual and social processes of making sense of one's interactions with others in the here and now (Stacey & Griffin, 2005). Clinicians practicing reflexivity reflect upon their own experience of simultaneously being formed by and forming the collective identity of the work group when applying evidence to clinical practice. In this process of forming and being formed by identity, the clinician is influenced by power relations, such as norms and values of those in their work group and their client or patient, as well as the authors of evidence-based practice guidelines, for example. A clinical practice utilizing reflexivity means that the clinician is conscious in the present moment of the power dynamic that is enacted when he or she is presented with evidence to guide practice. In the power dynamic, identity is both formed by and forms the local interactions where practice emerges on the edge of evidence.

By paying attention in the here and now to emergent processes of individual and group formation in the interactions around them, clinicians are practicing reflexivity. It is what occurs in the local situation, at the point of service, where the clinician's identity forms and is formed by interactions. A clinician responding to evidence to guide his or her practice is necessarily making explicit his or her way of thinking that is both formed by and forming the evolving relationship with patients or clients, other clinicians, and the authors of the presented evidence.

With a CRP lens, there are many opportunities to explore change in organizations using reflexivity. The opportunities for change lie in the dynamics of human interaction. Power relations are ongoing processes that nurses participate in as they negotiate with each other regarding what they do or do not do. In these processes, some nurses may find that by using persuasive language, they are in, or accepted, and others may find themselves out, or not accepted. Reflexivity is practiced in the processes of accounting to one another on the basis of power relations that includes norms and values. In the process of accounting to one another, nurses' individual and collective identity is formed, so is difference. Change occurs in human interaction. Organizational change may be noticed in one single human-to-human interaction, or the change may emerge after many iterations of interacting together. In the end, the emergence of new patterns based on evidence occur in human interaction.

When new evidence is presented to improve clinical practice in an organization, implementation is simultaneously a social and an individual process. It is an individual and social process as the clinician's identity is formed by and forms interactions with others in response to the evidence-based practice guideline. The clinician may value the evidence and change his or her practice according to the guidelines; the clinician may also feel the voluntary compulsion to follow the practice guideline to contribute to the formed collective identity with other practitioners of having an evidence-based practice.

Influenced by power relations, including norms and values, the clinician is formed by and forming identity in the here and now. Quite possibly, clinicians may find that the evidence-based practice guideline needs to be adapted to the local situation, and patient needs and preferences. Thus, the clinicians may also form and be formed by patterns of relating that are patient centered. The clinician's response to evidence in clinical practice occurs through this dynamic of the clinician being formed by and forming identity with others by paying attention to identity (individual and collective) in the here and now.

▶ New Lens, New Opportunities for Change

Here, we present a case study to demonstrate nurses paying attention in the here and now processes of formation for individual and collective identities in their clinical practice that was influenced by evidence-based guidelines. In this case study, nurses demonstrated interdependence and identity as they worked together on a medical–surgical–telemetry unit. These nurses were engaged in self-organizing nonlinear interactions. They embraced uncertainty and diversity in workflow solutions, and as a result they were able to respond rapidly and creatively to environmental changes. Ultimately this led to the nurses being able to safely administer ordered medication to patients. A second mini case study is presented that explores the interplay between leadership and health service innovation and organizational identity.

This first case study describes nurses formed by and forming identity while endeavoring to improve patient outcomes with a medication administration process. Nurses administer medications after verifying the five rights: right patient, right drug, right route, right dose, and right time (Federico, 2011). According to the evidence, the use of bar code medication administration (BCMA) improves patient outcomes with medication administration; thus, it should be implemented in hospitals to enhance the quality and safety of patient care (Institute of Medicine, 2001; Koppel, Wetterneck, Telles, & Karsh, 2008; Poon et al., 2010).

🔍 CASE EXAMPLE: IMPROVING PATIENT OUTCOMES WITH BCMA

To improve the medication administration process, a Magnet hospital in the southwest United States implemented BCMA technology. On one medical–surgical–telemetry unit of the hospital, the nurses found that the BCMA technology did not function as they had been shown two months prior to the technology going live in their training sessions. Several of the nurses said the way they were shown to use the technology was to take the medication into the patient's room, scan their employee identification badge, and look at the top bar of the computer screen to ensure they were in the correct clinical application. Then they were to use the handheld scanner to pick up the bar code on the patient's wristband to confirm the right patient to receive the medication. Next, the nurse was to review the medication administration screen on the computer to ensure the correct screen was displayed because there are two different computer modules: one for documenting medications and another for intravenous fluids. If tablets were to be administered, the nurse would then look at the screen to confirm that the correct medication module of the electronic medication record was displayed. Then the nurse would scan the bar code on the medication package, look at the computer screen for alerts (such as not on medication list or administering too early), then the medication would be automatically highlighted in yellow on the screen to indicate that the five rights were aligned. The nurse would then give the tablets to the patient and select OK on the screen to save the information.

However, the nurses found that the technology did not operate as they expected. The nurses scanned the bar code on their employee identification badge to record who was administering the medication. Then they scanned the bar code on the patient's identification band, but the patient's electronic medication record did not appear on the computer screen. When a nurse first experienced this obstacle, she stopped the medication process and located a coworker to ask for help. In the interaction between the two nurses, they found that they experienced the same problem in the BCMA process. One nurse called the in-house help desk while the other nurse asked a more experienced nurse about his experience with BCMA. The help desk technician was unable to guide the nurse through the BCMA process because he did not understand the designed process from a clinician's point of view. From the interaction among the three nurses at the patient's bedside, they found that they could use the computer keyboard and mouse to highlight the patient's name. Then, instead of scanning the bar code on the patient's identification band, the nurses used the keyboard and mouse to highlight the patient's name and scanned the bar code on the medication package. The nurses looked at the computer screen for any alerts before administering the medication to the patient.

The nurses agreed that the technology was not bringing up the patient's electronic medication record as expected. It was a norm on this unit for nurses to place patients' needs at the center of their activities, including administering ordered medication to patients at the scheduled time. Each nurse in this interaction valued efficient and safe medication administration. The nurses consulted with another nurse and tried again to follow the designed process for BCMA.

In the interaction, the nurses found that if they responded to the designed process in their local situation, they could highlight the patient's name in the electronic medical record using the keyboard and mouse, then highlight the patient's electronic medication record. After the patient's electronic medication record was on the computer screen, they could scan the bar code on the medication package and look for alerts on the computer screen, such as a violation of the five rights. If no alert was on the screen, the nurse would administer the medication and press the Enter key three times to record the medication administration. A new practice pattern emerged in the current situation as the nurses were forming and formed by individual and collective identity. As other nurses experienced this same problem with the BCMA, they asked their coworkers for a solution, and the use of the keyboard and mouse became the standard of practice within this unit.

The emerging medication process came out of the nurses' interactions that were influenced by norms, values, and power relations. The nurses worked on a unit where efficient and safe care was a norm. Each nurse in this medical–surgical–telemetry unit had an individual compulsion to find a way to administer the medication using BCMA in what they believed was an efficient and safe manner. The work-around to pull up the patient's electronic medication list using the keyboard and mouse became the standard process because their actions were influenced by power relations, including norms and values. The nurses, who were respected by their peers and who used persuasive language to respond to the evidence to improve medication administration safety with the designed process in their local situation, were forming the in group with the revised way to use BCMA. In these interactions, the nurses were formed by and forming identity while working on the edge of evidence.

Identity Forming in the Absence of Relationship

As demonstrated in this case example, it was in the interactions that identity was formed by and forming. There are occasions when workers do not interact, yet identity is formed by and forming in the absence of relationships. For example, consider a

(continues)

🔍 CASE EXAMPLE: IMPROVING PATIENT OUTCOMES WITH BCMA
(continued)

manager who does not engage in discussion with workers but puts out a memo describing a future state and directions for workers to achieve that future state. This manager may find himself in the "out" group while the more persuasive workers of the "in" group envision a different future state. The persuasive "in" group of workers will be engaged in interactions to advance the future state that is more aligned with norms and values of the workgroup rather than what was presented in a memo. The power, in this scenario, is held by the "in" group forming and being formed by identity that may possibly exclude the manager.

Questions

1. How did evidence stimulate a practice change?
2. Describe a situation in which you participated in a discussion with coworkers to find a better way to achieve the desired outcome.
3. Was a better way to achieve the outcome met? How was the outcome received by those outside the discussion? Who else do you think should have been involved in the discussion?
4. How many times a week do you think you participate in such discussions?

🔍 CASE EXAMPLE: ORGANIZATIONAL IDENTITY REFORMATION AS INNOVATION

The previous case example demonstrated the process of change within a work team within a healthcare organization. The following case explores the path taken as an organization undergoes significant transformation as it reinvents itself. This is a good time to introduce the case study organization because it is this story that exemplifies the dynamic tension between the necessity for organizational stability in competition with an equally necessary need for transformation of the organization during turbulent times in its history. Although the story might be related from any number of lenses, it is in a discussion of the process of organizational identity reformation that brings these discussions to life.

As is the case with any organization that succeeds in sustaining its presence over years, there had been transitions and changes throughout the twenty-year history of the community-based health organization. However, a change like this one had not been previously encountered. The change agenda was highlighted by the departure of the organization's one and only chief executive throughout its years of operation. A significant number of the organization's staff had worked together with the chief executive since its inception. Others still had been employees over many years. Kjaergaard (2009) has opined it is important to acknowledge that organizational identity is regarded as a key variable in shared beliefs, the emotional processes associated with sense making, and the actions undertaken by organizational staff leading ultimately to the success of the organization itself. Indeed, over the years of establishing the organization, the staff had collaborated in the development of established routines, practices, and mythologies through relationships during their history together. The origins of many of these were unknown at this point in the history. People simply knew what were organizational norms and values that informed relationships and practices.

To complicate matters, not only were staff dealing with the emotionally charged departure of their only chief executive, they would also be required to work with a chief executive hired with whom they did not have a previous relationship. Adding to the already palpable anxiety was the emergence of major government policy mandating the transformation of service delivery processes. The specific manner by which these changes were to be deployed remained ambiguous. It was regardless another departure from the past. The response of people in the organization might be categorized as predictable. The tremendous anxiety being experienced in the staff group created conditions that encouraged the clustering of staff around strong themes or stories to stabilize (Stacey, 2001) against the perceived internal and external threats to the prevailing organizational identity.

What Is a Leader to Do?

Davidson (2017, pp. 308, 444) proposed that adopting complex responsive processes is, in essence, adopting a view of "organization as conversation." Pragmatically, this then focuses attention on how communication occurs within the organization. More specifically, there is a focus on the themes that are organizing discussions throughout the organization (Stacey, 2001). In the organization being discussed, officially there were formal and conscious legitimate conversational themes within the organization acknowledging the new chief executive as the leader of the organization. Yet simultaneously, there were informal fully conscious, in-the-shadows communicative processes (Stacey, 2001) that were preserving stories and cultural artifacts to sustain the old organization.

Reflexively, the newly implanted chief executive understood the power differentials and the likelihood of failure of exerting energy to enforce formal, conscious and legitimate communications and actions to create a new organizational identity. Such practical judgment (Stacey, 2012) provided the chief executive an alternative to being organized by boundaries that would pit him against the staff, thereby creating a lose-lose scenario. Instead, the chief executive opted to move the organization forward deliberately utilizing communicative action based within an informal yet consciously acknowledged legitimate process of power dynamics.

According to Stacey (2012), the best use of power dynamics is to engage in processes that will open rather than close down conversations that move too quickly to solutions. This is a deliberate process view of emergent change. Within the organization, the chief executive engaged managers in conversations identifying the kind of organization desired. These transformative conversations were shared with staff through long-serving managers who were able to elicit their preferences for the future. These discussions that identified/verbalized staff ideas for the organization capitalized on the trust present in those long-term relationships. An example of this process is exemplified by a manager holding individual conversations with each staff member to explore what was good in the organization and what needed to change, and also sought aspirations of the staff for the future. These conversations were assimilated into aggregate feedback around themes that emerged that were, in turn, shared with staff. At the conclusion of the feedback, interactions occurred forming identity around shared organizational goals so that members knew how to interact with others to live the new reality. In these interactions informal shadow communication became part of the formal legitimate conversation of the organization. This action represents a robust example of power relations through complex responsive processes.

(continues)

🔍 CASE EXAMPLE: ORGANIZATIONAL IDENTITY REFORMATION AS INNOVATION *(continued)*

The introduction of an evidence-based practice that would formulate treatment delivery across the services provided by organizational staff created powerful norms that has brought staff together through common language and that has habituated behavior through which organizational identity is being formed. Power was shared through interactions by those who were accepted by the in group. These power relations created influence across the organization through coaching practices. The consistent messaging delivered through these communicative acts encouraged the formation of an organizational identity as these practices were embraced by clinical staff. These coaches engaged colleagues to embrace changes as the new identity of the organization emerged. The organization emerging from these practices is one shaped through spontaneity and continuous transformation while sustaining the core of its mandate and purpose. Increasingly, there is emerging an organizational identity that celebrates creativity and innovation. The organization continues to deliver the service for which it was created and is also expanding the identity of the organization internally and externally as it diversifies offerings.

Questions

1. Organizations experience both formal—conscious—legitimate and informal—conscious—shadow (gossip) communicative acts. As a leader, how might you contend with these competing processes?
2. Recall a time when there was tension and perhaps conflict in an organization in which you worked. If the leadership opted to create space for dialogue, how do you believe that shifted the relationships of the personnel? Alternatively, if leadership opted to shut down conversation, how do you believe that shifted relationships? What impact might both have upon the relationships of the personnel?
3. In what ways does a leader pay attention to the presence or absence of anxiety in the workplace?
4. How does reflexive process inform your practice?

▶ Organizational and Human Patterns Advance Innovation

Organizational patterns made up of human interactions advance evidence into practice. Leaders who hold the CRP perspective on organizational change recognize the practice pattern response to evidence occurs in human interactions in the present moment and that these interactions are influenced by norms, values, and power relations. To be part of the practice pattern response to the evidence, leaders will put themselves in relationships—in interactions with other members of the organization at the point of service. The leader understands the power relations dynamic that is influenced by norms and values of the work group. This leader will have a practice based in reflexivity because he or she knows to pay attention to interactions including evidence, the patient or client, clinicians, professional practice communities,

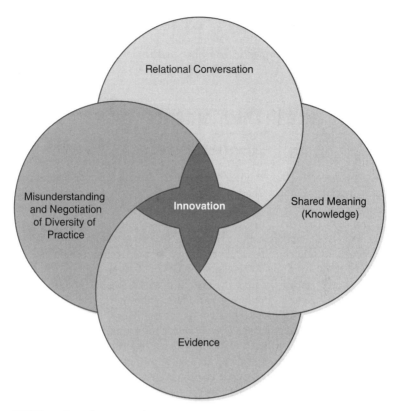

FIGURE 3-2 Four elements in the innovation process.

researchers or authors, and other members of the organization. Conversations with those who are most persuasive will influence when and how evidence advances practice that forms and is forming identity.

FIGURE 3-2 schematically depicts the processes involved in emergent meaning (innovation) creation and implementation of innovation from the lens of CRP. This depiction of a Venn diagram demonstrates that the processes associated with innovation in the moment, relational conversations, knowledge, evidence, and negotiation of diversity interact with one another in a pattern that has no definitive direction or order. The processes are iterative as the experience of energy and anxiety ebb and flow as the conversational processes progress. The diagram also depicts meaning emerging with the confluence of these practices, also calming anxieties that are associated with such transformation. Alternatively, should any of the four processes be underdeveloped so that anxiety prevails, the core of the process, emergent meaning, will remain an elusive target and the previous process will persist. The best hope that there will be sufficient awareness of the potential for innovation in the moment is the presence of reflexive processes by the members of the team. Through such action, sensitivity to the identity of each member as a team and of the team itself will pave a pathway grounded in the trust built in relationships to implement new practices.

A leader who practices reflexivity is conscious and pays attention to the present moment, knowing innovation in the form of local response will emerge in human interaction. Emergence of new patterns and the disruption of ineffective patterns occurs in local interactions of clinical practice. As clinicians, patients or clients, professional practice communities, researchers or authors, and other members of the organization interact to respond to the evidence, the human patterns emerge from each individual and the collective by paying attention to their experience in the here and now.

▶ Emergence in the Moment

Such attentiveness to the micro-level processes that are occurring in the living present give rise to the potential for innovation in practice to become known. Through interactional processes that honor the presence of divergent perspectives, potential new practices are emerging. There is no necessity for there to be a coordinated overseer to direct the process. As conversations are undertaken, people's identities are being formed as they are forming identity with others and the organization overall. Such generative interactions capture the energy that flows from power relations that emerge, shift, and churn as possibilities present themselves from thematic conversations that transpire. Should expressions of anxiety become pronounced through repetitive commentaries extolling the benefit of sustaining old practices, slowing the speed of change to ensure integrity of identity through conversation can calm mounting fears and will ultimately lead to successful change. This is aptly described in the work-around case presentation in which nurses remained tethered to the value and identity of providers of safe and efficient patient care as they collaboratively responded with novelty to a technological process that did not provide the promised process. The safety extended by the presence of a secure identity created a social context through which ingenuity transformed a potentially dangerous situation into a successful innovation to practice. Alternatively, the case of the leader who did not develop relationships to advance change highlighted the emergence of a powerful identity of the group that potentiated a different view of the workplace transformation.

To be highlighted is the acknowledgment that through conversation, meaning occurs only in and through the interactions of people. The patterns of interaction organize us as we conduct our business. When the diversity is sufficient and anxiety (although present) is contained, it becomes possible to transform meaning, knowledge, and practice.

▶ Leveraging Relational Practices to Create Change

For those of you who have engaged in a process similar to those that have been described in the case examples, you are familiar with the activity that is occurring during these interactions. Just as we have suggested in the previous discussion, you are no doubt aware of the multiple relationships that you are engaged in during the moments of interactions with the patient or client. In addition to the relationship with the evidence-based practice that has formed and is forming your identity and practice, you are processing information from your professional body, your disciplinary college, codes of conduct, and policies and procedures in your organization while simultaneously engaging with the person or people with whom you are interacting. No doubt there are numerous other relationships that are influencing you at the same instant. The interactions we all participate in every day influence our identity, individual and collective, and our response to evidence. Often we are not aware of how interactions form and are forming our identity. The interactions are not merely a conduit for an evidence-based practice that is formed by and informing identity, but in this collaborative process meaning is created, which is practice-based evidence.

Recall that in an earlier section of this chapter, we referenced Gergen (2009), who spoke of the need to appreciate that the effect be known before the cause can be identified. Extrapolating from this logic, it can be stated that the challenge that is being confronted is the source of innovation, which is found in interactions where meaning is created. Through reflexivity, practitioners incorporate views and perspectives that are formed by and forming with others. What becomes abundantly clear through such a process is the necessity for the development of a sense of trust within the variety of relationships. It is trust that is the basis of the relationship informing practice. With trust there is a foundation from which the possibility to engage in conversation that disturbs the status quo is established. A lack of relationships stifles the emergence of a practice based in evidence. Through a process of describing and amplifying new meaning, a credible innovative process with participants of the conversation emerges. Without the development of such trust, anxiety associated with the disruption of the power relationships that have persisted (Sarra, 2005) will threaten the cohesion that can thwart the change. Relationship becomes the vehicle by which power relations transition from an experience of power over to provide a pathway to experience power to promote new meaning and ultimately innovation (McNamee & Hosking, 2012). Our ability to relationally engage with each other provides opportunity for multiple perspectives of meaning, perhaps one perspective for each participant, to be shared in a context of trust and openness. During such conversations, fresh understanding that is shared with colleagues introduces new frames that were previously unknown. Misunderstanding may result. Through this conversational sharing, the possibility is present for the introduction of novelty that potentiates fresh meaning and, ultimately, innovation. This collaborative meaning making through conversation creates the space for fresh ideas to emerge and provides opportunities to innovate in the present moment. This, in turn, creates space for collaboratively developing meaning through conversational processes on the edge of evidence.

References

Bennet, A., & Bennet, D. (2004). *Organizational survival in the new world*. Boston, MA: Elsevier.

Davidson, S., (2017). Evidence-based education for healthcare innovation, in S. Davidson, D. Weberg, T. Porter-O'Grady, & K. Malloch (Eds.), *Leadership for evidence-based innovation in nursing and health professions* (pp. 441–474). Burlington, MA, Jones & Bartlett Learning.

Dooley, K. J. (2004). Complexity science models of organizational change and innovation. In M. S. Poole & A. H. Van de Ven (Eds.), *Handbook of organizational change and innovation* (pp. 354–373). Oxford, UK: Oxford University Press.

Durrant, T. (2004). The strategic management of technology and innovation. In T. Durrant, O. Grandstrand, C. Herstatt, A. Nagel, D. Probert, B. Tomlin, & H. Tschirky (Eds.), *Bring technology and innovation into the boardroom* (pp. 19–46). London, UK: Palgrave Macmillan.

Elias, N. (1978). *What is sociology?* New York, NY: Columbia University Press.

Federico, F. (2011). The five rights of medication administration. Retrieved from http://www.ihi.org/knowledge /Pages/ImprovementStories/

Flinn, K. (2018). *Leadership development: A complexity approach.* London, UK: Routledge.

Fonseca, J. (2002). *Complexity and innovation in organizations.* New York, NY: Routledge.

Fredrik, B., Gunnar, A., Lars, E., Annica, L., & Kerstin, N. (2016). Uncovering paradoxes from physicians' experiences of patient-centered ward-round. *Leadership in Health Services, 29*(2), 168–184. http://dx.doi.org/10.1108/LHS-08-2015-0025

Gergen, K. J. (2009). *Relational being: Beyond self and community.* New York, NY: Oxford University Press.

Homan, T. H. (2016). Locating complex responsive process research in the approaches of theorising about organisations. *International Journal of Business and Globalisation, 17*(4), 491–513.

Institute of Medicine. (2001). *Crossing the quality chasm: A new health system for the twenty-first century.* Washington, DC: National Academies Press.

Kjaergaard, A. L. (2009). Organizational identity and strategy: An empirical study of organizational identity's influence on the strategy-making process. *International Studies of Management and Organization, 39*(1), 50–69.

Koppel, R., Wetterneck, T., Telles, J. L., & Karsh, B. (2008). Workarounds to barcode medication administration systems: Their occurrences, causes, and threats to patient safety. *Journal of the American Medical Informatics Association, 15,* 428–423. http://dx.doi.org/10.1197/jamia.M2616

Lindberg, C., Nash, S., & Lindberg, C. (2008). *On the edge: Nursing in the age of complexity.* Bordentown, NJ: Plexus Press.

Lock, A., & Strong, T. (2012). Discursive therapy: What language, and how we use it in therapeutic dialogues, matters. In A. Lock & T. Strong (Eds.), *Discursive perspectives in therapeutic practice* (pp. 1–22). Oxford, UK: Oxford University Press.

Marion, R. (2008). Complexity theory for organizations and organizational leadership. In M. Uhl-Bien & R. Marion (Eds.), *Complexity leadership* (pp. 1–15). Charlotte, NC: Information Age.

McNamee, S., & Hosking, D. M. (2012). *Research and social change: A relational constructionist approach.* New York, NY: Routledge.

Mead, H. G. M. (1934). *Mind, self and society.* Chicago, IL: University of Chicago Press.

Mereth, T., Aasen, B., & Johannessen, S. (2009). Managing innovation as communicative processes: A case of subsea technology R&D. *International Journal of Business Science and Applied Management, 4*(3), 22–33.

Plowman, D. A., Solansky, S., Beck, T. E., Baker, L., Kulkarni, M., & Travis, D. V. (2007). The role of leadership in emergent self-organization. *Leadership Quarterly, 18,* 341–356.

Poole, M. S., & Van de Ven, A. H. (2004). *Handbook of organizational change and innovation.* Oxford, UK: Oxford University Press.

Poon, E. G., Keohane, C. A., Yoon, C. S., Ditmore, M., Bane, A., Levtzion-Korach, O., & Gandhi, T. K. (2010). Effect of bar-code technology on the safety of medication administration. *New England Journal of Medicine, 362,* 1698.

Porter-O'Grady, T. & Malloch, K. (2015). *Quantum leadership: Building better partnerships for sustainable health* (4th ed.). Burlington, MA: Jones & Bartlett.

Sarra, N. (2005). Organizational development in the national health service. In R. D. Stacey & D. Griffin (Eds.), *A complexity perspective on researching organizations: Taking experience seriously* (pp. 173–200). New York, NY: Routledge.

Shotter, J. (2012). Ontological social constructionism in the context of a social ecology: The importance of our living bodies. In A. Lock & T. Strong (Eds.), *Discursive perspectives in therapeutic practice* (pp. 83–105). Oxford, UK: Oxford University Press.

Snowden, A., Schnarr, K., & Alessi, C. (2014, February). *"It's all about me": The personalization of health systems.* London, Ontario: Ivey Centre for Health Innovation, Western University.

Sproedt, H. (2012). *Play, learn, innovate: Grasping the social dynamics of participatory innovation.* Sønderborg, Denmark: Books on Demand.

Stacey, R. (2001). *Complex responsive processes in organizations: Learning and knowledge creation.* London, UK: Routledge.

Stacey, R. (2012). *Tools and techniques of leadership and management: Meeting the challenge of complexity.* New York, NY: Routledge.

Stacey, R., & Griffin, D. (2005). *A complexity perspective on researching organizations.* London, UK: Routledge.

Stacey, R. D., Griffin, D., & Shaw, P. (2000). *Complexity and management: Fad or radical challenge to systems thinking?* London, UK: Routledge.

Swisher, A. K. (2010). Practice-based evidence. *Cardiopulmonary Physical Therapy Journal, 21*(2), 4.

Uhl-Bien, M., & Marion, R. (2008). Introduction: Complexity leadership—a framework for leadership in the twenty-first century. In M. Uhl-Bien & R. Marion (Eds.), *Complexity leadership* (pp. xi–xxiv). Charlotte, NC: Information Age.

Uhl-Bien, M., Marion, R., & McKelvey, B. (2008). Complexity leadership theory. In M. Uhl-Bien & R. Marion (Eds.), *Complexity leadership* (pp. 185–224). Charlotte, NC: Information Age.

Wheatley, M. J. (2006). *Leadership in the new science.* San Francisco, CA: Berrett-Koehler.

CHAPTER 4

From Organization as Machine to Organization as Conversation: Making Sense of Complexity in Health Care

Sandra Davidson

▶ Worldviews: If We Believe It, We See It

Our perspectives and beliefs about organizational life are predicated on our overall worldview. A worldview is a connected set of beliefs and assumptions about the form and function of the world coupled with beliefs about how best to investigate

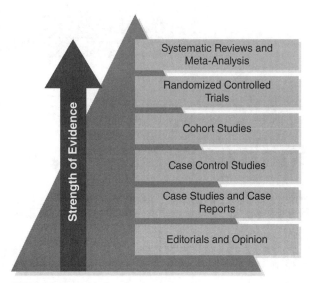

FIGURE 4-1 Pyramid of evidence.

it (Kuhn, 2007). The predominant paradigm and habits of thought about organizations are still largely rooted in the mechanistic, empirical, and rational ways of being. As such, objectivity and linearity also form the ways we conduct research as we seek to understand the world around us. This has implications for what we believe counts as useful or strong evidence. One of the clearest examples of this is the well-known levels of evidence pyramid (**FIGURE 4-1**).

Now, I must be clear here. I am not taking an antiempirical stance in this chapter. Far from it. There are many clinical and research questions that are best answered by the use of rigorous quantitative and empirical methods. And indeed, the levels of evidence pyramid does provide a useful framework for clinicians to use in appraising and making evidence-informed decisions about patient care. We will further explore the concepts of evidence and evidence-based practice (EBP) later in the chapter. For now, let us acknowledge that EBP is always enacted within an organizational context (primary care office, hospital system, public health district). Often, in such complex organizational settings, initiatives fail and preferred outcomes are not achieved, even when the evidence initiatives were based upon suggests that improvement should occur. From a complex relational perspective, there is much more to EBP than simply following the steps outlined in the latest clinical practice guideline. However, given our proclivity for viewing the world as linear, rational, and mechanistic, we seek to control and minimize the extraneous factors that constantly confound our plans. We often do not pay attention to the ever-present relational dynamics that seem to defy our best planning. Hassan (2014) used an excellent analogy for why empirical, rational, and predictive methods often do not work in complex adaptive contexts. "Imagine the difference between throwing a rock and throwing a live bird" (2014, p. 19). To take this a step further to the complex relational view, imagine releasing a flock of doves from a box, like at an outdoor wedding (**FIGURE 4-2**).

Each dove is an individual, but it also relates to all the other doves. They must negotiate and coordinate their movements and actions as they take to the sky. There

FIGURE 4-2 Relational complexity takes flight.
Courtesy of Pamla Wright.

is no predetermined, predictable path that every dove follows. Granted, they may all share the goal of returning safely to their roost, but each dove takes its own path. There are the doves that are first out of the box and lead the way home, and others that might need encouragement to take flight and leave the box. So too are our organizations made up of individuals that are in relation to each other. We must negotiate and coordinate our actions to reach our common goals. Personality, free will, and choice are ever present as we go about our day-to-day work together.

The Value of Seeing Differently

For every complex problem, there is an answer that is clear, simple, and wrong.

—H. L. Mencken

Widening our perspectives to consider more than just the dominant worldview presents different ways of thinking about human experience, and this often counters many of our taken-for-granted habits of thought. Because of this, it can be met with skepticism and scrutiny in both practice and research communities. However, it is precisely this novelty that makes complexity informed and relational perspectives useful frameworks for innovation in health care. As Kuhn suggests, "That complexity counters many commonplace assumptions means that there can be a re-noticing of ourselves and our world: a re-thinking and questioning of taken for granted, no longer tested assumptions" (2007, p. 160).

Many analogies have been used to describe and explain what happens in organizations. As we mentioned previously, the predominant view of the 20th century was organization as machine. **TABLE 4-1** presents an overview of three different organizational perspectives. Organization as organism is a popular perspective that has been applied and developed in the latter part of the 20th century and early 21st century. I have included it here as a midpoint perspective between the machine

TABLE 4-1 Comparison of Organizational Perspectives			
	Organization as Machine	**Organization as Organism**	**Organization as Conversation**
Theoretical perspectives	Newtonian physics, industrialization and scientific management	Complex adaptive systems, biological sciences, behaviorism	Social construction theory, complex responsive processes, pragmatism
Structural characteristics	Linear, hierarchical, closed system	Boundaried, organized functionally, aim is homeostasis, open system	Cocreated, pattern making, socially constructed and shared
Change is . . .	Controllable, introduced to a system from outside (cause and effect)	Evolutionary, adaptive, observable, and measurable	Local, emergent, participatory, and pragmatic (getting things done together)
System is . . .	Simple	Complex	Complex and relational
Leadership is . . .	Top-down, positional, exerted from outside the system, strategy and plan driven	Decentralized, formal and informal, enacted from various positions but still considered outside the system, outcome driven	Reflexive, enacted in participation with others in day-to-day interactions, relationship driven

and conversational perspectives because it illustrates the incremental shifts toward embracing organizational complexity rather than controlling or ignoring it. However, this perspective still retains many of the linear and rational characteristics of the machine model. The third view is organization as conversation. The remainder of this chapter will focus on this perspective.

▶ Organization as Conversation

In this section we will set the stage for thinking about and working within organizations using a complex relational perspective. The foundations of this perspective are found in complexity science (specifically complex responsive processes). The complexity principles of emergence and self-organization are the basis of understanding organizations as formed by patterns of meaning and patterns of relating (Stacey, 2012; Suchman, 2011a).

Patterns of meaning are specific themes that exist in an organization. For example, an organization's mission and vision serve as a pattern of meaning that informs the collective organizational identity. A mission driven by fiscal responsibility and profitability would influence the priorities and actions of every individual within the organization in a way that would be very different than an organization with a mission focused on patient safety.

Patterns of relating, or how people interact with each other, form an organization's culture (Suchman, 2011a). There may be habits of relating, such as a preference for e-mail communication, that result in specific patterns of relating that are different from that of an organization with a preference for face-to-face conversations. Maybe there are rituals around meetings (the unit manager always sits at the head of the table, or it is taboo to be late for a team meeting). These examples of patterns of relating illustrate culturally embedded understandings about power dynamics that are ever present in organizations (Davidson, 2015).

Emergence is an important aspect for leaders to understand. The patterns just described are emergent and evanescent. That is, they are enacted in the moment-to-moment interactions among people as they go about their work. As such, patterns must be perpetually recreated in each interaction or they cease to be. The flipside of this is that with every interaction or conversation, there is an opportunity for a new pattern to emerge. The living present is filled with potential—to recreate and perpetuate existing patterns or to bring into existence new ones.

To summarize, an organization can be understood as a temporary stabilization of themes and habits that serve to organize the experience of being together that takes place locally and in the living present (Fonseca, 2002). Organizations are paradoxical places where ideology and values-based human relating can manifest both stability and the potential for transformation (Booth, Zwar, & Harris, 2013). Making sense of what happens within organizations from a conversational stance necessitates a very different view of leadership. If leadership does not reside in the realm of planning, command and control, or otherwise exerting power to effect change in the system, what is the role of leaders?

Relational Leading

Just as the mainstream mechanistic, linear, and rational ways of being have shaped our organizations, so have they shaped our concept of leadership. A leader is traditionally thought of as an individual who is separate and stands isolated from others. From this perspective, a leader is an individual who possesses internal knowledge about how to be a leader or the personal ability to apply leadership skills to a given situation. Much of the discourse and literature on leadership is based on this perspective. There is the long-standing premise that leaders are made, not born, and its corollary, some people just have "it" and are born leaders. Both of these arguments are based on rationalist or bounded assumptions that "leadership potential resides within the individual person" (Gergen, 2009, p. 331). As I asserted in previous sections, if we choose to look at our world from the lens of relational complexity, we find different answers. Exploring the concept of leadership is no different.

Gergen observed, "None of the qualities attributed to good leaders stands alone. Alone, one cannot be inspiring, visionary, humble or flexible. These qualities are achievements of a co-active process in which others' affirmation is essential" (2009, p. 331). Fonseca (2002) suggested that an organization is a temporary stabilization of themes or habits that serve to organize our experience of being together. In essence, an organization creates the context in which the relational process of leadership happens. From the complex relational stance, leadership patterns emerge in the relational process that occurs among people in the living present, where the potential for novelty and change always exists (Walker, 2006).

If leadership is a relational or conversational process that emerges in the living present, then the essential role of the leader is to be present and participatory from moment to moment in his or her interactions with others. Leadership becomes improvisational in nature rather than relying on learned tactics or skills. Walker (2006) suggested that it may be more appropriate to speak of leadership potential rather than skill; potential carries with it a sense of movement, whereas skill seems to be a static construct.

New language is a powerful tool for creating the potential for novelty and change. If we want to transform leadership into something beyond our mainstream, mechanistic, and boundaried understanding, a change of language may be useful in generating new ways of leading. Gergen suggested that we consider replacing leadership with relational leading:

> Abandoned are the endless and often contradictory lists of what it takes to be a good leader. In their place we find increasing emphasis on collaboration, empowerment, dialogue, horizontal decision making, sharing, distribution, networking, continuous learning and connectivity . . . While leadership denotes the characteristics of an individual, relational leading refers to the ability of persons in relationship to move with engagement and efficacy into the future . . . To be sure, individuals may be designated as leaders, but the process of leading is ultimately relational. (Gergen, 2009, p. 333)[1]

If we start with this perspective of relational leading, what are the patterns of meaning and patterns of relating that generate the conditions for relational leadership? How do we individually and collectively engage relationally in ways that move us toward the preferred future of health care?

▶ Complex Relational Being

This section will present an overview of the philosophical roots and key concepts that support the complex relational way of understanding organizations. These iconoclastic ideas provoke us to reconsider and reimagine our organizations and the ways in which we contribute (or not) to the themes and habits that constitute them. Taking a relational perspective of healthcare organizations is a bit like putting on X-ray goggles. We may be looking at the same people, environment, and challenges, but suddenly we see new focal features and aspects that were previously obscured

---

[1] By permission of Oxford University Press, USA. www.oup.com

from our sight. The beneath-the-surface view opens new possibilities and the potential for transformation.

Ways of Being Together and Making Meaning

The complex relational viewpoint builds on the theoretical foundations set forth by American sociologist and pragmatist George Herbert Mead (1863–1931). Mead's concepts of gesture and response are important in understanding the process of meaning making within organizations. Meaning is born out of the experience of conversation that occurs in the living present. The abstractness of human interaction can be more fully understood if we choose to view human interaction as the unit of analysis rather than viewing the system or its agents as the unit of analysis, as is the case in systems thinking. Meaning arises in the living present, as do choice and intention (Stacey, Griffin, & Shaw, 2000). Our choices and intentions in the present moment are shaped by our past experiences.

Meaning, then, is a social construction. According to Mead (1934), meaning arises in the gesture–response interactions among people that occur in a medium of symbols. A gesture is a kind of symbol (an emotion, personal reflection, or explanation, for example). Mead understood the word *symbol* to be derived from the Greek words *symbolon* (a mark or token) and *sym-ballein* (thrown together). A gesture made by one person that is responded to by another is a symbol (Mead, 1934; Stacey, 2001). Meaning is created in the *response* to the gesture. This triadic relationship of gesture–response–meaning arises out of the social act of communicating (**FIGURE 4-3**). As such, any collaborative human interaction is made possible through the use of symbols. Together, the gesture and response symbolize or constitute a meaning.

In this way of conceptualizing meaning making, knowledge is not something that resides in the minds of individuals; it is created through the social act of relating. As such, knowledge is perpetually created by people interacting with each other in the living present. From a complex relational perspective, knowledge is simply the thematic patterns that emerge to organize the experience of the ongoing process of relating (Stacey, 2001). Mead purported that the self and society are always co-occurring. If this is so, it becomes pointless to ask whether organizations learn or people learn because the process is the same (Stacey, 2001). Human interaction or the process of responsive relating is simply people weaving together their actions to accomplish joint endeavors successfully (Stacey, 2001).

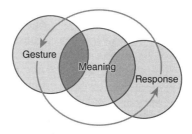

FIGURE 4-3 Gesture–meaning–response triad.

Power Dynamics: Complex and Relational

All human interactions and processes of relating include elements of power. Drawing on the work of Elias (1998), Stacey (2006) viewed power not as something possessed by any one person, but as a feature of all human relating: "In order to form, and stay in, a relationship with someone else one cannot do whatever one wants. As soon as we enter into relationships, therefore, we constrain and are constrained by others . . . we also enable and are enabled by others" (2006, p. 134).

Power is this enabling and constraining way of relating. The balance of power is often tilted in favor of one person based on the need the two individuals may have for one another, and this may shift over time or vary by context (Stacey, 2006). If we frame power relations in terms of Mead's idea that the individual and social are at once forming and formed by each other, there is no distinction between I and we identities (individual and social). Power relationships form groupings or patterns in which some are included and others are excluded. These patterns evoke a powerful feeling of belonging in which an individual identifies and resonates with the we of the group (Elias, 1998). Again, if the I and we are inseparable, then the larger patterns of inclusion and exclusion reflect the complex, conflictual, and cooperative patterns of power relating (Stacey, 2006). Understanding power relating within an organization as the patterns of inclusion and exclusion that create and sustain relationships is key.

If organizations are temporary stabilizations of a set of themes and habits (Fonseca, 2002), then the patterns of power are always present within organizations. Elias (1998) suggested that power figurations are sustained by ideologies, which in turn are sustained by gossip and processes of shame. Furthermore, power relationships and an organization's dominant patterns are made to feel natural and are stabilized by the unconscious and underlying ideology (Stacey, 2006). Ideology is a patterning process in which themes of inclusion and exclusion are perpetually reproduced. It follows, then, that "ideology exists only in the speaking and acting of it" (Stacey, 2001, p. 153). Often, the speaking of ideology takes the form of gossip in day-to-day interactions, as described by Stacey:

> The gossip builds layer upon layer of value-laden binary pairs such as clean-dirty, good-bad, honest-dishonest, energetic-lazy and so on. In less obvious form, the same point applies to the "in-out" dynamic created by particular ways of talking, for example, talking in terms of complexity, in terms of psychoanalysis, in terms of management control, and so on. Such gossip and other ways of talking attribute "charisma" to the powerful and "stigma" to the weak, so reinforcing power differences. (2001, p. 153)

Within organizations, the enabling and constraining forces that people use often take the form of emotions. Shame, jealousy, empathy, and compassion are all interwoven into the complex pattern of themes that make up organizations. Cooperation, conflict, politics, and negotiation are all elements of ordinary everyday communication that are lived out moment to moment (Stacey, 2006). Paying attention to the ordinary watercooler conversations and sidebar comments at staff meetings provides a way to understand the patterns of power and ideology within organizations.

🔍 *CASE EXAMPLE: PAGING DR. FRICK*

Organizations are defined by the stories that are told. Stories are expressions of our shared culture that can either stabilize (perpetuate) or potentially transform an organization. I see this clearly represented and supported by the organization as conversation perspective. Humans are, by nature, social beings, and storytelling is a powerful means to communicate, share, and perpetuate the values and norms (ideology) of any given culture. I first remember experiencing the power of stories to shape culture when I was a new nurse.

As many beginning nurses do, I worked on a casual basis on several different units within the same hospital. One weekend I picked up a Friday evening shift on a medical unit and then a Saturday evening shift on the adjacent surgical unit. Back in the early 1990s, overhead paging was still one of the most effective ways to contact physicians and surgeons who were on rounds throughout the hospital. In this particular hospital, nurses and other staff members who needed to reach a physician would call down to the switchboard, and the operator (who had a lovely English accent, by the way) would then page the physicians overhead along with the extension numbers that they were to call.

On Friday evening, two physicians, Dr. Frick and Dr. Hebert, were needed by staff of the same unit. The operator announced, "Dr. Frick and Hebert, please call 4295." Of course, to the casual listener it sounded like she was paging Dr. Frick'in Hebert! I happened to be at the nursing station on the medical unit writing in a patient chart at the time. Several of my nurse colleagues and the unit clerk were also there. After hearing the page, we all looked at each other and laughed. One of the nurses said, as she continued smiling, "I know Dr. Hebert seems serious, but he has a great sense of humor—I bet he's getting a good laugh out of that!" Several others at the desk nodded in agreement, smiling, and then we went about our work.

The next evening, I was waiting for report to start on the surgical unit. One of the nurses burst into the room and said, "Did you hear that overhead page last evening?" She went on to say, "I heard that Dr. Hebert was so mad that he went down to the switchboard and told that poor operator off!" She continued by saying, "He's still on call this evening, so we'd better be careful not to tick him off!" I was struck by the two very different interpretations of this event. On the medical unit, it was a story of an honest mistake, which anyone with a sense of humor could easily laugh off. On the surgical unit, the story was of retaliation, belittlement, and fear of being the next person to incur the wrath.

As I continued to work on both units over the next 6 months, I came to realize that the interpretations of this event were emblematic of the overall culture of each unit. On the surgical unit, everyone always felt on edge, and there was an intense fear of making mistakes. When a mistake inevitably happened, it meant that humiliation and shame followed for the unfortunate perpetrator. In contrast, the medical unit was a place of teamwork, camaraderie, and learning. If a mistake happened, the entire team supported the people involved, and it was an opportunity to improve our communication and processes. Eventually, I was offered a regular position on both units. I bet you can guess which one I chose.

Questions

1. Do you have an example organizational story that you have experienced? What is it?
2. Think about the last time you were in the cafeteria or lunchroom with colleagues. What were the themes of the conversations? What might this tell you about the culture?
3. How might you change the story within your work unit, organization, or group? Think about how you could purposefully use patterns of relating, patterns of meaning, and new language to introduce ways of being (for the better!).

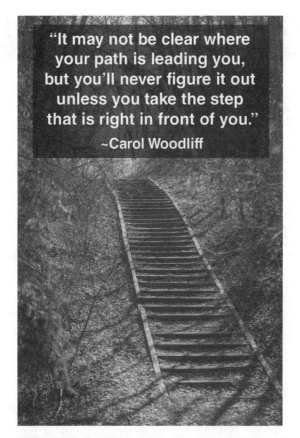

FIGURE 4-4 The future emerges as we move toward it.

Used with permission. Photo credit: James Davidson.

Living Present: Here and Now

From a complex relational perspective, the future is unknowable and therefore un-predictable (**FIGURE 4-4**). This means that many of our traditional ways of planning and communicating within organizations (such as long-range planning, setting carefully projected targets, and executing detailed implementation guides) are not particularly useful or relevant from a complexity view. Rather, the point of impact and influence that we have in organizations occurs in the living present (here and now). The living present provides a starting point for conceptualizing causality dif-ferently. Rather than thinking of causality as we ordinarily do, in a linear way (such as an organization moving toward a mature state or realizing a prechosen goal), from a complex relational aspect the future is under perpetual construction rather than predetermined. This means that human interaction that takes place in the liv-ing present perpetually modifies and shapes the future based on the more-or-less immediate past. The past, present, and future are all mutually enacted in the living present. Although the future may be unpredictable and unknowable as our day-to-day conversations move us into the future, it becomes somehow more recog-nizable (Stacey et al., 2000).

Strategic Plan or Conversation Guide?

As discussed previously, our individual choices in everyday dialogue that build upon organizational patterns of meaning and relating are at the crux of organizational change and potential. Taking up this premise (that relationships and coaction that take place in the living present are the inflection point for organizational change) means that we must reexamine the utility and value of long-range and strategic planning.

Almost every organization is engaged in some type of long-range or cyclical strategic planning process (e.g., 5-year plan). This practice is deeply rooted in our linear and mechanistic view of organizations. From an organization as machine stance, it is reasonable to have a group of managers, operators, and leaders set targets and, with some degree of certainty, be able to predict outcomes. Imagine that a line manager in a factory wants to produce a million widgets in the next 3 years. Based on the number of widget machines available and the speed (rate of production) and availability of raw materials, she determines that each machine will need to run for at least 12 hours per day with a production rate of 10 widgets per hour to meet this long-range target. The application of this type of mechanistic planning to human organizations is the legacy we retain from Taylor's *Scientific Management* (1911). Complex human organizations are not predictable, nor are they linear, yet we still feel compelled to create 5- and even 10-year strategic plans born of a management theory that is more than 100 years old.

Stacey (2006) proposed that from a complex relational stance, strategic plans are grand organizational fantasies that function primarily as social defenses against the anxiety of not knowing and not being in control. Managing our collective human anxieties and fears about the unknown and the uncontrollable provides a very plausible rationale for why strategic planning has endured. From the organization as conversation stance, at best, strategic plans can function as an organizational conversation guide. That is, the goals, strategies, benchmarks, and projections of the organization that are detailed in such a plan may be taken up by local teams and form the basis for dialogue about how the local team will contribute to and act in ways to move the organization closer to the future aspirations. At worst, strategic plans can blind individuals and teams to the possibility of more generative and improvisational behaviors that might emerge. Recall that design and planning at an organization-wide scale (generalizations) can only ever be enacted in local, specific, and particular contexts (Stacey, 2006).

Grand organizational plans often come in conflict with local emergent themes, expectations, and intentions, and thus strategic planning, when taken too seriously or enacted militantly, can hamper team functioning. The conflict that can arise between the strategic plan (what we are supposed to do over the next 5 years) and the on-the-ground realities (what is really happening here and now) must then be negotiated by the team, and this can mean precious time and energy are wasted on figuring out what to do when things do not go according to plan. This begs the question, How do we organize and coordinate our work if not through planning? Stacey suggested that grandiose planning does not mean abandoning purposeful actions and movement toward organizational improvement. "It simply means taking a humbler stance and working realistically in our own local interactions to improve what we can" (2012, p. 127).

Our ways of talking together can enliven and engage us or control and alienate us. Becoming more aware of our organizational habits, patterns, and norms enables us to purposefully choose the ways in which we talk, listen, and attend to each other. The next section will introduce ideas that can help us focus on local interactions in the living present.

The only thing we know about the future is that it will be different. Trying to predict the future is like trying to drive down a country road at night with no lights while looking out the back window. The best way to predict the future is to create it.

—Peter Drucker

▶ Working Live: Improvisation

Our ability to pay attention to our experiences with others in the living present becomes a critical skill in organizational life from a complex relational stance. The capacity to dwell in the present moment and to respond in emergent ways to what is taking form is something we can all develop. To many of us, this way of being is commonly understood as the ability to improvise. In organizational contexts, improvisation is perhaps less theatrical in nature than the metaphor of jazz musicians or an improv comedy performance. Rather, it is more the distinction between the raw and honest quality of witnessing a live (real-time) interview and watching a prerecorded and skillfully edited interview (Shaw, 2006). The latter has a hollow and rehearsed quality to it that is less authentic.

In any organization, there are well-used and routinized scripts (patterns of meaning and relating) that organize and stabilize our day-to-day ways of being together. This might take the form of a standardized clinical pathway, for example. In some instances, we may not want novel patterns to be created. In health care there will always be situations where precision, replicability, and a high degree of reliability are warranted and valuable (Suchman, 2011a). One example is the surgical sign-in, time-out, sign-out checklist (World Health Organization, 2009). Such standardized scripts are imperative for patient safety. However, we must also realize that each time a script is enacted, there are subtle differences because of the unique emergent and contextual conditions. This means that team members are paying attention to the present moment and adapting and modifying their interactions in a way that is appropriate to the unique current situation. This is different than the dogmatic (unthinking) adherence to a protocol that becomes robotic and acontextual.

Imagine that a surgical team is in the midst of the presurgical time-out, and they are introducing themselves (and their roles) to Mr. Johnson (the patient). The nurse begins to pick up on nonverbal cues from Mr. Johnson (he looks confused and does not seem to understand what they are saying). The nurse then realizes that Mr. Johnson has already removed his hearing aids and cannot hear the team members. The nurse adapts to this context by handing Mr. Johnson his hearing aids so he can put them in for a moment to ensure that he hears and understands what is being said to him. This is different than a surgical team that is simply going through the motions and introducing themselves to the patient, per the checklist, and failing to pick up on Mr. Johnson's cues that he does not understand what they are saying.

DISCUSSION

Improvisation is very commonly linked with creative and artistic endeavors, such as jazz music and improvisational theater. How might you learn from and adopt best practices and strategies from these genres and use them in your own conversations and relationships?

Reflect on the concepts that have been discussed in this chapter, such as the following:

- Organization as conversation
- Working live (present moment)
- Innovation
- Relational leading

What opportunities do you see in your own practice for integrating these concepts and practices? What challenges might you face in adopting such practices? What are some ways you might mitigate these challenges?

Paying attention to and discerning the most appropriate patterns (stabilizing or emergent) for any given situation is a form of improvisation. It simply means that we need to tap into the present moment (the gestures being made) and respond in a way that creates resonant meaning for those involved. This is the essence of working live; there is no rote or automatic default setting or response. Instead, it is about actively sensing the future as it emerges in the present moment. Sometimes that calls for perpetuation of existing patterns in our meaning making; other times we are called to break a pattern and open up the possibility for new ways of being. Our capacity for this type of improvisation is enhanced as we seek to develop and use practical judgment (Stacey, 2012). Practical judgment is made possible by reflexivity.

The goal of reflexivity is to be able access and use knowledge and situational awareness in real time to respond to the emerging present moment. Over time, and with practice, our ability to be in the moment and respond improvisationally within it (reflexivity) becomes familiar to us, and we begin to build practical judgment.

This is similar to what has been described as *habitus* in healthcare settings—the situated use of tacit knowledge within an emergent and complex clinical situation (Benner, Sutphen, Leonard, & Day, 2010; Bourdieu, 1990). Likewise, Benner, Hooper-Kyriakidis, and Stannard (1999) described the concepts of thinking in action and reasoning in transition as essential components in the development of clinical expertise. Thinking in action is the pattern of thought in action that is directly tied to responding to the demands of a changing situation and noticing the nuances of the interaction in the present moment (Benner et al., 1999). This is again similar to the ideas of working live and developing practical judgment that are being presented here, although we are extending and connecting these ideas beyond clinical experiences to a wider organizational and leadership context.

The work of relational leaders is to use practical judgment and distinguish among situations where stability and reliability need to be assured and other situations that call for novelty and creative emergence, then act accordingly.

Otto Scharmer's *Theory U* (2016) is an excellent resource for anyone seeking additional description and guidance about how to do and be in complex relational organizations. **TABLE 4-2** summarizes Scharmer's five movements that in essence move us through the U. An additional column highlights some of the concepts and

TABLE 4-2 Scharmer's Five Movements

Theory U Movements	Descriptions (Scharmer, 2016)	Complex Relational Competencies and Activities
Coinitiating	Listen to what life calls you to do, connect with people and contexts related to that call. Convene constellations of core people, then coinspire common intention.	■ Mindfulness and reflection ■ Relational leading ■ Creating new local patterns of relating ■ Enacting generative ways of talking and making meaning
Cosensing	Teams take deep-dive learning journeys that bring them to places of greatest potential. Observe and listen with an open heart, mind, and will.	■ Relational leading ■ Dwelling in the living present ■ Cocreating new local patterns of meaning ■ Reflexivity, practical judgment
Copresencing	Dwell in a place of individual and collective stillness. Open up to creativity and presence, and link to the future that wants to emerge.	■ Relational leading ■ Dwelling in the living present ■ Mindfulness ■ Improvisation and reflexivity
Cocreating	Build landing strips for the future by prototyping living microcosms to explore the future by doing.	■ Creating and experimenting with novel patterns of meaning and relating locally ■ Innovation through emergence and improvisation
Coevolving	Codevelop a larger innovation ecosystem that connects people and actions beyond boundaries. Seeing and acting from the whole.	■ Relational leading ■ Moving local innovation to the wider organization ■ Stabilizing new themes and patterns of meaning and relating (become the organizational ways of being)

relational competencies from this chapter that resonate with each of Scharmer's movements.

In the previous discussion we have talked about improvisation within complex relational organizations. In essence, working live is a particular way of being and relating in our day-to-day interactions that opens up the potential for meaning to emerge from the living present. In the sections that follow, we will delve deeper into two aspects of relational being that influence how patterns of relating emerge: ways of talking and ways of listening.

Ways of Talking

As we have previously discussed, our ways of speaking in organizations are patterns that can reinforce and stabilize culture. Social norms and values are taken up and become the ideology of the larger social group. However, humans possess the wondrous capacity for free will and choice. This means that each conversation presents an opportunity for reinforcing existing group values and norms, or for novelty and change. Over time, the choices we make in daily conversations result in a pattern of speech or habitual ways of talking.

How aware are we, from moment to moment, of how we are speaking? It is easy in the busyness of our work to fall into familiar and comfortable language and to then perpetuate and reify patterns we may not consciously intend (or want). By contrast, by being aware of our words and choosing language intentionally, we can purposefully perpetuate themes and ideology that are resonant and useful to us; or we can take up new language and new ways of speaking with others that are more authentic and meaningful. Language serves to form, and can transform, meaning. Emergent new meaning can transform our ways of being.

From a traditional mechanistic view of organizations, language is used in particular ways. Skilled leaders have always used language to persuade, motivate, and even control. The art of rhetoric has been employed in a vast array of contexts, from political campaigns to marketing a new breakfast cereal to large-scale social change initiatives. Even the daughter of friends skillfully used rhetoric to sway her parents in her quest to acquire a family dog.

"Rhetoric may be understood as the techniques of prose composition or speech which enable one to influence the judgment or feelings of others. It is the art of using language effectively" (Stacey, 2012, p. 119). So, then, what does rhetoric look like when we view the organization as conversation? **TABLE 4-3** shows some rhetorical devices for consideration.

These examples serve as a starting point to assist us in being more aware of the language we choose and how we use rhetoric in our organizations. If we take up the complex relational view of organizations, the power to transform our workplace comes from the quality of relationships that we engage in. We are at once formed by and forming the future as we talk about it together.

Ways of Listening

Communication is a collaborative process. It is enabled by both gestures (speaking and nonverbal cues, such as facial expressions and hand movements) and responses to those gestures. Taken together, gestures and responses create a kind of collective understanding, or shared meaning. Listening, attending to the conversation, and generally paying attention is an important aspect of this collaborative communicative process. Recall the earlier discussion of meaning that emerges out of the communicative process of gesture and response. To offer our response, we must be attuned to the gestures another person (or group of people) is making. Gestures include nonverbal cues and verbal communication. Sometimes it is as crucial for us to listen between the lines as it is to listen to the words themselves to fully apprehend the meaning that is being transmitted.

TABLE 4-3 Rhetorical Devices in Organizations		
Rhetorical Device	**Traditional Hierarchical**	**Complex Relational**
Influence the path of a conversation	Let's stay on target here	What might that look like?
Destabilize	There is no appetite for this	Does this process add value?
Construct urgency	There is a short turnaround	The faster we share this with other teams, the sooner all patients will benefit
Metaphor	Organization as machine	Organization as conversation
Irony	Doing more with less	Focusing on what works helps us find energy to fix what is wrong
Influence beliefs about what is true or real	Evidence shows	This worked for us

Modified from Stacey, R. (2012). *Tools and techniques of leadership and management: Meeting the challenge of complexity.* New York, NY: Routledge.

Just as we can choose the way in which we talk and make use of language, we can also purposefully choose how we listen and attend in conversations. We all know how it feels when we have another person's full attention and they are listening to us intently and without distraction. We also know what it is like to be in conversation with someone who is preoccupied and only half listening to what we might be saying. The quality of these interactions is distinctly different. As such, the possibility of what might emerge from them is also divergent.

TABLE 4-4 illustrates a variety of ways of listening that can dramatically change the way in which meaning emerges in interactions. Certain ways of listening may be more appropriate in some situations than others. We can work to develop practical judgment around our ways of listening by purposefully choosing to attend to conversations with a particular quality.

Mindfulness

Much of this chapter has discussed and stressed the importance of developing the capacity of dwelling in the living present. I am sure many readers have already been thinking about mindfulness because this is indeed a practice that focuses on being present moment to moment.

Mindfulness is described as the energy of being aware and awake in the present moment. To be mindful is to be present and at one with those around you and with

TABLE 4-4 Ways of Listening

Ways of Listening	Characteristics/Quality	Example
I already know that	Downloading. We listen to reconfirm habitual beliefs, judgments, and values. We deny or discount what does not fit with what we already know.	The evening news program reports that more stringent gun laws reduce violent crimes.
Wow, look at that!	Object-focused listening. Paying attention to facts and novel data that disconfirms current ways of thinking/doing. Empirical and cognitive in nature (objective).	A clinical expert is talking about the results of a new study that suggests a new treatment is beneficial.
I know how you feel	Empathic listening. Real dialogue; we are less aware of our own agenda and are focused more on connecting with the other person.	A patient is sharing his or her difficult but hopeful story of recovery from a life-threatening illness.
I cannot describe it, but I feel I am part of something larger	Emergent listening. Generative and focused on the emerging edge of the present moment. Listening from a state of flow or grace. Authentic, coming into being.	In a team meeting, you and your colleagues are in the zone and on your way to developing a shared vision for a patient-centered culture.

Modified from Scharmer, C. O. (2016). *Theory U: Leading from the future as it emerges* (2nd ed.). Cambridge, MA: Society for Organizational Learning.

what you are doing (Plum Village, 2015). Developing one's mindfulness practice is an excellent opportunity to cultivate the ability to participate and contribute to the organization as conversation, not to mention that the significant physical and emotional benefits of mindfulness practice have been well researched and documented (Luken & Sammons, 2016; Parsons, Crane, Parsons, Fjorback, & Kuyken, 2017).

LEARNING ACTIVITY: EXPLORING MEANING AND COCREATION

1. Take a few minutes for each person in the group to individually read William Stafford's poem "A Ritual to Read to Each Other."
2. Reflect on the poem and try to relate it to the main concepts in this chapter, such as the following:
   - Organization as conversation
   - Patterns of relating

(continues)

LEARNING ACTIVITY: EXPLORING MEANING AND COCREATION *(continued)*

- Patterns of meaning
- Ways of talking, listening, and being
- Innovation
- Other concepts and ideas that emerge for you

3. If you wish, make a few notes about your reflections (there is no right or wrong here; focus on the personal meaning you take from the poem).
4. Have a volunteer from the group read the poem aloud as everyone else listens.
5. Take another moment for self-reflection. Did hearing the poem read aloud by another person change the way you experienced the words and meaning? If so, how? If you were the reader of the poem, what was your experience of reading the poem out loud to others?
6. Now invite group members to share in a discussion about the experience. Here are some questions that might guide the sharing:
   - What concepts from the chapter did individuals find reflected in the poem?
   - What past experiences, emotions, images, or questions surfaced in the reading of the poem?
   - Was it difficult to fully listen or attend to the person who was reading the poem aloud? Why or why not?
   - What is our experience (right now) of talking about this activity? What meaning are we making? How are we talking together? Are themes and patterns emerging?
   - Has the individual meaning we found in the poem shifted as a result of the group dialogue? How? Why?

"A Ritual to Read to Each Other"

If you don't know the kind of person I am
and I don't know the kind of person you are
a pattern that others made may prevail in the world
and following the wrong god home we may miss our star.

For there is many a small betrayal in the mind,
a shrug that lets the fragile sequence break
sending with shouts the horrible errors of childhood
storming out to play through the broken dyke.

And as elephants parade holding each elephant's tail,
but if one wanders the circus won't find the park,
I call it cruel and maybe the root of all cruelty
to know what occurs but not recognize the fact.

And so I appeal to a voice, to something shadowy,
a remote important region in all who talk:
though we could fool each other, we should consider—
lest the parade of our mutual life get lost in the dark.

For it is important that awake people be awake,
or a breaking line may discourage them back to sleep;
the signals we give—yes or no, or maybe—
should be clear: the darkness around us is deep

In this section we have explored the improvisational nature of working from a perspective of organization as conversation. To be present in the moment and to purposefully choose how we speak, listen, and generally show up in conversations are competencies that we can all work to cultivate. Earlier in the chapter we discussed the overall implications of what it means to take up a complex relational view in our day-to-day work, such as how this view leads us to think differently about leadership and planning. Now we will turn our attention to specific topics of EBP and innovation. Building on the ideas presented earlier in this chapter and our growing understanding of what it means to take up the complex relational perspective, let's explore further.

▶ Complex Relational Health Care: Beyond Instrumentality and Either/or Thinking

One of the critiques of the EBP movement is that it leads to cookbook medicine or overly prescriptive guidelines that do not leave room for consideration of context, patient preference, and other local conditions (Romana, 2006).Yet many of us who work in the area of complexity and innovation are often asked to provide tools or recipes to assist leaders and practitioners to make changes in their organizations (Patton, McKegg, & Wehipeihana, 2016; Patton, 2011; Stacey, 2012). The pull of our habitual mechanistic and empirical ways of talking and acting is strong. Indeed, part of the conundrum is language based (Gergen, 2009). What commonly understood language do we have that allows us to communicate to others that we are seeking guidance about how to do things differently? We ask for tools, guides, manuals, or instruments. The organization as conversation perspective can create an opportunity to introduce new ways of talking together and to create a new vernacular that moves beyond tools to something else that resembles relational processes or ways of being, for example. What would it look like to be an evidence-based healthcare team? How can a complex relational lens assist us in this process?

Evidence and EBP

Clinical decisions should be informed by evidence, but it is the role and responsibility of the clinician to critically appraise and then apply that evidence in a manner that is contextually appropriate.

The application of evidence within a specific context brings us back to an earlier point about practical judgment. Recall that in practical judgment, two aspects are brought to bear. First, our past accumulation of knowledge (including research-based evidence), experience, and praxis provide us with an array of possible actions. Second, the unique contextual tapestry of the present moment must be sensed and discerned. Practical judgment happens at that point of convergence between the past and the emerging future in the living present. This way of understanding contextual appropriateness is intensely particularized (local). Before we move on to discuss how EBP happens in teams and organizations, let us take a step back to consider what counts as evidence.

What Counts as Evidence?

Kuhn (2007) reminds us that our predominant worldview consists of a connected set of beliefs and assumptions about the form and function of the world coupled with beliefs about how best to investigate it. As previously discussed, our Western habits of thought are still largely rooted in the mechanistic, positivistic, and rational ways of being. As such, objectivity and linearity also form the ways we conduct research as we seek to understand the world around us. This has implications for what we believe counts as useful or strong evidence.

We largely believe that measuring things (such as blood cells, antigens, outcomes, effects) means quantifying them. We seek to isolate, control, and randomize in an effort to ensure validity and rigor. In other words, the predominant discourse about evidence and what is good or bad, weak or strong, is based in rationalism, positivism, and linear thinking. This either/or way of thinking, coupled with a strong affinity for valuing positivistic inquiry as strong, sets us up for a false dilemma between quantitative and qualitative inquiry. The false dilemma becomes this: if quantitative evidence is strong or good, then qualitative evidence must be weak or bad.

A more balanced view of these two types of inquiry is that they both have merit and value, and depending on the question or phenomena we seek to investigate, one may be more appropriate than another. Again, we arrive back at the issue of contextual appropriateness. Just as it would be considered inappropriate to design a phenomenological study to discern the efficacy of a new proton-pump inhibitor in an adult population, it is likewise as ludicrous to use a randomized control trial to determine the usefulness of an innovative care delivery model implemented in a multihospital care system. What might be more beneficial in addressing our complex, multifaceted, and often chaotic healthcare system is a healthy dose of both, and thinking.

This means that we are open to the idea that there may be more than one right way, that there may be multiple right answers. It provides a basis for synergy among ways of thinking. **TABLE 4-5** presents an array of research methods that align with two of the perspectives we have discussed in this chapter (organization as machine and organization as conversation). The table is meant to illustrate the value of both/and thinking when it comes to evidence. Rather than falling prey to the false dilemma

TABLE 4-5 Worldviews and Research Methods	
Worldview	**Resonant Research Methods**
Modernism, rational, positivistic, empirical EBP Organization as machine	Rational scientific inquiry, such as experimental and quasi-experimental studies, randomized control trials, meta-analysis, case-controlled studies
Complex relational Practice-based evidence Organization as conversation	Qualitative inquiry, such as grounded theory, action research, metasynthesis, phenomenology, narrative inquiry, organizational ethnography, autoethnography

and feeling pressed to choose one or the other, imagine the possibility of holding both perspectives as different but useful and valuable.

To use a comfortable (albeit mechanistic) analogy, imagine that you are using a computer program, and one window provides you with a spreadsheet view of data with raw numbers and averages. Another window presents this same data organized by theme and category. Both views use the same data but portray it in very different (and useful) ways. The most complete understanding of the data or phenomena comes from being able to toggle between the two screens.

Let us return for a moment to the issue of language and specifically how it relates to evidence. Any one of us who has read research articles can attest that quantitative and qualitative researchers use different language. Many of us are fluent in one language, and some of us may even be bilingual. For discussion purposes, let us suppose that quantitative is the predominant language spoken in health care. How much more varied, challenging, interesting, and inclusive would our conversations be if we challenged ourselves to learn a new language? Granted, we may not become fluent, but seeking to understand, or at the very least appreciate, a different way of speaking can be very enriching.

EBP

A publication is a complex abstraction of the actual activities that were undertaken to address a research or clinical question. Based on the aims and focus of the journal, the value judgments made by the authors about what data and results are most important or salient, and the assessment of the peer reviewers and editors about the overall quality and merit of the study, the reader finally receives a 15- to 20-page glimpse into the complex undertaking of the original study.

After a study, systematic review, or meta-analysis is completed, published, and finds its way into the hands of practitioners, it enters a complex milieu of health care. There is a wide array of unpredictable and highly relational dynamics that influence the dissemination, implementation, and local value judgments about the usefulness and value of the evidence.

From a complex relational perspective, EBP is a specific theme that serves to help us organize our work together in health care. Specific patterns of relating and patterns of meaning emerge as the generalized theme of EBP is taken up. Here are some examples:

- Patterns of relating in EBP:
  - Journal clubs
  - Clinical practice guideline implementation committee
  - Latest clinical practice guidelines are embedded in electronic medical records
  - Dedicated computer on each unit for database searching (CINAHL, MEDLINE, and other EBP-related resources, such as clinical practice guidelines)
  - Shared governance monthly meeting agenda has a standing item for EBP updates
- Patterns of meaning in EBP:
  - Organizational vision is adapted to include a statement about high-quality, evidence-informed care
  - Award is developed to recognize teams that exemplify or demonstrate excellent patient outcomes based on the use of EBP

- Clinical staff who have completed an intensive 2-day training session about EBP are given unique lapel pins that identify them as EBP champions
- EBP expert is invited to be keynote speaker at organization-wide clinical care conference

The specific patterns of meaning and relating are taken up (or not) in local clinical settings. Recall that the organizing theme and patterns are enacted or perpetuated only in the speaking and doing of them. What conversations happen at the local level that might stabilize the theme of EBP? Perhaps a well-respected nurse practitioner enthusiastically shares a new meta-analysis that supports the use of cognitive behavioral therapy as an effective secondary prevention strategy for patients with coronary heart disease. The team may then decide to explore cognitive behavioral therapy programs they could use in a pilot project.

All of the constituent aspects of complex responsive processes come into play in the complex, conflictual, relational activities of day-to-day organizational life. Consider the potential influence of the following aspects of complex responsive processes in relation to EBP:

- Ideology (organizational values and norms)
- Power dynamics (in group versus out group dynamics; processes of shame)
- Dance between stability and transformation of patterns and themes

FIGURE 4-5 illustrates evidence generation and the flow of evidence into a healthcare practice that eventually may be taken up and form EBP. The bottom half of the diamond

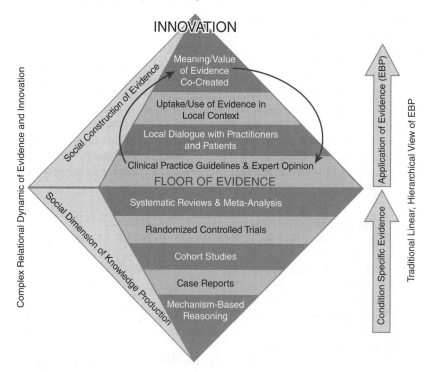

FIGURE 4-5 EBP diamond.

Data from Lefkowitz, W., & Jefferson, T. C. (2014). Medicine at the limits of evidence: The fundamental limitation of the randomized clinical trial and the end of equipoise. *Journal of Perinatology, 34*(4), 249–251. http://dx.doi.org/10.1038/jp.2013.172

represents the pyramid of evidence that we generally use to appraise and make sense of condition-specific evidence. After this accumulated high-quality evidence reaches practice environments, it becomes the basis for practice (the floor of evidence).

What occurs, then, is the complex relational process that I have called the social construction of evidence. This is the process of making sense of evidence in local interactions, which is iterative and ongoing. Sometimes the sense-making process results in the introduction of novelty (local tweaking of evidence to better meet the needs of patients and providers) or stability (the adoption of EBP that the team experiences as valuable and useful).

In some instances, the process of meaning making may result in the identification of a gap in the evidence or a misalignment of the evidence to the practice setting. This may result in the introduction of novel conversations, themes, and patterns that can lead to transformation and innovation. Innovation, then, can represent practice-based evidence (Gergen, 2015). The creation of new knowledge and practices emerges as novel patterns and serve to organize our way of working together differently.

▶ Innovation as Transformational Conversation

Earlier in this chapter we discussed both/and thinking as an alternative to the either/or false dilemma. Both/and thinking can also enable innovation. The *both* of the statement recognizes the need and value of holding multiple perspective as useful and viable. The *and* is innovation and represents the yet-to-be-formed idea, process, or product that may emerge from ongoing conversations and the introduction of sufficient novelty.

Fonseca (2002) suggested that innovation is the emergence of dissipative structures of meaning and that a certain level of misunderstanding (redundant diversity of meaning) is required for innovation to occur. Different ways of talking or new patterns of relating can lead to misunderstanding. In the ensuing conversations, people probe and question each other to attempt to stabilize meaning and understanding. In this process, new (shared, coconstructed) meaning may emerge that becomes a new pattern. This is the complex relational process of innovation.

There are a myriad of organizational dynamics that can either coalesce to enhance the potential for innovation or dynamics that conspire to minimize the potential for novelty and change. **FIGURE 4-6** illustrates the hurly-burly blend of relational dynamics from which innovation may emerge.

If I were to ask you to name someone you know who is innovative, you would probably quickly come up with a name. It might be someone from popular culture, like Steve Jobs or Mark Zuckerberg, or a historical figure such as Thomas Edison or Leonardo da Vinci. It might just as easily be Dr. Jones who works in the office two doors down from you. Whoever came to mind, we could agree that innovators have a capacity or habitual ways of being that emancipate innovation. From a complex relational perspective, people who are skilled in innovation have habituated ways of talking and attending in conversations. Further, they may leverage or create novel patterns of relating that bring together a constellation of coconspirators in a way that introduces sufficient novelty, misunderstanding, and diversity to produce innovation. Each one of us can build our capacity for innovation, for leadership, for improvisation.

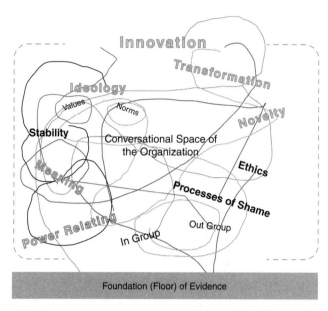

FIGURE 4-6 The mess of healthcare innovation.

Many ideas for this have already been highlighted in this chapter (such as ways of listening and talking, and dwelling in the present moment). In the final section, we will discuss several ideas that relate specifically to our capacity for innovation.

▶ Say Yes to the Mess

Frank Barrett wrote a wonderful book, *Yes to the Mess: Surprising Leadership Lessons from Jazz* (2012), that brings together his experience in organizational behavior and development and as a jazz pianist. In the book, he provides helpful perspectives and insights that leverage the capacity for improvisation in the service of relational leadership and innovation. Many of the principles in Barrett's book resonate with what we have discussed in this chapter.

Figure 4-6 illustrates the messiness of healthcare organizations as conversations. Looking at the figure may induce anxiety, uneasiness, and even panic in some readers. Often our initial reaction (based on our habitual mechanistic and linear ways of thinking) is to simplify, control, and organize. Stacey (2012) suggested that this craving for order and planning is a very human reaction to the anxiety evoked by not having control. Innovators, however, have developed a capacity to say yes to the mess and to dwell in the disorder and see the potential that emerges.

I am reminded of a technique that is used in improvisational theater. When a fellow actor leads with a line that you have no idea how to respond to initially, actors use the rhetorical device "yes, and . . .". This values and honors the creation from the other actor and allows an addition to the scenario without derailing, controlling, or closing off the potential for what might emerge from the collaboration. Yes, and . . . can be a useful way of talking together that invites emergence and allows us to build on the ideas of others.

Another attribute of skilled innovators is their ability to build and maintain trusting relationships. For people to be okay dwelling in the messy present moment, not knowing and even misunderstanding, there must be a sense of trust (Fonseca, 2002). Trust is the relational antidote to our anxiety of not knowing. Creating a sense of relational safety and trust allows people to stay engaged in the evolving conversation, and the ebb and flow of misunderstanding and new meaning.

Curiosity is also a potent tonic for innovation. In my experience, taking up an attitude of curiosity has allowed me to move beyond downloading and object-focused listening in challenging conversations. Rather than dismissing what someone is saying or looking for only the facts, curiosity keeps us engaged and we are able to attend to the conversation at a higher level. The next time you are in a conversation and you feel anxiety mounting, or if you find you are switching into download mode, try moving beyond the emotion of anxiety by asking yourself a curious question: why would someone think that way or do what they did? Pursue the answers with a curious attitude.

Brené Brown is a researcher who specializes in shame and vulnerability. In *Daring Greatly* (2012), she explores shame and vulnerability within organizational contexts. In her book, she recounts a conversation with a Silicon Valley CEO in which she asked him what he believed the greatest barrier to innovation was. He replied, "I don't know if it has a name, but honestly, it's the fear of introducing an idea and being ridiculed, laughed at, and belittled" (2012, p. 186). What this man is describing is shame. In our earlier conversations of complex relational organizations, we have identified that processes of shame are a powerful social sanction enacted to maintain stability and the dominant organizational ideology. He goes on to say that "the problem is that innovative ideas often sound crazy and failure and learning are part of revolution" (2012, p. 186). Brown identified that for innovation and creativity to flourish and create positive change, there is a need to rehumanize our workplaces—to invite and welcome vulnerability as an essential element of innovation.

The concept of rehumanization brings us full circle to the two metaphors of organizational life that we began this chapter with: moving away from the organization as machine and toward a vision of organization as conversation. (What is more human than talking together about our day-to-day work?) This means having the courage to have honest conversations about shame and daring to shine a light into dark corners that we would rather leave unexplored or ignored. Brown (2012) calls these kinds of conversations disruptive engagement, which is wonderful new language for creating patterns of meaning that move the conversation forward.

References

Barrett, F. J. (2012). *Yes to the mess: Surprising leadership lessons from jazz*. Boston, MA: Harvard Business School Publishing.

Benner, P., Hooper-Kyriakidis, P., & Stannard, D. (1999). *Clinical wisdom and interventions in critical care: A thinking-in-action approach*. Philadelphia, PA: Saunders.

Benner, P., Sutphen, M., Leonard, V., & Day, L. (2010). *Educating nurses: A call for radical transformation*. Stanford, CA: Jossey-Bass.

Booth, B. J., Zwar, N., & Harris, M. F. (2013). Healthcare improvement as planned system change or complex responsive processes? A longitudinal case study of general practice. *BMC Family Practice, 14*(51), 1–12.

Bourdieu, P. (1990). *The logic of practice* (R. Nice, Trans.). Palo Alto, CA: Stanford Press.

Brown, B. (2012). *Daring greatly*. New York, NY: Avery.

Davidson, S. J. (2015). Shifting the balance: Relationship as power in organizational life. *Nursing Forum, 50*(4), 258–264. http://dx.doi.org/10.1111/nuf.12115

Elias, N. (1998). *On civilization, power, and knowledge*. Chicago, IL: University of Chicago Press.

Fonseca, J. (2002). *Complexity and innovation in organizations*. London, UK: Routledge.

Gergen, K. J. (2009). *Relational being: Beyond self and community.* New York, NY: Oxford Press.

Gergen, K. J. (2015). *An invitation to social construction* (3rd ed.). Thousand Oaks, CA: Sage.

Hassan, Z. (2014). *The social labs revolution: A new approach to solving our most complex challenges.* San Francisco, CA: Berrett-Koehler.

Kuhn, L. (2007). Why utilize complexity principles in social inquiry? *World Futures, 63*(3–4), 156–175.

Laloux, F. (2014). *Reinventing organization: A guide to creating organizations inspired by the next stage of human consciousness.* Brussels, Belgium: Nelson Parker.

Lefkowitz, W., & Jefferson, T. C. (2014). Medicine at the limits of evidence: The fundamental limitation of the randomized clinical trial and the end of equipoise. *Journal of Perinatology, 2014*(34), 249–251. http://dx.doi.org/10.1038/jp.2013.172

Luken, M., & Sammons, A. (2016). Systematic review of mindfulness practice for reducing job burnout. *The American Journal of Occupational Therapy, 70*(2), 7002250020p1–7002250020p10. http://dx.doi.org/10.5014/ajot.2016.016956

Mead, G. H. (1934). *Mind, self and society.* Chicago, IL: Chicago University Press.

Parsons, C., Crane, C., Parsons, L., Fjorback, L., & Kuyken, W. (2017). Home practice in mindfulness-based cognitive therapy and mindfulness-based stress reduction: A systematic review and meta-analysis of participants' mindfulness practice and its association with outcomes. *Behaviour Research and Therapy, 95*, 29–41. http://dx.doi.org/10.1016/j.brat.2017.05.004

Patton, M. Q. (2011). *Developmental evaluation: Applying complexity concepts to enhance innovation and use.* New York, NY: Guilford Press.

Patton, M. Q., McKegg, K., & Wehipeihana, N. (2016). *Developmental evaluation exemplars: Principles in practice.* New York, NY: Guilford Press.

Plum Village. (2015). The mindfulness bell. Retrieved from http://plumvillage.org/the-mindfulness -bell/

Romana, H. W. (2006). Is evidence-based medicine patient-centered and is patient-centered care evidence-based? *Health Services Research, 41*(1), 1–8. http://dx.doi.org/10.1111/j.1475 -6773.2006.00504.x

Scharmer, C. O. (2016). *Theory U: Leading from the future as it emerges* (2nd ed.). Cambridge, MA: Society for Organizational Learning.

Shaw, P. (2006). Introduction: Working live. In P. Shaw & R. Stacey (Eds.), *Experiencing risk, spontaneity and improvisation in organizational change: Working live* (pp. 1–18). New York, NY: Routledge.

Stacey, R. D. (2001). *Complex responsive processes in organizations: Learning and knowledge creation.* London, UK: Routledge.

Stacey, R. D. (2006). Complex responsive processes as a theory of organizational improvisation. In P. Shaw & R. Stacey (Eds.), *Experiencing risk, spontaneity, and improvisation in organizational change: Working live* (pp. 124–138). New York, NY: Routledge.

Stacey, R. (2012). *Tools and techniques of leadership and management: Meeting the challenge of complexity.* New York, NY: Routledge.

Stacey, R. D., Griffin, D., & Shaw, P. (2000). *Complexity and management: Fad or radical challenge to systems thinking?* New York, NY: Routledge

Suchman, A. L. (2011a). How we think about organizations: A complexity perspective. In A. L. Suchman, D. J. Sluyter, & P. R. Williamson (Eds.), *Leading change in healthcare: Transforming organizations using complexity, positive psychology and relationship-centered care.* London, UK: Radcliffe.

Suchman, A. L. (2011b). Organizations as machines, organizations as conversations: Two core metaphors and their consequences. *Medical Care, 49*(12), S45–S48.

Taylor, F. (1911). *Scientific management.* New York, NY: Harper.

Walker, D. (2006). Leading in the moment: Taking risks and living with anxiety. In P. Shaw & R. Stacey (Eds.), *Experiencing risk, spontaneity and improvisation in organizational change: Working live* (pp. 97–123). New York, NY: Routledge.

World Health Organization. (2009). *Surgical safety checklist.* Retrieved from https://www.who.int /patientsafety/safesurgery/checklist/en/

SECTION 2

Organizations/ Systems

Evidence-Based Practice and the Dynamic of Innovation: A Model for the Advancing Practice Excellence

Tim Porter-O'Grady and Kathy Malloch

The secret of change is to focus not on fighting the old but on building the new (p. 113).[1]

CHAPTER OBJECTIVES

Upon completion of this chapter, the reader will be able to:

1. Define and outline the key components of a cybernetic dynamic model of evidence-based practice and innovation.
2. Outline the critical interdependencies between evidence and innovation that are indispensable to creating appropriate action and achieving sustainable outcomes.
3. Identify the essential processes associated with linking evidence and innovation that are vital to advancing positive change.

---

[1] Spoken by the character Socrates in Millman, D. (1984). *Way of the peaceful warrior: A book that changes lives.* Tiburon, CA: HJ Kramer.

▶ Introduction

One of the most challenging issues related to intersecting evidence and innovation is the perception that they are fundamentally different. Evidence and innovation are critical partners in a relationship continuum, and their interaction is essential to accurate and sustainable outcomes (Melnyck & Overholt, 2019).

It is easy to differentiate evidence-based practice (EBP) and innovation by definition. EBP represents a more solid and factual foundation that is the product of deep study or research incorporating all related elements derived from multiple sources, from disciplined research to experiential applications (Spencer, Detrich, & Slocum, 2012). Innovation, on the other hand, demonstrates a more generative but just as rigorous process that leads to something new and changes our circumstances and lives (Morrar, 2014). Clearly, both are dynamic processes with clear structures, stages, and disciplines that lead definitively to an impact or a product. Each relates to the other insofar as one (evidence) serves as the foundation for the other (innovation) (Hofbaur, Murawski, Karlsson, & Freddie, 2013).

This notion of evidence and innovation as a dynamic is critical to understanding the multidimensional nature of both. Dynamics suggest that there is an element of both interaction and impact (Rook, 2013). Also implied is the continuous nature of this interaction as indicated by a cybernetic (closed loop) process that ultimately changes the environment, the system, and people (Pickering, 2014). The assumption here reflects the level of complex interactions between elements and components of a process in a way that influences what those processes do, how they work, and the future change the action of this relationship creates on processes and products (Kluever, 2015) (**FIGURE 5-1**).

FIGURE 5-1 Evidence and innovation dynamic.

▶ Why Evidence and Innovation?

Much transformation and essential change is occurring in the healthcare delivery system. The very foundation of the delivery of health care is shifting from a volume foundation to value drivers (Shaw, Asomugha, Conway, & Rain, 2014). Elements of a new concept associated with Triple Aim objectives are now forming the cornerstone of the future delivery of health care. These Triple Aim objectives reflect the shifting change in the broader landscape of technology and clinical science and are radically altering the context and framework for health service delivery (Costich, Scutchfield, & Ingram, 2015). These products of the digital age now create the possibility for generating and managing big data in a way that provides a high level of usefulness and applicability never seen in the history of human experience, especially in the healthcare system (Simpao, Ahumada, Galvaz, & Rehman, 2014). One of the aims of value-based health care is to ensure that there is a strong relationship between clinical and patient outcomes. Increasingly there is a need to evaluate the effectiveness of care delivery with the number and kind of resources essential to obtain it. In this scenario and the objectives related to advancing it, it is important that the strength of the relationship between process and outcome delineate a specific and intentional determination of the most effective cost-benefit relationship existing between the two (Ikhwanuliman, 2017) (**FIGURE 5-2**).

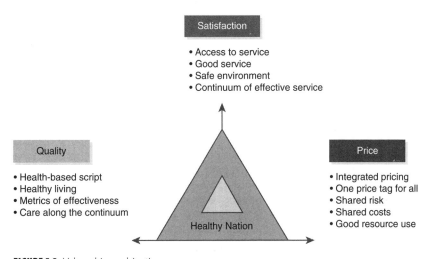

FIGURE 5-2 Value-driven objectives.

One of the most dramatic impacts of this digital reality is the ability to aggregate, integrate, and coordinate huge composites of data and to sort through it in meaningful ways to obtain significant information that provides value in defining, interpreting, and evaluating the vast variety of healthcare activities in an unlimited array of arrangements. The larger the data pool becomes, the more difficult it is to manage, yet the more vital it is to systematically organize it and accelerate its usefulness in making decisions, taking action, and evaluating the impact. Management of these huge pools of data now becomes a significant, indeed vital, challenge in the appropriate provision of health care and the evaluation of its effectiveness (Wills, 2013).

It is out of these foundations that evidentiary dynamics have emerged. EBP is a formal process associated with this notion of evidentiary dynamics, which serves as the complex driver of the fluidity necessary to understand the interactions and relationships embedded deep within the evidentiary process. *Evidentiary dynamics* is merely a term that suggests that there is a complex array of individual elements (agents) that must operate in concert to produce a value that is both meaningful and useful in making decisions and taking action. In evidentiary dynamics, it is the confluence of the full range of facts, factors, elements, and influences that, when converged, deliver a message that has meaning and value for the receiver (Malloch & Porter-O'Grady, 2010).

▶ What Is Evidence?

Evidence is simply the accumulation of facts and factors that provide conclusive insight into the legitimacy, accuracy, and viability supporting a particular process or action (Davidson, Weberg, Porter-O'Grady, & Malloch, 2017). Because of the veracity of the evidence and its generalizability, it serves as a foundation or the floor of an action that establishes a rational and justifiable basis upon which to undertake the action and to utilize it as a standard for performance. An EBP serves as the foundation of our actions in health care for patients by ensuring that the minimum standards of viability, appropriateness, and safety have been established and can be replicated with a high level of assurance such that consistent impacts and outcomes can be achieved (Magnavita & American Psychological Association, 2016). Until such evidence is eclipsed by newer and more relevant data to suggest a change in practice and behavior, the current evidence in practice serves as the standard (C. Brown, 2014).

However, since evidence is dynamic, a static or permanent foundation for practice is never created in an evidence-based environment. Evidentiary dynamics suggests the continuous exploration, discernment, and ultimately creation of new information, insights, and practices (Schmidt & Brown, 2015). These processes imply an ongoing currency—a continual production of data that suggests an aggregation of existing practices and the generation of new knowledge that emerges from those practices. This knowledge-based practice evolves into new research outcomes and changes that are suggested by enhancements and best practices drawn from both experience and new interpretations of data (Porter-O'Grady & Malloch, 2014).

In evidence-based processes and practices, a mosaic of actions and interactions become necessary to ensure both relevance and viability in a way that positively influences clinical practice. Structures of EBP are grounded in effective data systems that demonstrate a high degree of interoperability, fluidity, flexibility, and portability (Prescott, Maeschalck, Miller, & American Psychological Association, 2017). All these elements or characteristics are associated with the capacity to make just-in-time decisions and undertake dynamic and continuously modified clinical practice. To do so, both the information system and the practitioner must find that the components of the information and the characteristics of clinical practice have the capacity to change quickly in ways suggested by emerging evidence. Two dynamics must occur in concert to make these practices real. First, the evidence-driven data systems must yield accurate, immediate, and relevant data related to particular practices in a relatively short period of time and in a useful manner. Second, the users' approach to practice must be fluid and flexible enough so practice processes can be immediately adjusted and changed in a way that incorporates these changes into the normative delivery of specific patient care. Both of these objectives are highly problematic if the information systems are not sufficiently responsive to the data or if people tend to perpetuate ritual and routine instead of embracing relevant and immediate recommended changes to practice. Our clinical history is grounded in volume that is certified and sanctified by an endless array of mechanisms founded in ritualistic protocols, procedures, and practices that almost prevent individuals from being available to recommend improvements in practices without a great deal of personal and organizational drama and trauma (McNelis, Ironside, Zvonar, & Ebright, 2014).

▶ Evidence as a Requirement for Practice

EBP implies a generalized availability and practitioner readiness to incorporate sometimes substantive adjustments into practice in relatively short periods of time as an ordinary operational mechanism for undertaking clinical work (Lubejko, 2014). This is precisely the reason that evidence-based processes must be incorporated into the structural components of operating clinical practices so they become the prevailing format for clinical work activities and the normative way of doing clinical business.

🔎 *CASE EXAMPLE: DESIGNING AND IMPLEMENTING EBP*

Sally Brown, RN, MSN, has just become the new director of medical–surgical services in her hospital. An initial assessment of the clinical structure supporting care indicated that much of practice in a medical–surgical setting was grounded on policy and procedure, historic practice routines, and individual nursing experience. Recently the organization had committed to lean strategies to minimize practice variability and errors in clinical practice. The staff members had not robustly engaged these efforts and seemed lost in bridging their own nursing approaches in a more formal process that set new parameters for their practice.

Sally believed that EBP was essential to build solid practice foundations that would lead to more data-based practices, reduce variability, strengthen professional and

(continues)

🔍 CASE EXAMPLE: DESIGNING AND IMPLEMENTING EBP

(continued)

patient care relationships, and advance quality nursing practice on all medical–surgical units. She knew she would have to initiate an effective plan in a series of steps to structure EBP and to gain staff engagement in its implementation.

Prior to a process of implementation, Sally knew that a structured approach to EBP would be required to formalize EBP as a part of nursing clinical work. The first steps of implementation were grounded on the plan function beginning with three steps—ask, acquire, and appraise, to include the following:

- Raise key questions with staff regarding the safe care of individual patients, episodes, populations, and communities.
- Define and search legitimate sources of data regarding these questions of care.
- Select care priorities and processes that are most important to particular patient care activities or interventions.
- Clarify specific and definable goals with regard to care and intervention and the intended impact and outcome the related activities would produce.
- Clarify and study existing evidence related to effective EBP programs elsewhere, as well as interventions and standards specifically related to aligned patient care events, episodes, or interventions in other settings.

As Sally and her design and implementation team pursued building a framework for EBP, the following key questions related to effective implementation needed to be specifically addressed by the clinical leaders:

- How are the insights, views, and experiences of providers and patients included in the EBP considerations?
- How was the implementation design specifically tailored to the unique characteristics of units and care groups, including consideration of role, competencies, unit culture, patient characteristics, and past practices?
- How were successful models from other organizations and institutions accessed and analyzed to determine their relevance and viability in informing the development of EBP at Sally's institution?
- How was the design and implementation team educated, supported, and resourced, and how was their work communicated to all stakeholders?
- Were metrics established to measure progress and challenges ahead of understanding, commitment, and application of strategies for EBP implementation?
- When adjustments were made in the implementation plan, were they noted and evaluated for effectiveness and impact?
- Is evaluation continuous, does the produced data inform and influence subsequent action and provide an opportunity for necessary change, and does it include staff engagement?

Sally recognized that these are simply initial essential steps and stages in designing and creating the beginning structures for a dynamic evidence-based process for each unit. Guided by a consistent and systematic approach for the medical–surgical services as a whole, each unit of service and clinical team is able to adapt the processes and questions to their unique culture in specific patient populations. Continuous evaluation of the framework helps Sally make sure that EBP plan is appropriate and effective and that the implementation achieves the intended impact.

As organizations become more amenable to value drivers and responsive to the Triple Aim of service excellence, metrics of high-level quality, and affordability, they will have to increasingly embed deeply within their cultures an operating milieu that requires an accelerating level of responsiveness to just-in-time practice changes that demonstrate their availability to evidence that points to an immediate change.

Also of immediate interest in relationship to particular significance of evidentiary dynamics in the clinical workplace is the increasingly necessary and growing emergence of transdisciplinary care models in patient-centered delivery systems (Nandan & Scott, 2014). Each discipline brings its own clinical culture, practices, and applications to patient service in a way that is clearly and uniquely valuable in meeting patient needs. However, it is becoming increasingly evident that value is influenced and moderated by the degree of integration and goodness of fit between the activities of any one discipline and the actions of all disciplines involved in patient care (Pilon, 2015). Current research suggests that the interface of clinical activity of each discipline with the work of other disciplines is fragmented, often not aligned, and may even represent divergent goals for care (Starck & Rooney, 2015). Past mechanisms for communication among disciplines have been highly compartmentalized, vertically oriented, and structured in ways that often make it cumbersome and difficult. Research has shown that these mechanisms significantly reduce the ability of practitioners and organizations to change practices or create innovative solutions to improve care (Weberg, 2013).

From the patient's perspective, individual increments of care and service operate at a low level of comprehension. The only interest is that all essential stakeholders' clinical activities converge in a way that positively affects the patient experience, improves the patient's condition, and advances the patient's healthcare experience (Olson, Young, & Schultz, 2016). What individual practitioners provide for the patient, from the patient's perspective, is often amorphous and indeterminate. The patient hopes that all the practices of key stakeholders demonstrate a high level of synthesis that, when coalesced, results in improvement and moves the patient to a higher likelihood of health. It may be a good thing that the patient is not aware of how limited communication is among providers and how difficult it is to coalesce clinical goals, interactions, and communications in a way that ensures a concerted, tightly woven clinical alignment rather than a patchwork quilt of somewhat isolated clinical events.

One of the significant challenges of EBP is the centrality of communication and integration of clinical stakeholders around an interfaced clinical plan of action. This plan should be clearly enumerated—to provide significant opportunity for demonstrating how well-grounded in evidence the individual and collective clinical action is, and to demonstrate how mutually supportive both the evidentiary data and clinical action is in practice. Lack of coordination is certainly becoming less acceptable as evidentiary principles now more broadly drive practice planning and decision making. Yet improving tool sets and mechanisms must be refined in the practice environment in a way that reflects a strong foundation in team-based clinical practices that are subjected to well-defined models of care delivery and ongoing mechanisms for evaluating impacts and effectiveness (Sheikh, George, & Gilson, 2014).

Sustainable EBP will increasingly be dependent on the capacity of team-based practice to ground itself in collective efforts to link and integrate discipline-specific practices in a community of practice for the convergence of effort that yields direct patient-centered benefits and impacts. Evidence of the degree of interface

TABLE 5-1 From Volume to Value to Practice	
Yesterday:	**Tomorrow:**
■ Procedural	■ Evidence
■ Positional	■ Mobile
■ Subordinated	■ Partnered
■ Task/ritual/routine	■ Impact/making a difference
■ Volume of work	■ Value of practice
■ Hospital-based	■ Continuum-focused
■ Treatment/intervention	■ Health, patient-centered

and goodness of fit of clinical effort will be as critical a part of the dynamics of evidence-grounded processes as will the clinical activities themselves. Transdisciplinary evidence-based mechanisms and processes are quickly becoming the foundation for future practice and the tool set for viable value-based practices.

A good part of establishing EBP as a foundation for future practice is eliminating rituals and routines that reflect the linear and procedural orientation to practice and moving to value-based practice that demonstrates clinical impact, care outcomes, and sustainable health (**TABLE 5-1**). Evidence suggests the capacity for meaningful change. The meaningfulness of change requires the ability to understand the foundations for decisions and actions, comprehend the shifts that are occurring in real time, and translate those shifts into relevant response and action. The commitment to past practice and well-established activities and routines simply because they have been proven effective is a direct impediment to using those same processes as a reference point for improving practice. If emerging evidence coming out of improvements or revelations in the science—or the failure or success of current practices, or even emerging innovations that elevate practices and outcomes—fails to change past practice, it then ceases to be relevant and viable (Belar, 2014).

Many practitioners hold to the values of what they were taught or believe that if it was good enough for them to learn, it is still good enough today, along with similar beliefs that suggest a sort of dictatorship of history. This notion that good practices are fixed and finite results in a rather strident connection to functionalism. At the institutional level, the same behaviors are represented by the infrastructure of policy, procedure, protocol, standardization, and so forth. From either the personal or institutional perspective, these patterns of behavior represent practice as a series of tasks and checklist items that, if completed properly, can ensure safe patient care activity and positive outcomes. They assume that basing the plans and processes of care on metrics that suggest value and positive impact is a stronger and more sustainable approach to obtaining and advancing health. The issue here is not one of value for these tasks and practices; instead, it is an issue of perspective.

▶ Standardization and Evidence

Certainly, the use of safe practices, routines, and protocols provide significant value to good and safe patient processes and positive impacts. However, such standards need to be seen as foundations for practice in a way that establishes the foundation of practice upon which all practitioners firmly stand. These protocols suggest an agreement of knowledge-driven professionals of basic practices and processes that reflect minimum expectations for relevance and safety that simply cannot be transgressed or violated. These foundations suggest to the practitioner that good practice is grounded in solid principles and that, as long as those principles remain valid, the foundation simply represents the ground of practice upon which all professionals stand for their individual and collective professional work.

It must be posited, however, that establishing the base of the foundations of practice does not itself ensure practice excellence. Safety, for example, is a minimum right of expectation of every patient. Maintaining a safe environment for patient care should not be considered a measure of excellence. A safe environment is a basic expectation and right of patients in their interactions and experiences with the health system. A high level of safety is a low level of measure for patient care because it is a basic expectation that every practitioner should demonstrate at all times in all actions. Regardless of the principle or the foundation promulgated, patient care providers must clearly recognize that upholding those principles and foundations with a high level of consistency does not imply excellence; instead, it simply reflects both understanding and compliance with basic practice principles.

This same insight holds true for the process of standardization. Standardization reflects a basic set of principles or protocols that are proven effective and adhered to consistently in a way that demonstrates a good measure of value and positive impact for the patient (Merry & Hamblin, 2012). Recognizing that, no one should suggest that organizations or individuals can standardize their way to excellence. While standardization represents the consistent application of the foundation of our practice, excellence represents the stretch toward the ceiling of our practice. Standardization represents the ground we stand on, and excellence represents a reach to different higher levels of service and care delivery that, once achieved, become the new foundation of our practice—a new foundation upon which to reach anew toward a ceiling (excellence) that raises our practice and enhances the patient experience. Excellence requires the understanding that simply repeating the actions of standardized practice never leads to obtaining and sustaining practice excellence. The inherent action of excellence suggests a different expression of practice, a new notion and understanding informing emergent practice, ultimately resulting in a transformed practice.

▶ Evidence as Movement

As stated at the beginning of this chapter, EBP is a dynamic. As such, it suggests constant activity and movement. Such practices indicate that when foundations are laid and principles are established, the work of practitioners is to use those foundations as a premise for setting out on a journey that ultimately challenges these practices in a way that will result in advancements, improvements, and enhancements of patient care practices and clinical outcomes. While evidence is predominantly about establishing principles and foundations through dynamic activity, it creates the drive—the urge, if you will—to grow, improve, and advance action and impact. Therefore, deeply implied in evidentiary dynamics is the suggestion for creativity and innovation, which are forces that are essential to enhancement and advancement.

The leader in EBP environments is challenged to create a context where evidence-based processes serve as the dynamic impetus for mindfully reflecting and analyzing professional practices and clinical behavior as an ongoing requisite for data-driven patient care. The evidence-grounded leader recognizes that an environment essential to evidence is energized by rigorous and methodological, yet creative and imaginative, relationships and processes that move beyond existing evidence as professional staff reach for improvement, enhancements, and innovative opportunities for advancing practice (Aarons, Ehrhart, Farahnak, & Hurlburt, 2015). This notion of "movement" is fundamental to the understanding of EBP. Movement, in a complexity framework, suggests that nothing remains static or the same. The universe is in constant motion, both continuously constructing and deconstructing energy and matter everywhere (Grady, 2016). Therefore, nothing in existence can remain static or unchanged. The forces of this positive and negative energy are constantly operating to both create and deconstruct. The same can be said for human dynamics, including clinical practice. If practice is not always changing and improving, it is not simply doing nothing (remaining static). Because practice is itself a dynamic, if it is not improving, it is regressing. This regression is ultimately seen in accelerating levels of risk; diminishing rates of improvement; and continuing challenges to patient safety, care relevance, and positive outcomes. There is ample evidence to suggest that the slavish addiction to permanent ritual and routine, policies and procedures, tasks and processes, ultimately results in diminishing performance and decelerating metrics of value and patient impact (Grimmer, Dizon, Milanese, King, & Beaton, 2014).

DISCUSSION

How do we understand this notion of movement in light of clinical practice? Is movement always either negative or positive? What do we mean by the statement that there is nothing static in the universe? How do we keep EBP from becoming negative (ritual, routine, nonrelevant, etc.)? How does EBP lead to the potential for creativity and innovation?

▶ Innovation and Evidence

Evidence and innovation are dynamic partners within the same continuum. The innovative practice leader is always grounded in the evidence and uses that evidence as the footing from which creative energies are generated to advance and change the care experience. At the same time, the evidence-grounded innovator values and respects both the discipline and the rigor of the scientific process for its use and the translation of its products into practice. This attachment to the exactitudes of analysis guides the evidence-based innovator in validating good processes, disciplining the translation of innovation in ways that represent a high level of relevance that result in a strong demonstration of positive impacts (Porter-O'Grady & Malloch, 2014).

The relationship between evidence and innovation can be described as cybernetic. The definition of *cybernetic* is the science of communication and control that looks at the controlled yet interactive and continuous relationship of elements within a system and their dynamic influence on each other. Cybernetic systems are usually closed-system mechanisms that loop continuously, determined by how processes move within them and the relationships among elements in the system. Cybernetic systems are generally cyclical, dynamic, and highly interactive. Each component or part of the system is interdependent, with other parts representing a continuous flow that begins at one place, loops through other elements of the process, and ends up where the process began. It is this cybernetic relationship between evidence and innovation that is described subsequently in this chapter and forms the foundation for the interdependent interaction between evidence and innovation (Porter-O'Grady & Malloch, 2015).

The evidence-based innovator understands the relationship among the firm foundation of principles, protocols, and standards supported by the evidence. At the same time, he or she recognizes that this foundation represents only half the work of good practice. The other half of the work of good practice is represented by faithful commitment to the movement from firm principles and foundations toward new, emerging, and innovative practices that produce new technologies, models of care, and clinical activities that advance both the experience and the health of the patient. Furthermore, the evidence-based innovator acknowledges the overriding need for the commitment and engagement of the practice community and represents in his or her own attitudes and practices a constant mobilization toward the creative, the innovative, and the new as the innovator grapples with the improvement and advancement of practice.

The innovative milieu grounded in evidentiary dynamics provides the kind of context that frees practitioners to discern, debate, and delineate new insights, practices, collaborations, technologies, and configurations for patient care. Rather than being constrained by evidence-based structures and processes, the evidence-grounded innovator represents both the commitment to the rigors of evidence and the freedom to embrace the generativity embedded in exploring opportunities for enhancement, enrichment, change, and invention. For example, EBP with regard to patient falls establishes a set of principles and processes that best demonstrate safe foundations for limiting the dangers and risks of patient falls in particular circumstances. These safety protocols establish a consistent floor for the practice of all professionals and generate a standard that influences everybody's action and serves as the foundation of their relationship with high-risk patients. Assuming this standard is in place, the emergence of a new digital device or software that helps practitioners remotely monitor and follow these patients and alerts providers of the potential risks of falls or compromises in safety changes the landscape of practice. This innovation therefore calls into question existing standards and protocols related to falls and patient safety and asks practitioners to create a new framework or foundation that now includes the application and utility of the new technology in establishing future safe fall-prevention practices. Here, existing EBP standards served as the floor (some would say, impetus) for good practice, and the emerging innovation created the challenge for the stretch away from existing practices that caused the need to reexamine and recalibrate evidence-based foundations to reflect the application of the emerging technology. While evidence provided the floor of good practice, innovation created the opportunity to stretch toward a new ceiling for good practice.

Where evidence demands grounding in the rigors of scientific process and analysis, innovation requires an environment that is open, responsive, reflective, challenging, and enabling (Bleich, 2014). The innovative practice leader needs to reflect on his or her skill set regarding the capacity to be responsive, discursive, flexible, and challenging. Both the discipline of evidence and the requisites of innovation push the leader to create an environment in which practitioners can fully experience their autonomy and represent it in patterns of practice that are themselves open, discerning, discursive, responsive, and collaborative, representing a sustainable culture of innovation and creativity. Indeed, the environment must be truly professional, representing a full engagement of the professional practice community in both defining the foundations of its practice (evidence) and exploring the rich possibilities of the future of practice (innovation). More often than not, organizations that have embraced shared governance and the Magnet Recognition Program have demonstrated the best partnership between organization and profession. The mutual commitment between healthcare organizations and healthcare professionals to affirm the foundations of good practice (evidence) and advance the interests of excellence and creativity (innovation) serves as the best frame for sustainable positive impact on the patient healthcare experience.

None of these dynamics or practices can be sustained, however, without an appropriate context and infrastructure that provides the medium for ensuring fluid and meaningful movement along the evidence–innovation continuum. Just as shared governance ensures autonomy in professional practice and creates a structure that advances the ownership of each professional in his or her own practice and in the obligations of the profession, the evidence and innovation relationship needs good structure to support it (A. Brown, 2014). As in all human activity, there is an overarching need for a strong interface between structures that create the vessel supporting action and a process discipline that provides a rigorous yet progressive vehicle for advancing practice, adapting to change, and creating the new and different. This model further provides the essential interface between evidence and innovation that accurately enumerates the action of each and the contribution of both to advancing good practice and to improving the nation's health care.

▶ The Cybernetic Model for Evidence and Innovation

A model that is cybernetic demonstrates an approach to systems analysis that describes its elements, characteristics, and relationships within a closed loop structure that continually feeds back upon itself (Paul, Muller, Preiser, Neto, & Marwala, 2014). These cybernetic structures are dynamic and in continuous movement, wherein the relationship among each and all of its constituents is continuously interacting. This dance of interaction describes the life of the system and shows how that system functions and interacts in a way that creates meaningful emerging and growing change. This same cybernetic infrastructure operates in the relationship between evidence and innovation, demonstrating their inherent interface and the part each plays individually and with the other in a way that advances and changes practice.

DISCUSSION

Value-driven practice has created a catalyst for fundamental changes in practice transformations. The convergence of sociopolitical, technological, and economic forces evidencing the need for service change in the U.S. healthcare system created the conditions that make existing approaches to care decreasingly relevant or useful. As a result, healthcare leadership has been stimulated by the demands for deconstructing a volume-based approach and creating a value-based system. Embedded inside the demand for change is the need for the inclusion of new healthcare databased infrastructure, technologies, delivery models, metrics, and person-centered clinical approaches. All these emerging demands and opportunities have forever and radically shifted the foundations for building the sustainability of health care.

In these circumstances, how does value-based health care act as a catalyst for shifting your own organizational and clinical foundations toward new service structures and clinical practices? How did the architecture of your clinical practice change to meet the demands of the more person-centered and mobility-based care delivery system? What personal impact has the catalyst for advancing the health of the nation had on your own practice and service delivery?

Gather a team of four to seven colleagues and explore the following questions:

- What are the short-term and immediate shifts in clinical practice that must occur now as the foundations for evidence-driven and value-based future service changes?
- What kind of clinical partnerships will need to emerge to address a more integrated and value-driven model of clinical service for episodes of care, populations, and the continuum of care?
- How do you communicate the demands for changes in clinical practice and the need for innovating approaches to health service delivery to colleagues and clinical partners in a way that helps them engage the requisites of a truly value-grounded, patient-centered health system?

Context describes the frame within which all action and change occur in a cybernetic process. Although the process is a closed-loop dynamic, it occurs within a larger environment in which the forces that create the conditions for change are in constant flux. This vortex of continuous, cyclical, and dynamic interaction at the environmental level creates the landscape within which organizational and individual action unfold. In human dynamics, there is a constant interface between sociopolitical, technological, and economic forces that are interchangeably congruent and discordant and create the conditions within which the agents of change operate (Porter-O'Grady & Malloch, 2010). At times in this complex environment, these sociopolitical, technological, and economic forces converge to create conditions that require a concerted response and force communities and individuals to address their impact and give substance to their actions. This is no less true in the relationship between evidentiary dynamics and innovation. Here, as at any point of convergence in response to the environment, the aggregation of the evidence provides a critical demand for change and transformation in the structures, processes, and impact of human activity. In health care this means that the complex dance among health system, provider, and user (including individuals, populations, communities, and society as a whole) requires a constant awareness of the impact of these broad environmental forces that are particular and specific in order to grow, improve, and advance change—in short, to innovate (Schartinger, Miles, Saritas, Amanatidou, & Giesecke, 2015).

▶ The Cybernetic Process and Risk as Fuel for Evidence and Innovation

Much of the energy fueling EBP comes out of the significant knowledge deficit and wide variability in clinical practices in nursing and other healthcare professions. This wide variability creates a high degree of risk. Further, variability implies a wide latitude of permissible behavior that fails to reflect and demonstrate already well-defined parameters for safe and appropriate practice in a wide variety of clinical settings. This variability is perhaps one of the most concerning in dangerous aspects of nondefinitive care practices that result in high patient risk every year.

These gaps in professional practice create not only a high degree of risk, but also questions with regard to exactly what practices are appropriate, meaningful, and viable. The assumption is that we know little about which particular foundations produce or influence specific outcomes. The truth is, however, that we know much more about these relationships than is often evidenced in the wide variety of practice settings across the nation. This lack of a uniform, disciplined, and aligned set of foundations for practice that are clearly and specifically enumerated across institutions and environments is not only a great threat to effective health care but also provides a great opportunity for healthcare leaders (Kaplan, Witkowski, Abbot, Guzman, & Higgins, 2014).

The development of an organized and systematic approach to managing knowledge is a critical effort to actually successfully handling it (Swapna, 2017). Knowledge regeneration and application approaches require a comprehensive framework that can be used regularly and stands the test of time. Not only that, the model or approach must be able to adapt to the continuing influences that unfold in the environmental, developmental, strategic, tactical, and priority-setting activities of systems and people today, especially in this digital, value-driven age. There is a fundamental demand to ensure that there is a strong cause-and-effect relationship between action and consequences. The value equation requires that there be a meaningful relationship between the actions undertaken and the impact desired. This critical relationship defines the constant focus and activity of clinical leadership as the leaders begin to unfold, first, foundations that ensure a set of solid principles that ground clinical action and, second, the capacity to change practice as quickly as the evidence indicates a need for change.

Because of the activities that must be centered at the point of service, organizational support structures and activities that enable this point-of-service locus of control must be designed in a way that ensures that practice is nimble, fluid, and flexible. Ownership of the obligations of practice must be deeply embedded in the practitioners. This ownership must be evidenced by their capacity to make decisions, take action, evaluate impact, and change actions quickly to accommodate the need for accuracy and relevance. The further away from the point of service the decisions related to these activities are made, the slower the response time, the greater the opportunity for error, and the less likely that the response will be accurate and appropriate (Cristofoli, Markovic, & Meneguzzo, 2014).

In addition to the need for point-of-service-driven responses is the requirement for increasing the accuracy and veracity of clinical action and data. The more specific and detailed information is with regard to the appropriateness and viability of clinical activity, the more useful it is. The ability to assess metrics specifically and clearly is critical to determining their veracity and impact on the patient experience. Also, the clarity of specific actions help define in a uniform and precise way how those actions perform. Furthermore, as we become clear about the performance of specific clinical actions, we can also get a stronger sense of the interface of those individual actions with other related actions in a way that helps us assess the comprehensive impact of these interfaced and related actions. Keep in mind that from the patient's perspective, that interest is in impacts and outcomes on the patient experience. The patient is generally unaware of the particular and unique activities of any one discipline or provider. The patient is aware, however, of the impact of the collective action of all providers on his or her clinical experience. Therefore, it becomes critical that clear and specific clinical behavior enumerated by any one discipline be strongly correlated, linked, and integrated with activities of other providers in a way that demonstrates the comprehensive impact of the collateral and collective contribution of all providers. This is a fundamental characteristic of the cybernetic process. It is also a central element of good EBP management and demonstrates the essence of seamless patient-centered care (Davis, Mahanna, Joly, Zelek, & Riley, 2014).

In addition, any cybernetic evidence–innovation model requires that the intersections and relationships among components demonstrate a flow of effort that is progressive, reflects the value of each component in subsequent steps, and ultimately demonstrates the seamless interface between each component. This must occur in a way that creates a systematic approach to addressing knowledge creation, generation, application, evaluation, and adaptation. Furthermore, it is essential that the innovation process be applicable at any stage of the cybernetic process so that whatever variables or variances that require particular responses can be addressed in those places where action is necessary. Here again, the more specific and particular the application is in each phase, the more utility it demonstrates in addressing the particular issue at a given point in the cybernetic process. Such a cybernetic model must also have embedded in it the flexibility necessary to adjust and adapt timing, intervention, dramatic environmental shifts, or the products of evaluation in a way that moves to quick resolution and sustainable solutions. The cybernetic process must also be understood and have high utility at the point of service where practitioners of all kinds can use it, understand its application to their own practice, and tease out its mechanisms and use them as a vehicle for assessing and adjusting their own practices (Yolles, 2010). In short, the model must make sense and have a high degree of utility in the practice environment. At the same time, it must be relevant to the organization at large and useful at the senior levels of the organization where environment and system meet, providing an opportunity for the system to make the same kind of adjustments that are expected to be seen in practice decisions at the point of service.

▶ Cybernetic Evidence and Innovation Model

Models serve as a composition of integrated and interacting concepts and elements. The use of models helps both capture and encapsulate whole notions that are comprised of particular elements, components, and phases. A cybernetic model demonstrates the action of the integration and interface among elements and components of the model, how they relate and interact, and how they feed back upon themselves to contribute to the dynamic (cybernetic) nature of the model. This modeling lends itself well to the evidence–innovation continuum insofar as it enumerates their essential relationship, the characteristics that lend utility to processes and applications of EBP, and the innovation enterprise.

In the case of the evidence–innovation cybernetic model, the forces driving human activity—enterprise, social, political, and economic—create the contextual framework for all the activities influenced by and responsive to those environmental forces. These forces can be seen as a series of continuous winds that blow out of the broad contextual environment that influences human action and creates forces that require a specific response in a particular way, as evidenced in human action and continuous change. The degree of effectiveness of the action and change is directly related to the goodness of fit between the character of the forces (our so-called winds) and the impact of the action. This impact is visualized positively by resulting enhancement, improvement, change, or innovation. Because these winds are constantly blowing and carrying with them the seeds of change and adjustment that is generated out of immediate past and current creative thinking, ideation, formation, or production, they constantly influence knowledge creation and generation, which then initiates the cybernetic cascade through a system. In the case of evidence and innovation, cybernetic cascade begins with knowledge creation, research, and generation, and influences and informs practice, and advances particular expertise. This movement then forms and deepens clinical insights and values, which drives the creation of a strong culture. In the case of health care, it influences service and care, and provides the framework for clinical action, which ultimately creates an impact, outcome, or particular change.

Because this process is cybernetic all along the way, incomplete and unformed notions and actions demonstrate gaps in knowledge creation, generation, and application and require a response if negative results are to be minimized or avoided. Each of these gaps provide the engine for innovation out of which comes new ideas, processes, applications, and products that, when created, enhance, advance, or transform both process and product. And because this dynamic is cybernetic, it continues to feed back upon itself, unceasingly informing and advancing both knowledge and action (**FIGURE 5-3**) (Porter-O'Grady & Malloch, 2014).

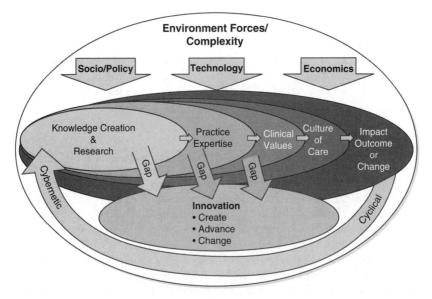

FIGURE 5-3 Cybernetic interface of innovation and evidence.

▶ Knowledge Creation and Research

Structure

Healthcare organizations, to be relevant, are in the knowledge management business. In patient care, it is critical that the most relevant and often most recent technologies, models, and mechanisms for delivering patient services be utilized to compete and thrive in the healthcare arena. Knowledge is therefore one of the central critical tools that is essential to the organization's work. The many types of professionals that work in concert related to any particular patient process depend both on their own capacity to generate and use contemporary clinical knowledge and the commitment of other disciplines to do the same. This mutual expectation with regard to knowledge currency, appropriateness, and viability is a critical assumption upon which the disciplines depend to successfully do their own work. Physicians assume that nurses are utilizing the most recent and relevant skills in caring for their patients in a way that facilitates clinical outcomes and positive impact. Nurses, on the other hand, expect that physicians, social workers, physical therapists, and other professionals are utilizing their own contemporary best practices in their roles to advance patient interests and ensure positive outcomes (De Bruijne, 2010).

The truth, however, lies somewhere short of the assumptions made by each discipline regarding its own practice and the practice of others. The precision associated with a tight fit between evidence-grounded best practices and the actual practices of professions does not necessarily demonstrate a strong cause–effect relationship between knowledge and practice. Questions are raised with regard to whether a large segment of practices are based essentially on assumptions, rituals, routines, or protocols that have simply stood the test of time but have never been rigorously validated through close examination that addresses viability and impact. The foundations of EBP over the past decade have raised the specter of how well structured this cause-and-effect relationship is embedded in the healthcare organization's expectations and in the normative practices of each of the disciplines.

Organizations and professions that are committed to relevance and viability recognize that embedded in the structure of the organization and its relationship to the professions must be a framework that makes knowledge creation and management a normative part of the relevant work of the organization. Creative design around laying the foundations of managing the generation, utility, and application of viable knowledge calls the organization to engage its professional members in a way that requires each to commit to a formal process related to the evidence-grounded management of knowledge. Creativity and innovation are embedded in the design of such structures; evidence-based insights and practices are the products of the work undertaken in such a structure.

Increasingly, collaboration among the disciplines in a way that reflects value-based principles and commitment to the Triple Aims of meaningful service, health impact, and price effectiveness are vital in today's environment (Hansen, 2013). The focus of each discipline will be evidenced in the character of the relationship with partner disciplines; the clarity of their interdependence; the specificity of their clinical partnership; and the collaborative and coalescing impact on the high reliability, high viability related to patient outcomes. The historic compartmentalized, segmented, and vertically siloed insulation of the disciplines from each other is not a sustainable premise upon which a viable knowledge management system can be built.

Embedded inside the knowledge management system is the information infrastructure that allows the organization to use just-in-time and highly mobile mechanisms to change and adapt practices in a way that reflects emerging clinical research and new knowledge generation. Many of the associated issues with the management of new and emergent knowledge and its generation and utility, such as big data, electronic medical records, supportive shared governance structures, innovation and failure, and so forth, are related to knowledge that is generated from the innovation process. The relationship between the emergence of knowledge affecting relevant practice and the capacity of practitioners to access and translate that knowledge in a relatively short period of time demonstrates the organization's capacity to innovate. The ability of the practitioners to utilize and apply that knowledge in their own practices demonstrates their commitment to be continuously relevant, current, and evidence-based (Dalkir, 2013). Here again, evidence and innovation are both points of reference along the same continuum. The organization's innovation in this scenario is reflected by a well-defined and systematic knowledge management structure and also by functional flexibility and adaptability that stimulate practice change in the face of new evidence. Practice change in the ideal infrastructure can be made easily and fluidly when the emerging evidence suggests that change is appropriate. Gone from that structure should be the long-term, ineffective, and pedantic policy and procedure process. In its place should be an effective, linked, interoperative, and continuous information management infrastructure that informs clinical team members at the point of service about the products of evidence and research generated by continuous small testing, comparative practices, and intersystem measures of comparative effectiveness. Adapting these mechanisms as a way of doing business creates an effective and useful operating infrastructure that is responsive to innovation, grounded in evidence, and dynamic in application.

These emerging evidence-grounded innovations will require a new compact within and among health professions. The often rote addiction to past practices, rituals, and routines found frequently in the disciplines must give way to a more reflexive and adaptive model of clinical practice that reflects a basic understanding that change is a fundamental attribute of the work of these professions and that, when validated as viable and appropriate, is evident in the processes and applications associated with that work.

The role of innovation in the evidence–innovation continuum is evidenced by a continuously systematic flexibility and personal adaptability that is apparent when the evidence indicates that there is a need for a change in practice. The trajectory of innovation is always an improvement in practice, a relevant new practice, and the continuous and growing positive impact on individual and population health. While evidence-based methodology is the means to improve and advance practice, innovation is the driver that requires the organization to develop mechanisms and focused testing of evidence-grounded approaches; draw comparisons; build practices based on best practices; and participate in a comprehensive, systematic, multisite undertaking of comparative effectiveness analysis to establish strong population-associated best practices (Grant, Guthrie, Entwistle, & Williams, 2014).

Institutional structures and methodologies linking innovation and EBP demonstrate their commitment to effective knowledge management through strong information-based systems that support ongoing research and clinical data management (Quinn, Huckel-Schneider, Campbell, Seale, & Milat, 2014). Fluid and flexible mechanisms, which make information availability and utility a systems

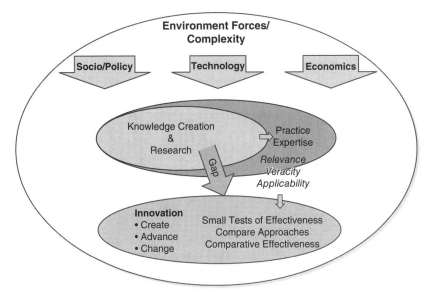

FIGURE 5-4 Environment forces/complexity.

characteristic for those delivering healthcare services, are critical components of effective patient care. Here again, evidentiary dynamics and methodologies are the means for ensuring best practices, and innovation is the medium that provides the enabling dynamic and impetus for continuously pushing the walls of currency in the organizations and the professions that continuously reach for practice excellence. The innovation framework in the organization stimulates the search for gaps between current practices and the potential for excellence. These gaps create the urge to analyze and examine current practices, products, and behaviors in the interests of refining, improving, or changing practice for advancing service excellence and health (**FIGURE 5-4**). It is out of these gaps that true innovation emerges, the results of which are to actually change or create new culture, practices, products, and behaviors.

▶ Practice Expertise: Translation to Impact

Evidence of viability and effectiveness is the constant driver for practice excellence. This continuous and dynamic journey is essentially a disciplined process that represents an intentional yet continuous march toward improvement, enhancement, and change (innovation). As previously indicated, practice change reflects the rigors of good knowledge management, research, and comparative effectiveness processes. At the same time, evidence-based dynamics also reflect the more relational interactional and experiential elements and characteristics embedded in the acts and interactions of practice. While the consistencies and rigors of the science of evidence are the essential platform upon which providers stand to make judgments regarding their practices, the relationships and interactions embedded in the dynamic of practice also provide relevant insights and information that positively or negatively affect the healthcare experience. Issues associated with the more subjective and relational aspects of health service driven by political, social, cultural, ethnic, regional, familial, and personal variables and vagaries strongly influence the viability and sustainability of health. Failure to incorporate these more collateral characteristics influencing the health service experience; quality metrics; and the social, emotional, and financial price of health care can clearly affect its positive viability and sustainability.

🔍 CASE EXAMPLE: INNOVATION AS THE CULTURE OF CARE

Ben Jones, RN, DNP, is a health system chief nursing officer (CNO). He recognized that, with all the changes that are unfolding in the health system while moving toward value-based care and accountable care models, many changes would have to occur in the structures and processes of nursing. He knew that many of the adaptations and changes in practice would have to be driven by clinical and management leadership very close to the point of service. His problem was that the organization has historically been very hierarchical and vertical, with a strong management-driven work environment. This clearly needed to change.

Ben realized that the significance of the change means that a shift in the culture would have to emanate from every place in the health system. He believed that nurses were positioned to provide leadership in making this cultural change because nursing is one of the central activities of the health system. He began to plan for systematically implementing a culture change that would support an environment of innovation throughout the nursing service.

Ben's first issues were as follows:

- Who do I need to include in the initial deliberation and design process to best strategize how we might affect the nursing culture?
- How would the nursing vision and mission need to change to give purpose and direction to the shift in the nursing culture of care?
- In a value-driven care model, patients and partners need to be at the table. How do we form this process so discussions and decisions are informed and competent?
- How do we avoid creating a department/office/center of innovation that is isolated and independent from the ownership of innovation at the point of service and engage the stakeholders?

The necessary elements for a structure of innovation are as follows:

- Ben realized, after detailed study, that some essential principles were needed to guide the leaders in their work of creating a culture that supports innovation. These principles include the following:
  - Wherever innovation occurs in a system, it must align with the system's environmental requirements and strategic priorities that guide and direct the innovation choices and actions anywhere in the system.
  - Successful innovation is never driven from the top of the system. Innovation is always generated from the work of the system and best engages stakeholders that are closest to the system's point of service.
- Formal structures must be developed for framing, informing, guiding, and rewarding innovation in a way that makes innovation a normative part of everyone's work and continually engages them.
  - Innovation is a discipline/process. Its various mechanics, stages, and phases can be defined and learned. A dynamic, available, and ongoing innovation

learning process must be incorporated into the development activities of the organization so that every stakeholder can access and understand the elements and applications of innovation.

- Recognition and reward are part of the lifeblood of innovation and must be structured into the dynamics of innovation. This critical element is utilized liberally to sustain energy, motivation, and commitment to innovation.
- Regular assessment and evaluation of the supported innovation mechanisms and processes in the organization help determine the viability of the innovation program, the effectiveness of innovation activities, the impact of innovation, and the required needs for adjustment or accommodation to accelerate the effectiveness of innovation.

Ben recognized that if the health systems innovation program is to be successful, particular themes must guide leadership to ensure that innovation is viable, effective, and sustainable:

- Innovation is tied to mission.
- Innovation must advance the success of the organization and the individual.
- Innovation is best directed from the point of service.
- Innovation requires recognition.
- Innovation is a team activity. No innovation is successful if unilaterally controlled.
- Innovation is a disciplined process and must be structured into the organization's way of doing business.
- Failure is a fundamental element of all innovation; it must be accepted, accommodated, and even celebrated.
- Innovation leaders must become comfortable with risk takers, brokers, contrarians, out-of-the-box thinkers, actors, and creative noise.
- A system of just-in-time communication, decision making, and movement accompanies the innovation process and requires an immediate response and quick turnaround from leaders and stakeholders.

Within the context of this practice framework, evidence-based dynamics support, indeed require, the inclusion of the collateral and collaborative mechanisms that generate insights, algorithms, and service approaches, experiences, and data that reflect evidence emanating from sociocultural contexts, population/group history and experience, collective wisdom, tradition, and regional practices (Sarkadi, Sampaio, Kelly, & Feldman, 2014). Keep in mind that the patient brings a set of beliefs and notions about health care, about him- or herself, and about his or her relationship to the world. This informs the patient's interaction with the healthcare system, health professionals, and family. All these elements combine to create a contextual framework for the patient that informs and guides his or her thinking and conversation with regard to personal health and his or her role and relationship with the healthcare system. Many of the concepts associated with this patient-centered dynamic create the frame for the relationship and interaction among the individual, the family, and health professionals. In addition, the patient brings past experiences related to personal health, his or her health journey, and the healthcare system. All these combine to create the conditions in which the patient and provider meet and operate under the rubric of the healthcare system. This complex array of interactions creates the frame within which all healthcare activities will unfold and guides the thinking, communication, and interaction among all these players (Damie, 2014).

For the care of professionals, evidence for practice expertise is a result of their own history, experiences, gained insights, shared wisdom, policies, and standards. Reliance on these factors is served as the backdrop to much of practice and has created a cultural overlay that values particular traditions, approaches, and practices that define the provider's role. As the social, political, and technological landscape change and produce a paradigm shift in a way that transforms these experiences within a new set of conditions, many of the traditions and established practices are challenged with regard to their relevance and viability. Still, they have stood the test of time, and dependence on them have provided some of the impetus and information that has ultimately generated new insights and emerging practices. This historical context creates another frame within which practice is defined, challenged, and changed and therefore must be valued. As it is valued, practice expertise and experience must be incorporated into the evidentiary dynamic as a part of lending insight, context, and wisdom to the host of other evidentiary factors driven by analysis, research, and data synthesis.

Experience too comes with its contribution to the gap between what we have done traditionally and what emerges out of the processes of knowledge management in EBP. Often the connection between practice experience and knowledge management creates the landscape for innovation. Additionally, the convergence or divergence between practice experience and knowledge management creates the catalyst for generating either validation or contest out of which will spawn emerging shifts in understanding and practice. The tension between what is known, what is experienced, and what is anticipated ensures that the evidentiary dynamic continually moves within the individual practitioner, resulting in the identification of gaps requiring the need for innovation. The elements of the patient's experience and insights, the provider's clinical practice experience, and the science associated with knowledge management each contribute to the other and collectively provide information that, when coalesced, leads to an understanding that enhances the patient experience, improves the quality of care, and affects the economics of service delivery (**FIGURE 5-5**).

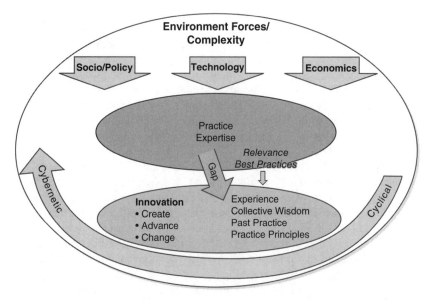

FIGURE 5-5 Cybernetic application of practice expertise.

▶ Individual, Personal, and Cultural Values and Practices

Health care is not provided in a sterile, scientific, evidentiary cocoon. Because health service is a human dynamic, it comes with individual, family, community, tribal, cultural, and societal beliefs, practices, and behaviors that have an equally significant impact on the healthcare dynamic, as do the clinical and scientific variables. These traditions are deeply embedded in faith, families, and cultures in a manner that often defines the fundamental characteristics of people in a way that influences who they are and what they do. Along with these characteristics come the personal attributes, tools, and processes they use for meeting the challenges, accommodations, and circumstances of their lives. All these devices are incorporated into health practices and influence personal and collective choices that ultimately influence individual and community health.

Many cultural beliefs and practices demonstrate some level of evidence about the impact on quality of life and health, but some do not. Yet all practices have some relevance to EBP when they are incorporated into the full range of understanding regarding persons and populations. Aggregating this information with more objective and data-driven sources of clinical evidence creates a composite frame of reference for the healthcare community that guides providers' partnership with the patient in a way that better informs both patient and provider about what is potentially viable and sustainable in relation to health.

Except for practices that are clearly dangerous or debilitating, evidence-based providers must accommodate in their data integration these personal and communal beliefs and cultural characteristics that more fully inform the caregiving community of all the circumstances that inform healthcare choice making in person-centered best practices. Insightful and culturally competent providers are aware of the synergy between culture and care and find ways to use tactical choices from both arenas in planning and executing the best care approaches. Out of this evidence-based foundation in the partnership among culture and care, personal practices, faith and belief, and healing processes emerge new and innovative paradigms. These new connections or insights, when added to the evidentiary foundations for care, may positively influence the creation of more effective models or approaches to advance health. Indeed, many of these culturally specific health practices may serve as the vehicle for gaining engagement and ownership for science-based, evidence-grounded clinical practices that may have otherwise been rejected if approached solely on their own merits (Napier, Ancarno, Butler, Calbrese, & Charter, 2014).

DISCUSSION

Many cultures provide alternative models or service supports as a part of their caring culture (e.g., doula, *promotora*, medicine man, shaman, *curandera*, etc.). As health care moves to more person-centered models and approaches, community, family, and culturally based healing and health support systems will become increasingly important. Partnerships among these various family and community health supports and formally trained health professionals will be critical to build a culture of health and healing.

(continues)

DISCUSSION *(continued)*

What kind of different thinking will help professionals bring to the interdisciplinary table other partners and health service delivery mechanisms? In what way is person-centered care different from patient-centered care, and what does it mean to providers? What is your organization doing to expand the inclusiveness of care partners, family, and community, and what is it doing to plan for continuum of care services?

In these circumstances the partnership between evidence and innovation becomes more definitive. Care providers and practitioners from the involved traditions now must meet on common ground to delineate and negotiate the most effective evidence-based choices that can be made within the vagaries and variables of a particular culture. The innovation arises out of this communion between the individual or community and the provider in ways that suggest unique negotiated approaches that both meet the cultural health norms of the user and incorporate the data-driven practices of the provider. This communication and interaction between person and provider demonstrate the best in both evidence and innovation. Evidence demands that both bring to the table a clear delineation of the impact of both culture and data and determine how each serves as a medium for the other in making effective health choices. Innovation, on the other hand, requires that the stakeholders deliberate and determine viable mechanisms or processes that link culture and care in a way that produces positive outcomes and advances personal and/or community health (**FIGURE 5-6**).

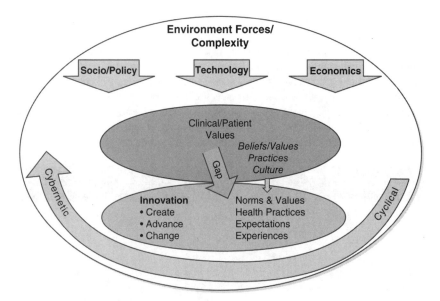

FIGURE 5-6 Cybernetic application of patient values.

▶ The Cultural Framework for Innovation and Care

Innovation is certainly more than the sum of its parts. In every system/organization, innovation occurs because there is both an environment and leadership that generate the context, conditions, and drive for innovation as a way of life (Rivenburgh, 2014). This context provides the vessel within which the vision and values of the system, opportunities for translating vision into action, and commitment of individuals at every level exists as a backdrop to the actions of innovation. Without a particularly definitive context that meets the fundamental criteria supporting innovation, the dynamics associated with innovation simply do not function. Although the contextual foundations are not complex, they are fundamental. When the foundations are not established, innovation is not possible.

Following are some of the critical cultural circumstances essential to providing the frame within which any innovation process is supported (**FIGURE 5-7**). Herein the relationship between evidence and innovation is affirmed, and the continuum that is necessary to sustain both is established and structured as a cultural requirement for each.

Creative Norms and Values

Leaders who are committed to establishing a strong relationship between evidence and innovation recognize that the organizational culture must demonstrate specific conditions that support innovation as the organization's way of doing business. This means that structure includes processes and mechanisms of shared rules in developing organizational strategies, models of shared decision making, locating the predominant locus of control for decisions and actions at the point of service. Additionally,

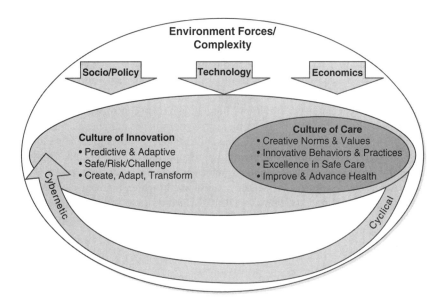

FIGURE 5-7 Culture of care within a culture of innovation.

shared rules support the creation of systems of reward for risk taking, out-of-the-box thinking, structural mechanisms that support innovation, and the legal and methodological components associated with the successful processes of innovation.

In addition, leaders recognize the inherent interaction between evidence and innovation, and recognize the indispensable organizational and leadership ingredients that support the associative thinking that links them. These associated mental processes demonstrate the capacity to determine the relationships and intersections among seemingly unrelated interactions, processes, and actions. The structures and culture of the organization and its leaders certify that innovation is embedded in evidence and is demonstrated by organizational members' capacity to merge past practices, protocols, and data generation (all sources of evidence) with different or challenging mental models, new modes of thinking and acting, and new insights and connections, all generated from the evidentiary platform and stimulated by the culture where expectations continually raise the bar (all elements of innovation).

Innovative Behaviors and Practices

Innovation takes life and form at the point of service where 90% of organizational life is experienced. Leaders in innovative organizations recognize that innovation is a collective enterprise, and no successful innovation was ever advanced through unilateral action (Yang, 2015). Culture supporting innovation must give way to behaviors and practices that demonstrate the processes and actions of innovation, ultimately leading to an innovative outcome. After the ground of evidence has been established and serves as the platform for subsequent action, innovative behaviors take precedence. The capacity of individuals to scan and give form to the changes generated out of the environment translate their impact on practice and process and recalibrate their definitive response in recognition of the need for a particular modification/adaptation that is essential to organizational sustainability. In a high-intensity environment and milieu of high-technological transformation, this innovative cultural overlay becomes an essential driver of organizational life at all levels (Marques, 2014).

Of increasing vital importance in this equation in health care is the role of the point-of-service provider. Here this translation from evidence to innovation is incorporated inside the clinical partnership between provider and patient and forms a good part of the substance of this relationship. Ultimately, viable and sustainable innovations must animate here because this is the predominant arena where health scripts are written and lived. Traditional models of vertical control and rigid hierarchical checks and rechecks along with managerial dominance must be realigned into a much stronger collateral, horizontal, and collaborative organizational calibration. Contemporary and mature operating models that promulgate a more adult setting of organizational membership, mutuality, engagement, and ownership, provide exemplars that demonstrate the essential context within which innovative behaviors and practices are stimulated (Nicoletti, 2015). Much of the content of this text includes a focus on the importance in the development of leadership in facilitating the dynamics of innovation.

Excellence and Care

The notion that EBP is demonstrated by rigid parameters, standardization rigidities, deterministic protocols, and judgment-eliminating routines is simply untrue. EBP is grounded in good science and methodology, validated clinical practices, and data-based practices. These characteristics provide the firm foundation that comprises the floor of good practice. In short, they establish the universal platform—measured, analyzed, synthesized, and clarified—upon which all providers stand. However, it is on this evidentiary foundation that the actions of innovation generate. From this place of clarity, the processes of innovation, discernment, creativity, insight, collective wisdom, and clinical practices moved to new heights. Again, evidence establishes the floor of clinical practice, and innovation reaches for its ceiling. Innovation efforts are not simply the act of trying something new; they are the practices and efforts that continually expand the foundational floor of practice and require the same research, diligence, refinement, and scrutiny that is afforded to the EBP process. This is how the discipline of innovation will affect care, practice, cost, outcomes, and organizational structure for better health.

Excellence and best practice are the goals of both evidence and innovation, yet they play different roles. While evidence validates the veracity of the foundations of practice, innovation challenges us on the trajectory toward excellence, obtained through transforming mental models, dialogue and discernment, creative design, and small yet transforming tests of change (Hildrum, 2014). Out of this partnership come new models and methodologies that advance health partnerships, practices, new approaches, and improved service and clinical outcomes. When linked, evidence and innovation provide the urge for improvement, transformation, and changes in structures and practices that advance the interests and conditions of health for people, populations, and society.

Improving People's Health

No activity in health care has meaning or value if it does not ultimately positively affect the health of those to which it is directed. All the methodologies, practices, and processes that exemplify high levels of service and care are pointless if there is no net aggregated positive impact evidenced in continuous evolving and improving levels of health. Evidence-based data suggest definitive, viable, and safe foundations for health; sustainable innovation suggests a continuous trajectory toward ever-increasing levels of excellence that advance health.

There is clearly a sufficient indication of the history of healthcare providers' addiction to trendy or catchy initiatives associated with notions of potential improvement in clinical processes or outcomes. If most of these notions actually demonstrated veracity in transforming sustainable improved outcomes, we would by now have seen a significant inverse trajectory in our contemporary quality–cost equation in U.S. health care. Not only is there a powerful need for a frank and unambiguous framework for health improvement, there is also a need to establish regional and national standards of practice measurement and payment that reflect the definitive data generated from sound EBP and well-validated service and care innovations in the U.S. healthcare system. Contemporary and prospective changes in the value-based effort at bundling care and payment around best practices for episodes of care, specific populations, and communities of care provide strong hope that the definitive and normative practices directed to improve and advance health can be more clearly established and their impact on advancing health more specifically demonstrated (Huang, 2015).

The emerging emphasis on creating networks of health service that will now operate across episodes, populations, and communities gets us all closer to the potential to truly improve and advance health. Besides connecting a particular array of health partners around specific episodes, populations, or communities of health service, the communication and interaction among them will help advance role clarity and the contribution to health care. Out of these communities of practice and health partnerships will come growing opportunities for using evidence-based methodologies and approaches to defining healthcare common ground and creating new opportunities for innovating relationships, interactions, processes, and the products of health care. There are most clearly gaps across the continuum of health that require innovation and evidence to close.

Culture and Sustainability

Leaders of evidence and innovation must realize that their predominant role is in creating a supportive culture and structure that sustains EBP and the processes of innovation. This means more than simply establishing continuous (some say, endless) initiatives that drive one or many elements of change. Over time, organizations and their people become weary of initiatives. The gimmicks and incentives necessary to generate sufficient interest become increasingly more extreme and ridiculous. Organizations, like all systems, are highly complex and dynamic structures in which the many agencies and forces converge to create the conditions and culture within which people work. The effective leader recognizes the necessity to create a synergy among all these agents whose converging effort is a central constituent of meaningful growth and change (Malaina, 2015). Driven by the organization's values and commitment to advancing health and accelerating the healthcare experience, a clinical leader ensures his or her own commitment to discipline-specific measures of excellence. These leaders also recognize a solid and generative interface between the actions of individual, discipline, and healthcare partners. This culture of personal and professional accountability, partnership, and shared obligation for health becomes the decisive framework for all choices and actions exercised by organizational members.

In evidence-grounded innovative organizations, the leadership capacity of alignment becomes an increasingly important skill as health systems recalibrate their structures and cultures inside a value-driven health service environment. The convergence necessary among all stakeholders provides a requisite for leaders to ensure that their roles, skills, capacities, relationships, and contributions reflect an alignment and synergy that, upon examination, have a specific and conclusive impact on the quality of health service and the net aggregate level of health. There are many activities that can be associated with improving advancing health service. For the leader, the issue is whether these individual sets of activities, when coalesced around patients and users, are integrated in a way in which the impact is substantive and clearly apparent in the positive results on health service and on a healthy community. If this develops into a healthcare way of life and the provider's way of doing business, it becomes the best evidence of the presence of an effective, supportive, and sustainable culture of care. Without the alignment and coordination of innovation activities, leaders risk further fragmentation, one-off solutions, and disconnected systems and practices that could have a negative impact on the organization and the care provided to individuals.

▶ Cybernetic Interface of Innovation and Evidence

Innovation is meaningless unless some change occurs. It is informed by purpose, which drives in the center of the innovation process and keeps the activities associated with it focused and directed. The innovation trajectory includes a series of stages that enumerate its various processes, all of which lead from idea to outcome. All innovation begins with the mechanics, metrics, and measures that provide the evidence that serves as the basis from which any innovation is generated.

Evidence and innovation reflect two ends of the same continuum. Grounded in solid metrics, research, culture, and practice, evidence provides the rationale and reason supporting the foundations that indicate the appropriateness associated with the potential trajectory toward innovation represented in any transformation, change, or new product. Elements of the cybernetic process operate across all of its components from knowledge creation; practice expertise; clinical values; culture of care; and impact, outcome, or change. The dynamic is always creative and reflects a cause-and-effect relationship demonstrated by a forward advance and resulting in some meaningful and viable change.

Driving each stage of the continuum is a relentless and faithful execution of all the components of the trajectory from vision and values, culture, leadership, data and evidence, process movement and measurement, and finally to the innovation, either for a new product or a transformation. Because the dynamic is continuous and cybernetic, the outcome or product reactivates the knowledge process and the metrics and measurements associated with evaluation of effectiveness and the impetus for the very next thing (Nan, Zmud, & Yetgin, 2014).

As the cybernetic cycle reengages the knowledge creation and generation phase, it further stimulates the organization to look at its own characteristics and culture to demand further assessment of the synergy among its culture, its processes, and its impact on transforming health or producing better means for doing so. This assessment is multilateral and multilayered—multilateral insofar as it involves all agents, components, relationships, structures, and functions in the organization at each level of operation, and multilayered because evaluation addresses decisions and directions from governance to the point of service, measuring their effectiveness and synergy at every intersection and interaction in the organization (**FIGURE 5-8**).

It is at this stage that the entire dynamic is viewed as an integrated whole. Questions related to the efficacy of each of the components in the synergy of all of them is a part of the evidence–innovation continuum and the tools and processes that move the system seamlessly among them. Here questions are related to the effectiveness of the cybernetic process and help drive evaluation of its utility and value:

1. Does the trajectory of the organization tightly reflect the demands and characteristics of the environment within which it exists and thrives?
2. Are the strategic priorities for health consistent with the needs and demands of the community the organization serves, and does it advance its level of health?
3. Is the culture and the character of the organization designed and supported in a way that encourages point-of-service ownership of decisions, actions, evaluation grounded in EBP, and driving innovation?

FIGURE 5-8 Cybernetic integration of innovation and evidence.

4. Do the organization and its providers demonstrate a high degree of partnership with patients, users, populations, and the community in advancing the health of all?
5. Are the values, beliefs, and cultural characteristics of patients and communities incorporated into health relationships and the practices of providers and their partners?
6. Is the health system faithful to its proven and validated evidence-based disciplines and processes, and can it demonstrate improvement and advancement of health as the product of its work?
7. Is the health of the community improving, and can the health system demonstrate a direct relationship between its own evidence-based practices and innovation?

▶ The Key: Leadership

Most leaders are disappointed by their capacity to stimulate and sustain long-term innovation. McKinsey and Company, in a survey of senior executives, found that 65% of them were disappointed in their capacity to stimulate real and sustainable innovation (Barsh, 2008). Although innovation has its unique characteristics, it is still a fundamentally human activity. To understand how to succeed in innovation, leaders need to know what it takes to create a solidly evidence-grounded, successful innovation process.

Innovation, like EBP, is essentially a discipline. It has elements and components, phases and stages, and processes and activities, and it is continually evaluated and adapted to reflect constantly changing realities. Through explication of the cybernetic interface of evidence and innovation model in this chapter, we have specifically pointed out how systematic and cyclical the continuum of evidence and innovation truly is. We also clearly indicated that if it is to be successful, leaders have to create and support a particular culture that is unique to the dynamics of innovation and requires particular leadership skill sets (Mockhber, Wan, & Vakilbashi, 2015).

A priority for leadership should be the understanding that evidence and innovation must be a structured, strategic priority for the organization. It must be an organizational way of life—a framework for the way it does business. Evidence and innovation depend on structuring the elements and components of the continuum between slices of the cybernetic model discussed in this chapter. Organizing and structuring the strategic activities of the board from environmental scanning to priority setting should be undertaken in a way that reflects the engagement of all stakeholders, from the boardroom to the patient experience. This high degree of inclusion with the right stakeholders signifies that senior leadership has the capacity to set a diverse table around which key stakeholders engage with each other in the processes associated with laying the foundations (evidence) and pushing the walls to create the future (innovation).

After the strategic framework is constructed in the organization, senior leaders must actively create the structures and processes that find and support the often untapped innovation resources at every level of the health system. These creators and innovators, when enabled, act as catalysts for others in the organization and help create a milieu where evidence, creativity, and innovation become a normative operating process. By stimulating the culture of innovation, and facilitating innovators and innovative action, leaders begin to create networks that develop around specific innovations and interface with other created agents generating communities of EBP and innovation that, when linked, exemplify a dynamic, engaged, creative milieu.

When the groundwork is laid for creating a culture of dynamic growth and development, evidentiary foundations, and creativity and innovation, a demand for high levels of trust in the organization emerge. People cannot risk, experiment, or stretch in an environment where they do not feel secure or embraced. Creativity and laying the groundwork for evidence and for advancing the elements of innovation is a noisy generative process filled with uncertainties, experimentation, and risk. Engagement in any of these activities will be limited to the extent that there is a sense of comfort and trust that the organization is a safe place for extending oneself and that leadership will support the related necessary innovative behaviors and practices. In this kind of environment, members of the organization feel that their efforts are valued, that the system is structured to support the generation and development of those ideas, and that there will be concerted and collective support throughout the cybernetic and dynamic continuum between evidence and innovation (Zia & Khan, 2014).

Ultimately, the commitment to evidence and innovation is demonstrated in how the leader embeds the dynamics associated with EBP and innovation practices in all the ways in which the organization works. The question for leadership is: How are the characteristics and elements associated with evidence and innovation embedded in board meetings, the senior staff priority setting, regular operational meetings, clinical standards and practices, discipline-specific and interdisciplinary meetings, deliberations, councils, point-of-service models of care, interdisciplinary interactions, and so forth? How do the new models of value-driven transdisciplinary and patient-centered health service delivery demonstrate the ownership and engagement of key creative stakeholders at the point of service? And finally, in truly innovative organizations: How do structures and infrastructure continually support a culture where the engagement of evidence and innovation is the prevailing organizational frame of reference? The expectation of every member in the organization is that he or she is a part of a continuous innovation dynamic, grounded in evidence and encouraged to continually stretch toward excellence. The ascending determinant of success in all of this will be found in how the health system's basis in evidence and reach for innovation and excellence result in enhancing the patient experience and advancing the health of the community. Without having done that, none of this will matter.

References

Aarons, G., Ehrhart, M., Farahnak, L., & Hurlburt, M. (2015). Leadership and organizational change for implementation: A randomized mixed method pilot study of leadership and organization development intervention for evidence-based practice implementation. *Implementation Science: IS, 10*(11), 1–12.

Barsh, J. (2008, January). Leadership and innovation. *McKinsey Quarterly*, 1–6.

Belar, C. (2014). Transformation through relationships. *Creative Nursing, 20*(2), 75–81.

Bleich, M. (2014). Developing leaders and systems thinkers. *The Journal of Continuing Education in Nursing, 45*(4), 158–159.

Brown, A. (2014). Organizational paradigms and sustainability in excellence: From mechanistic approaches to learning and innovation. *International Journal of Quality and Service Sciences, 6*(2), 181–190.

Brown, C. (2014). The Iowa model of evidence-based practice to promote quality care: An illustrated example in oncology nursing. *Clinical Journal of Oncology Nursing, 18*(2), 157–159.

Centers for Disease Control and Prevention (CDC). (2016). STEADI—Older adult fall prevention. Retrieved from https://www.cdc.gov/steadi/about.html

Clavelle, J., Porter O'Grady, T., Weston, M., & Verran, J. (2016). Evolution of structural empowerment: Moving from shared to professional governance. *Journal of Nursing Administration, 46*(6), 308–312.

Costich, J., Scutchfield, F., & Ingram, R. (2015). Population health, public health, and accountable care: Emerging roles and relationships. *American Journal of Public Health, 105*(5), 846–850.

Cristofoli, D., Markovic, J., & Meneguzzo, M. (2014). Governance, management and performance in public networks: How to be successful in shared governance networks. *Journal of Management & Governance, 18*(1), 77–93.

Dalkir, K. (2013). *Knowledge management in theory and practice.* St. Louis, MO: Elsevier.

Damie, N. (2014). Commentary by the American College of Physicians on the "Joint Principles: Integrating behavioral health care into the patient-centered medical home." *Families, Systems & Health: The Journal of Collaborative Family Healthcare, 32*(2), 151–152.

Davidson, S., Weberg, D., Porter-O'Grady, T., & Malloch, K. (2017). *Evidence-based innovation in nursing and health professions.* Cambridge, MA: Jones & Bartlett Learning.

Davis, M. M., Mahanna, E., Joly, B., Zelek, M., & Riley, W. (2014). Creating quality improvement culture in public health agencies. *American Journal of Public Health, 104*(1), 98–104.

De Bruijne, M. (2010). *Managing professionals.* London, UK: Routledge.

Grady, C. M. (2016). Can complexity science inform physician leadership development? *Leadership in Health Services, 29*(3), 251–263. http://dx.doi.org/10.1108/LHS-12-2015-0042

Grant, S., Guthrie, B., Entwistle, V., & Williams, B. (2014). In meta-ethnography of organizational culture in primary care medical practice. *Journal of Health Organization and Management, 28*(1), 21–40.

Grimmer, K., Dizon, J., Milanese, S., King, E., & Beaton, K. (2014). Efficient clinical evaluation of guideline quality: Development and testing of a new tool. *BMC Medical Research Methodology, 14*(63), 2–10.

Hansen, M. (2013). *Collaboration: How leaders avoid the traps, create unity, and reap results.* Boston, MA: Harvard Business School Press.

Hildrum, J. (2014). Turning stone into gold and silver into stone: On the importance of studying innovation. *The Innovation Journal, 19*(2), 1–5.

Hofbaur, M., Murawski, C., Karlsson, J., & Freddie, H. (2013). Innovation in orthopedic surgery as it relates to evidence-based practice. *Kneecap Surgery, Sports Traumatology, Arthroscopy, 21*(3), 511–515.

Huang, J. (2015). Bundled payment and enhanced recovery after surgery. *The Journal of Medical Practice Management: MPM, 30*(5), 349–353.

Ikhwanuliman, P. (2017). Redefining health: Implication for value-based healthcare reform. *Cureus, 9*(3), 1067–1078.

Kaplan, R., Witkowski, M., Abbot, M., Guzman, A., & Higgins, L. (2014). Using time-driven activity-based costing to identify value improvement opportunities in healthcare. *Journal of Healthcare Management, 59*(6), 399–413.

Kluever, A. (2015). *Dynamic systems: Modeling, simulation, and control.* New York, NY: John Wiley & Sons.

Lubejko, B. (2014). Improving the evidence base of nursing education programs. *The Journal of Continuing Education in Nursing, 45*(8), 336–343.

Magnavita, J. J., & American Psychological Association. (2016). *Clinical decision making in mental health practice* (rev. ed.). Washington, DC: American Psychological Association.

Malaina, A. (2015). Two complexities: The need to link complex thinking and complex adaptive systems science. *Emergence: Complexity and Organization, 17*(1), 1–9.

Malloch, K., & Porter-O'Grady, T. (2010). *Introduction to evidence-based practice in nursing and health care* (2nd ed.). Sudbury, MA: Jones & Bartlett Learning.

Marques, J. (2014). Closed versus open innovation: Evolution or combination? *International Journal of Business and Management, 9*(3), 196–203.

McNelis, A. M., Ironside, P. M., Zvonar, S., & Ebright, P. (2014). Advancing the science of research in nursing education: Contributions of the critical decision method. *Journal of Nursing Education, 53*(2), 61–64.

Melnyck, B., & Overholt, E. (2019). *Evidence-based practice in nursing and healthcare: A guide to best practice* (4th ed.). New York, NY: Wolters Kluwer.

Merry, A. F., & Hamblin, R. (2012). More for less: Best patient outcomes in a time of financial restraint. *Journal of ExtraCorporeal Technology, 44*(4), 178–185.

Mockhber, M., Wan, K. T., & Vakilbashi, A. (2015). Effect of transformational leadership and its components on organizational innovation. *Journal of Management Studies, 8*(2), 221–241.

Morrar, R. (2014). Innovation and services: A literature review. *Technology Innovation Management Review, 4*(4), 6–14.

Nan, N., Zmud, R., & Yetgin, E. (2014). A complex adaptive systems perspective of innovation diffusion: An integrated theory and validated virtual laboratory. *Computational and Mathematical Organization Theory, 20*(1), 52–56.

Nandan, M., & Scott, P. (2014). Interprofessional practice and education: Holistic approaches to complex healthcare challenges. *Journal of Allied Health, 43*(3), 150–156.

Napier, A., Ancarno, C., Butler, B., Calbrese, J., & Charter, A. (2014). Culture and health. *The Lancet, 384*, 1607–1639.

Nicoletti, B. (2015). Optimizing innovation with the lean and digitized innovation process. *Technology Innovation Management Review, 5*(3), 29–38.

Olson, K., Young, R. A., & Schultz, I. Z. (2016). *Handbook of qualitative health research for evidence-based practice.* New York, NY: Springer.

Paul, S., Muller, H., Preiser, R., Neto, F., & Marwala, T. (2014). Developing a management decision-making model based on a complexity perspective with reference to the Bee Algorithm. *Emergence: Complexity and Organization, 16*(4), 1–13.

Pickering, A. (2014). Cybernetic futures. *Technology and Culture Innovation Management Review, 55*(1), 245–248.

Pilon, B. (2015). Evidence-based development nurse led interprofessional teams. *Nursing Management, 22*(3), 35–40.

Porter-O'Grady, T., & Malloch, K. (2010). Partnership economics: Creating value through evidence-based workload management. In T. Porter-O'Grady & K. Malloch (Eds.), *Introduction to evidence-based practice in nursing and healthcare* (2nd ed., pp. 181–220). Cambridge, MA. Jones & Bartlett.

Porter-O'Grady, T., & Malloch, K. (Eds.). (2014). *Creating and sustaining a culture and an environment for evidence-based practice* (Vol. 3, 3rd ed.). New York, NY: Wolters Kluwer.

Porter-O'Grady, T., & Malloch, K. (2015). *Quantum leadership: Building better partnerships for sustainable health* (4th ed.). Burlington, MA: Jones & Bartlett Learning.

Prescott, D. S., Maeschalck, C. L., Miller, S. D., & American Psychological Association. (2017). *Feedback-informed treatment in clinical practice: Reaching for excellence* (rev. ed.). Washington, DC: American Psychological Association.

Quinn, E., Huckel-Schneider, C., Campbell, D., Seale, H., & Milat, A. (2014). How can knowledge exchange portals assist in knowledge management for evidence-informed decision-making in public health? *BMC Public Health, 14*, 443–444.

Rivenburgh, D. (2014). Creating a vibrant, thriving, responsible culture. *The Journal for Quality and Participation, 37*(1), 4–9.

Rook, L. (2013). Mental models, a robust definition. *The Learning Organization, 20*(1), 38–47.

Sarkadi, A., Sampaio, F., Kelly, M., & Feldman, I. (2014). A novel approach using outcome distribution curves to estimate the population level impact of the public health intervention. *Journal of Clinical Epidemiology, 67*(7), 785–792.

Schartinger, D., Miles, I., Saritas, O., Amanatidou, E., & Giesecke, S. (2015). Personal health systems technologies: Critical issues in service innovation and diffusion. *Technology Innovation Management Review, 5*(2), 46–57.

Schmidt, N. A., & Brown, J. M. (2015). *Evidence-based practice for nurses: Appraisal and application of research* (3rd ed.). Burlington, MA: Jones & Bartlett Learning.

Shaw, F., Asomugha, C., Conway, P. H., & Rain, A. (2014). The Patient Protection and Affordable Care Act: Opportunities for prevention and public health. *The Lancet, 384*(9937), 75–82.

Sheikh, K., George, A., & Gilson, L. (2014). People-centered science: Strengthening the practice of health policy and systems research. *Health Research Policy and Systems, 12*(1), 19–20.

Simpao, A., Ahumada, L., Galvaz, J., & Rehman, M. (2014). A review of analytics and clinical information in health care. *Journal of Medical Systems, 38*(4), 45–51.

Spencer, T., Detrich, R., & Slocum, T. (2012). Evidence-based practice: A framework for making effective decisions. *Education and Treatment of Children, 35*(2), 127–151.

Starck, P., & Rooney, L. (2015). Leadership for the integration of comprehensive care and interprofessional collaboration. *Clinical Scholars Review, 8*(1), 43–48.

Swapna, J. (2017). *Transitioning from fee-for-service to valuability.* (Master of Science). Utica College, Utica, NY.

Weberg, D. (2013). *Complexity leadership theory and innovation: A new framework for innovation leadership* (PhD Doctoral). Arizona State University, Phoenix, AZ.

Wills, M. (2013). Decisions through data: Analytics in healthcare. *Journal of Healthcare Management, 54*(4), 254–256.

Yang, U. (2015). Role of task characteristics in the relationship between technological innovation and project success. *International Journal of Innovation, Management and Technology, 6*(2), 100–104.

Yolles, M. (2010). *Organizations as complex systems: An introduction to knowledge cybernetics (managing the complex).* Charlotte, NC: Information Age.

Zia, Y., & Khan, M. (2014). Organizational trust: A cultural perspective. *The Journal of Humanities and Social Sciences, 22*(2), 127–134.

Exemplars of the Cybernetic Integration of Evidence and Innovation

C apstone projects from the doctor of nursing practice (DNP) are exemplars of this model as the DNP project focuses on the translation of current evidence into practice venues in new and innovative ways. DNP students systematically formulate a well-developed question based on a clinical problem or issue, review the literature to identify available evidence-based resources, assess the validity of the resources, identify the gap in evidence resources, and develop a plan to apply existing evidence to a new population to advance the evidence and close the evidentiary gap.

▶ Exemplar 1

In this project, the DNP student identified a gap in staff nurse knowledge about professional governance (Clavelle, Porter O'Grady, Weston, & Verran, 2016). The purpose of this project was to determine if the newly developed and published professional governance model could be used to increase nurse engagement in the ownership and management of the electronic health record (EHR) and increase nurse satisfaction with the electronic record. The DNP student educated and coached nurses about professional governance and reinforced the importance of nursing professional obligation, accountability, decision making, and relationships. After 3 months, the DNP student found positive statistical significance between pre- and post-surveys of nurse satisfaction. These results aligned with the literature, which supports the positive impact of professional leadership on nursing satisfaction and nurses' desire to participate in the design and sustainability of the EHR and close the gap between knowledge and practice related to professional behaviors.

▶ Exemplar 2

In this exemplar, the DNP student identified a lack of practice related to fall protocols for outpatient cancer patients. In particular, fall protocols are not routinely used in ambulatory settings, and the student identified an opportunity to close the gap and use an established national protocol in a unique way in a multidisciplinary oncology ambulatory center. The DNP student put the Centers for Disease Control and

Prevention (CDC, 2016) Stopping Elderly Accidents, Deaths and Injuries (STEADI) materials to music in a video with staff from the oncology clinic. The video is now used for staff and patient education. The STEADI protocol consists of three questions to identify individuals with balance challenges and refers those individuals to physical therapy and also provides education support for families. To date, an increase of 20% at-risk individuals have been identified. The gap in practice application of evidence is closing slowly.

CHAPTER 6

Assessing Your Innovation and Evidence Capacity: Essentials for Organizational Infrastructures

Kathy Malloch and Tim Porter-O'Grady

Life is not about waiting for the storms to pass . . . it is about learning how to dance in the rain.

— **Unknown**

© Everything Possible/Shutterstock

▶ Introduction

The passage of time necessarily brings new ideas, new people, and new expectations for all of us and, in particular, for the work we do in health care. Figuring out what to do to be relevant within a context that moves rapidly and with a mix of digital and manual processes can be overwhelming. What is important in this figuring out process is for each of us to reflect on where we are and where we can now move to as leaders in creating the conditions for the ultimate integration of high levels of evidence and innovative processes.

In this chapter, we discuss the current state of leadership, an overview of the driving forces for changing to higher levels of innovation, the impact of the Internet, new approaches that integrate the evidence–innovation dynamic, and behaviors to transform to the desired organizational infrastructure, with an emphasis on professional accountability. In particular, emphasis is laid on the importance of a dynamic organizational infrastructure that includes defined processes and authority designations, and this is also aligned with desired behaviors to optimize value.

▶ Historical State of Organizational Leadership: Sans Evidence

Historically, there has been a lack of evidentiary thinking and working in organizations. In the past decade, however, much has been made of the high level of judgment and assumptions-based clinical practices that characterize all of the healthcare disciplines (Freshwater & Rolfe, 2004). The attempt to build evidence-based practice has raised a number of significant concerns regarding the foundations of clinical practitioners' judgment (McNamara, 2002). The evidence indicates that much weight has been applied to past practices, individual experiences, and traditional foundations of learning used in the formation of the body of knowledge upon which most practitioners base their own clinical judgments and actions (Smith, 2004). This foundation for behavior is quite unstable and unreliable—the inadequacies inherent in the dependence on past practice and individual assumptions cannot be understated (McSherry, Simmons, & Abbott, 2002). Even so, for most practitioners, in contemporary clinical situations, the past remains the foundation of the vast majority of practice decisions and actions in the present.

This reality of uninformed and evidence-lacking decision making and action, which is readily apparent in clinical practice, is only extended and broadened when we consider leadership and management practices in health care. Indeed, much of management practice is based on an unbounded and wide variation of myth, whim, fancy, fad, and fashion (Malloch & Porter-O'Grady, 1999; Tourish & Hargie, 2004). In no area of human endeavor are there as many nonvalidated assumptions of practice and the management of human behavior as in the arena of management and leadership (Albrecht, 2003). Almost weekly, self-proclaimed management gurus announce new insights regarding leadership and management practice based solely on the expression of their own thinking and fantasy regarding what works and does not work in the leadership of people and organizations. Management and leadership are most bereft of any continuous aggregated and related body of knowledge that would in any way validate the foundations upon which many of the practices of leadership and management are based (Drucker, 2001; Drucker & Stone, 1998; Mintzberg, 1990).

Contemporary notions of accountability would require the resolution of such a difficulty. Yet new tomes appear weekly on the bookshelves attesting to emerging personal insights with regard to judgments of what makes effective leaders and what produces sustainable outcomes in business and service. At the same time, broad-based evidence of the lack of accountability and ownership with regard to personal decisions and actions in almost every arena is rife both in the United States and on the global stage, demonstrating the paucity of real and effective leadership. This lack of accountability and the corresponding lack of understanding regarding what accountability means underpins much of the problem associated with building an evidentiary foundation to leadership decisions and practices (McDaniel, 2004; Oliver, 2004; Price, 2006).

▶ Driving Forces That Are Shifting Organizational Structure

The rules of organizational engagement are changing significantly on the basis of the emergence of an informational and technological foundation for human experiences and practices as well as the increasing impact of globalization (Trompenaars & Hampden-Turner, 2002; Global Forces of 21st Century Leadership, 2017). These emerging realities are calling organizations and leaders into a different contextual framework for leadership and the management of work (Wolper, 2004). Goals of improved process times, lower production costs, improved coordination and management of functional interdependencies, and time reductions continue to push organizations forward (Davenport & Harris 2017).

Further, the information age is changing all the rules affecting structure and the processes associated with doing work, achieving outcomes, or producing products (Watkins, 2004). According to Scharmer (2017), Scharmer and Kaufer (2000), and Castells (1998), the changes occurring because of the information age are significant, most notably the Internet. There are now social structures based on networks, an economy tightly linked to information, and cultures steeped in virtual reality. These changes call for rethinking of just about everything a leader does, from visioning to planning to collaborating to implementing to evaluating.

The new world taking shape before us necessarily affects the very nature of health care and the ways in which healthcare services are organized, packaged, delivered, and evaluated. Specifically, the availability and sharing of information, the media used for knowledge transfer, the range and types of relationships among providers and patients, and the time required to transfer and share information now require new structures, principles for communication, and outcome expectations for leaders. In particular, the information infrastructure is now able to aggregate huge volumes of data, correlate that information, integrate it, and report it clearly and efficiently.

The changes in how information is communicated, who can access information, real-time availability of information on the Internet, and the availability of digitized media for nearly every bit of information have had a unique impact on traditional organizational structure. These structures serve to define levels of authority, communication pathways, and span of control. The organizational chart at one time

TABLE 6-1 Comparison of Traditional and Information Age Dimensions

	Traditional	Information Age	Advantages	Disadvantages
Structure for communication and authority designation Who is involved?	Organizational chart Vertical communication	Internet Social networks Open communication	Eliminates silos Increases integration of work products	Uncertainty with open communication Perceived loss of control and power
Media How is knowledge transferred?	Paper, books, video, audio	Digital	Consistency, quality of information	Lack of resources to implement
Space Where does it happen?	Physical buildings/ offices Local	Virtual Nonlocal	Space available for open collaboration	Perceived loss of privacy
Time When does it occur?	Business hours	No limits 24 hours/day	Decreases lag time across time zones and between individuals	Blurs the boundaries between work and personal time

defined clear lines of accountability and role relationships believed appropriate for organizational effectiveness and efficiency. Now with the widespread use of the Internet, digital device real-time communication, and self-organizing networks, these boundaries have become blurred at best and nearly invisible in most organizations.

Three areas have significantly changed the nature of work: media communication, location of stakeholders, and time. **TABLE 6-1** summarizes the description and impact in these areas.

Media Communication

The manner of communication among healthcare stakeholders has changed significantly with the availability of transportable and real-time Internet-available information. Communication media have evolved from physical to electronic and from isolated to interactive. The assumptions related to the media or vehicle for transfer of information, including written, oral, and video modalities as the primary vehicles, are challenged in nearly every venue. The availability of text messaging, instant messaging, and social networks has contributed greatly to the new model for organizational structure. Communication with anyone now reflects increasing complexity; communication occurs at any time and in any place. Power relationships are now dramatically reconfigured. Communications among executives, managers, and staff managers are now horizontal, vertical, and diagonal rather than up-and-down historical lines of authority and chains of command. According to Bennis, Goleman, and Biederman (2008), the effectiveness of an organization depends on the flow of information. Further, the organization's capacity to compete, solve problems, innovate, meet challenges, and achieve goals requires all the organization's intelligence—and this is directly related to the healthy flow of information. Attempts to formally control and limit communication are no longer effective.

No matter how well text is written, it is not an interactive medium. Paper was once the most reliable form for communication; now digital files are becoming the norm. Audiovisual media have also dramatically decreased the need for travel and physical presence. Physical presence has long been exchanged with a multiuser conference line. As global communication occurs quickly and efficiently with access to the Internet and a video camera, connections with multiple individuals in many locations are commonplace. With the introduction of affordable video conferencing, physical presence is less important. Heavy desktop computers have been replaced with flat-screen monitors and handheld devices. Data storage capacity is significant because sophisticated users have unlimited access to information on the Internet. Leadership roles have evolved to include roles of accessing, filtering, and interpreting information for others. With this rapid and prolific ability to instantly communicate comes further disruption of the organization requiring leaders to embrace the network of communications or attempt to maintain linear order. Both have advantages and disadvantages.

The changes in media availability will alter current work flows in the organization and require new ways to manage the decreased length of processing time, data storage, hardware, and software. Further, although media have been more readily available to others, it is nearly impossible for workers to access, interpret, and manage the information as quickly as it is now available. The limitations are now human personnel availability rather than the timely movement of media. Another interesting phenomenon is the challenges of privacy regulations and how to be compliant with them. In some cases, leaders are restricting access to text, web, and video media and are thus restricting information flow into the organization, reinforcing a linear model of communication rather than the complex reality.

Another example of evolving communication is the creation of social media accounts by most senior leaders, inviting members of the organization to share ideas and feedback continuously. Rather than the traditional, formal face-to-face meeting, leaders are now accessible to employees with Internet access 24 hours a day, 7 days a week. Based on these changes, new assumptions about the structure of organizations are needed. The new infrastructure is now based on openness and minimal lines of authority or divisions of work units. Behaviors and structures that support unconstrained communication and open relationships are redefining the roles and accountabilities of both leaders and staff. The increasing numbers of video applications for group communications that are readily available and often at minimal cost provide for face-to-face communication across distant locations. This further negates the need for and value of a physical presence.

Digital communication based on social network theory has also enhanced dissemination of healthcare information according to Solomons (2016). Solomons developed the relational model of communication and adherence to EBP from diffusion of innovation theory, social network theories, relational coordination theory, and quality improvement literature. She reported findings to provide empirical support for the role of social networks and relationships among staff in adoption of, and adherence to, evidence-based practice. These findings reinforced the importance of relationships and communication among hospital nursing (RN, LPN, CNA) and discharge planning staff on adherence to evidence-based practices (EBPs) for reducing preventable hospital readmissions.

Stakeholder Location

The location of both providers and users of the healthcare system changed dramatically with the introduction of the Internet. Providers are now often remote while providing assessment, observations, and robotic interventions. As a result, the role of physical space and location is changing. The functionality and utility of physical space in many settings has shifted from accommodating both providers and users of the healthcare system to accommodation for the user of the system and the technology to support virtual services. Further, both the provider and user may remain in their own settings while the technology equipment is stored in central locations. Gathering together at common sites is becoming the exception rather than the rule.

In the current context of large and complex facilities, the physical space among individuals, offices, and geographical locations that once resulted in a delay in communication between individuals, as well as a delay in the transmittance of paper documents, is now minimized and in some cases eliminated. The need for individual office space is now questioned regularly. The utility and purpose of individual private office space and the affordability of spaces used that are used less than 10% of the time provide an opportunity for new configurations. Space for teamwork rather than individual work space is preferred. What is not clear is the appropriate mix of face time on-site and off-site in which communication occurs using audiovisual technologies. Even with the best technologies, physical gatherings remain an essential part of the work processes. To be sure, there is nothing better than a welcome hug from a longtime colleague or a welcoming hand extended to a new member of the team. As the organization moves forward, efforts will continue to determine how best to optimize human gatherings and available technology. New consideration about the use of physical space will focus on value, flexibility, and multipurpose use for both individuals and teams. Current examples include the repurposing of waiting areas to healing spaces, multiuser access to examination rooms based on need rather than specific ownership of a room, and multipurpose telemedicine rooms supporting multiple providers. These changes require new approaches in managing virtual workforces and off-site clinicians to ensure engagement in the organizational vision and mission while supporting a work–life balance.

DISCUSSION: MEDIA, SPACE, AND TIME

The changes from the Internet affect different generations in different ways. Convene a group that includes representatives from as many generations as possible and explore the following topics:

- Ask each person how he or she has been affected (or not) by the changes in media, space, and time.

- What practice changes have been necessary to accommodate the ready access to individuals and data?
- What new connections among devices have changed or improved the quality and time lines of patient care services?
- Which devices have improved your ability to share and evaluate clinical information?
- What are the downsides of the increase in digital sharing?

Time

Traditionally, work was accomplished at the workplace during specified hours. With the Internet, the time parameters for availability and access to data are forever blurred. Shared files and social networks now make connections possible at any time in any location around the globe. Waiting time for global dialogue is nearly non-existent and often dependent only on the work and sleep schedules of individuals around the world. No longer is the individual waiting for the mail to arrive—an e-mail is waiting!

Further, traditional shift times and lengths may be even more flexible as virtual care is integrated with physical, on-site care. Research on caregivers' fatigue identified issues of compromised competence near 12.5 hours in a 24-hour period or 40 hours in 1 week (Geiger-Brown et al., 2012; Martin, 2014; Rogers, 2002; Stimpfel, Lake, Barton, Gorman, & Aiken, 2013). Different shift lengths or rest period intervals may be required with increased screen monitoring work.

▶ More Thoughts on the Impact of the Internet

To be sure, the unceremonious dismantling of traditional organizational structures and processes increases the chaos in healthcare organizations. Necessarily, the evolving organizational infrastructure is dynamic rather than static and stable. The available digital world requires leaders to continually challenge the expectations of turnaround time and access to individuals related to organizational communication, interdisciplinary collaboration, the location of providers and patients, and the time frames in which this work can occur.

While these advances are exciting to many individuals, some individuals are resistant to the shifts to the digital world. The resistance is part of the transformation to a new paradigm and necessarily increases chaos and complexity for the leader. The resistance to advancement of an evidentiary paradigm may be driven by the historical absence of focus on evidentiary thinking and processes.

It is important to remember that the role of leaders in an evidence–innovation dynamic is relatively new but critical to organizational effectiveness. Creating evidence to support the evolving organizational structure dynamic is an imperative for successful organizational performance.

If your actions inspire others to dream more, learn more, do more and become more, you are a leader.

—John Quincy Adams

▶ Moving Forward: Rethinking Organizational Structure and Role Accountabilities

The transformational work for leaders begins with an end in mind—a desired state that is believed to achieve value for the users of the organization. An assessment and gap analysis on the basis of organizational context and professional roles begins the process. In the next section of this chapter, new thoughts on the foundational framework for this work and specific changes in role obligations and behaviors are discussed. Necessarily, this work must be fully sensitive to and carefully integrated into the organizational culture—the underlying assumptions, defining values, and artifacts that embody the organization. The behaviors and norms supportive of new expectations include a vision and infrastructure that continually support and develop the capacity to change, the capacity to evaluate and integrate changes resulting from digital innovations, increased communication access, media management, and expedited work flow. **FIGURE 6-1** reflects the proposed evidentiary dynamic and the intersecting components.

Stability is no longer the goal for the healthcare leader; the goals now support continual evaluation of new ideas while ensuring that competent and safe patient care is provided. The emphasis on high-reliability organizations is now more actively tempered with the notion of focus and accountability on the work being done with the understanding that procedures necessarily will change. The emphasis must not be on completing high-reliability checklists and redundancies; the emphasis, or time out, needs to focus on defining the team's goal: what is the team doing, and is it the right thing? Are we using the most contemporary, evidence-based approach for the work we are doing?

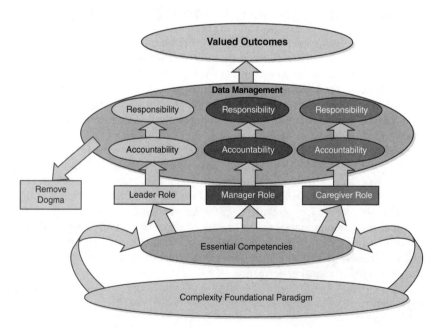

FIGURE 6-1 Evidentiary organization: Dynamics and intersection components.

Now, the challenge for the leader is how to facilitate the development of essential roles, accountabilities, competencies, and expectations in team members for excellence in patient care services and simultaneously ensure flexibility and openness to new and emerging processes. The desired healthcare culture is no longer able to solely support cultures of rote performance based on standards, practices, and technology developed yesterday and achieve the optimal outcomes of today and tomorrow. The continual evaluation and introduction of new work processes and technology require higher levels of presence and engagement than ever thought possible.

In addition to the expectations for evolving work processes, an increase in diversity competence is expected. Patients are now from a global, virtual world that is increasingly diverse. Caregiver knowledge of multiple cultural traditions, beliefs, and values is foundational. An increasing challenge is for the caregiver to sublimate personal values in deference to the patient's unique values. Providing patient care services from the perspective of one's social obligation as a provider now assumes more significance in the global world. Preferences are for treatment modalities, family involvement, and life and death rituals, and so the role of the caregiver varies more widely now, based on the individual patient. Now more than ever the provision of person- and family-centered care is essential (Barnsteiner, Disch, & Walton, 2014). The best decisions for the patient based on his or her beliefs and values must now be supported by structures and processes in the healthcare system as the norm rather than the exception.

As such, leadership staff is called to skillfully and persistently transform the organizational culture from one less reliant on traditional static authority-based communication structures to a more dynamic infrastructure that recognizes interrelated and intersecting roles and communication across complex networks. These changes are only now possible because of our increasing capacity to apprehend organizational complexity brought about by the Internet. Necessarily, the traditional box-and-line organizational diagrams need to go by the wayside because there is no information to be gained from them. The Internet, as previously noted, has eliminated hierarchies and standard lines of communication; thus the historical diagrams do not provide direction or information for members of the organization.

This endeavor requires a series of steps that begin with personal and organizational reflection and a call to the table of the most senior leaders to generate both a framework and a set of expectations with regard to evidence-based decision making and action taking (Giacco, 2003; Wager, Wickham, & Glaser, 2005). Reflection at the highest levels of the organization and the construction of evidentiary foundations upon which strategy, tactics, performance, and outcome measures can be based create a foundation from which data that builds evidence-driven practices can emerge. Further, their relationship to positive impacts and outcomes can be established. These steps include transformation to a complexity-driven foundation, creation of clear accountability expectations for role performance, and development of a sophisticated data management infrastructure.

▶ Complexity: Moving from a Static to Dynamic Paradigm

Recognition of the nature of the complexity in organizations is an important step in beginning the transformation. In quantum thinking and within complexity-defined systems, change is a constant, a fundamental dynamic of existence. In this circumstance, change is an existential condition, uncontrolled, beyond human manipulation; it is also a fundamental characteristic and operation of the universe (Blum, 2006). Complexity and complex systems thinking and research have provided a strong contemporary foundation for rethinking and reconfiguring the leadership and management and caregiver roles in complex organizations (Murphy, Ruch, Pepicello, & Murphy, 1997; Shan & Ang, 2008; Suh, 2005; Zimmerman, Lindberg, & Plsek, 1998). Thus, the organizational structure must now be influenced by these complexity attributes.

Accomplishment will prove to be a journey, not a destination.

—Dwight D. Eisenhower

The most important element to shift to an evidentiary framework for the leader is the recognition that past leadership practices have been guided by linear, cognitive, and rational processes that reflect rather predictable changes in processes and outputs. In the new environment, decision making and action must reflect more nonlinear and quantum influences in human dynamics and behavior. The evidence-based leader understands that human (and therefore health) behavior is such that change is better conceptualized, understood, and addressed through the lens of complex adaptive/responsive processes (Ang & Yin, 2008).

The attributes of nonlinearity, self-organization, uncertainty, emergence, interaction, intersection, and limited span of control describe the nature of complex organizations. The complex systems literature has demonstrated the power and influence of self-organization and emergence within organizations (Miller & Scott, 2007). This new research is revising the foundations for understanding leadership practices and behavior and even reconceptualizing the role and application of leadership in organization decision making and actions (Morrison, 2007).

Much of the work on complex systems sciences emerged from the biological, social, and physical sciences. The convergence of those data revealed patterns of behavior that emerged from examples of interacting and intersecting human societies, e-systems, ecosystems, the human brain, and bee colonies, among others (Rouse, 2007). These various exemplars of systems now serve to inform our understanding of the leader's role and leaders' interactions with and within the systems of which they are a part (Stacey, 2007).

A larger question related to complex systems is how much control should be exercised by the agent of control (the manager) within systems—in this case, within the healthcare system. We know that varying levels of agency control are evident in a variety of systems. For example, on the Internet, almost no central control is exerted. In contrast, in the military and the solar system, high levels of control are exhibited. In the human body, intermediate interacting levels of control are evidenced.

Degrees of criticalness also influence level of agent control. In highly critical circumstances, where the life of an organism or system is directly and dramatically threatened, high levels of control are necessary to stabilize the system and bring it back into balance. By comparison, in systems with a high level of equilibrium and good responsive interface between external environmental challenges and demands, and internal mechanisms of response, low levels of critical condition exist and therefore there is a reduced need for levels of agent control (Solow & Szmerekovsky, 2006).

Within the frame of complexity, there is the understanding that complex adaptive systems represent a highly complex dynamic of interacting and intersecting forces operating externally and internally, constantly affecting the life of the system

(Yin & Ang, 2008). For example, the management of a patient in a critical care unit requires much more agent intervention surveillance and intensity than does the management of a patient in a long-term care facility or hospice setting. In many day-to-day nursing activities and work flows, increased control by management can actually inhibit the ability for the frontline care provider to use the best evidence, exercise clinical judgment, or practice at the top of his or her license. Excessive control and micromanagement removes adaptability from the system.

The degree of agent control and manipulation of circumstance and relational variables leads to different agent roles and relationships with respect to the amount of control needed or desired. Evidence-based management perceives this relationship in terms of the complex network of intersections and interactions and the degree of internally generated locus of control or the degree of external management of control. In broad terms, the incidence of emergent leadership and its influence on decision making and action may be directly related to the level of agent control, ranging from highly critical (greatest agent control) to highly self-managed (least agent control). For example, the greatest agent control would be for a leader to assign a project and the project plan to the team to complete the work; in the least control situation, the leader would assign problem resolution (outcome) to the team to determine what the process and approach should be to address the problem. The next area of assessment for the leader is ensuring the presence of an evidentiary dynamic—a dynamic that fully integrates operations and innovation as well as the transformation between them.

Integrating Operations and Innovation

In current organizations, increasing efforts to address complexity are seen in the establishment of innovation centers or departments to support and assess new products and processes—processes that are congruent with a complexity paradigm in which uncertainty is the norm, and emergence and highly interacting and intersecting relationships are present. **BOX 6-1** includes common strategies currently used by organizations to generate new ideas and processes. The contemporary organization requires an infrastructure that effectively supports both the linear, predictable, evidence-based processes in routine operations alongside the integration of innovations to replace outdated operations at the appropriate time as well as an openness to testing and implementing new ideas. This often seems contradictory; however, in an evidentiary dynamic model, both the evidence-based work and the creation of new evidence from innovation must be supported in an ongoing process. Traditional organizational models have segmented innovation from routine operations and limited the flexibility and responsiveness of the organization.

The accelerated velocity of the introduction of new ideas further supports the need for an integrated approach to an advancement of innovation and an emphasis on the transition from innovation to operation. More importantly, there is a need to integrate the work of innovation with the work of each particular role. New ideas should be generated and developed in ways that take into account the perspectives of point-of-care knowledge workers. In a complexity-driven organizational model, the lines among operations, innovations, and transformation become blurred as responsibility and accountability behaviors are elevated and particularized for each role in the organization.

In an evidence-based framework, engagement and involvement inside the innovation process reflect the least intensity of agent control, allowing the greatest

---

BOX 6-1 Tools to Advance Change and Innovation

- Deep dive: A particular area is selected for observation in multiple ways. Work flows, photos, interviews, and observations are gathered by a team to analyze current processes and brainstorm new ways of doing the current work processes (Kelly, 2005).
- Directed creativity: A situation is proposed to encourage and advance new ideas. For example, individuals are presented with the following scenario and directed to respond: A new unit is being designed for medical–surgical patients. If there were no limits on space, technology, resources, staff, or financial resources, how would you design the unit for the future in a way to dramatically improve the cost and quality of the healthcare experience (Plsek, 1997)?
- Mind mapping: Mind mapping is a software tool for collecting, organizing, and synthesizing large amounts of data in layers, with complex relationships. It is a very useful tool for documents connectivity, interdependencies, and emerging phenomena in health care.
- Innovation space: An innovation space is a place or laboratory where inquiring minds collaborate to create a more livable and sustainable world focused on developing products that create market value while serving real societal needs—products that are progressive, possible, and profitable (Boradkar, 2010).
- Brainstorming: A collective exercise process to generate ideas. A good exercise generates 100 ideas. This is different from directed creativity in that brainstorming focuses on suspending judgment and criticism, encourages freewheeling thinking and quantity of ideas, and builds on the ideas of others (Endsley, 2010).
- Disruptive innovation: An innovation that cannot be used by customers in mainstream markets. It defines a new performance trajectory by introducing new dimensions of performance compared to existing innovations. Disruptive innovations either create new markets by bringing new features to nonconsumers or offer more convenience or lower prices to customers at the low end of an existing market (Christensen et al., 2004, p. 293)

---

freedom in an environment that fosters successful innovation. Ready access to all of the supports, resources, tools, and processes that facilitate the energetic and free-flowing activities of creativity would be essential to innovation. The manager in this case would create conditions and circumstances that permit this more open dynamic to thrive. By contrast, emergence of this type of control would be less likely in a situation where the variables need to be tightly manipulated and managed with narrowly defined but clearly applied manager (agent) control, such as in situations involving employee discipline, critical interventions, system control (such as in a prison), or terrorism. The next section presents a discussion of the transformation of three essential professional roles.

▶ Leaders, Managers, and Direct Care Provider Roles in an Evidentiary Dynamic

Three major roles are required in an evidentiary organization: leader, manager, and caregiver. Each of these roles has distinct descriptions. **TABLE 6-2** provides an overview of the essential elements of each role and the supportive accountability, responsibility, and value for each role. Note that each of these roles is considered a knowledge worker's

TABLE 6-2 Evidentiary Organization: Key Roles and Accountabilities

		Knowledge Workers[a]	
	Leader Role	**Manager Role**	**Direct Care Provider Role**
Accountable for: ■ **Doing the right work** ■ **Focusing on the product and results of work; the actual difference the work makes**	■ Creates the context for accountability, responsibility, and value creation ■ Recognizes the action of complexity and the value of establishing new roles responding to current circumstances ■ Recognizes the confluence and consonance of interaction between external environmental forces and internal relational, operational, and behavioral response to an ever-changing set of circumstances ■ Ensures there is support necessary for appropriate decisions and actions, resourcing ■ Integrates an evidence-based value set ■ Creates the data infrastructure	■ Facilitates the planning and construction of designs for creating infrastructure and processes that support point of service, evidence-based data integration and translation of its utility into clinical practice ■ Applies contemporary research and theory of complex systems, and translation and use of this information in the workplace ■ Develops the infrastructure for evidence-based processes through the analysis of patterns within the system ■ Applies clinical research and theory of complex systems and translation, and use of this information in the workplace ■ Manages data relationships—establishes the attachment between data and clinical decision making at the point of service; data are available and integrated for effective decisions	■ Accountability for performance and achievement of clinical outcomes rests exclusively and solely with the competent practitioner ■ Seeks out and uses all available evidence/data to make decisions and provide care

(continues)

TABLE 6-2 Evidentiary Organization: Key Roles and Accountabilities   *(continued)*

| | Knowledge Workers[a] | | |
	Leader Role	Manager Role	Direct Care Provider Role
Responsible for: Doing the work well	■ Provides effective systems, structures, and resources for the work to be done	■ Provides effective infrastructures for patient care recognizing complexity, interrelationships, and current evidence within patient care dynamics	■ Provides evidence-based, state-of-the-art patient care that results in the desired value to the patient and family
Valued Outcomes	■ Increased health of populations served ■ Increased evidentiary resources ■ Goodness of fit between desired outcomes (value) and effective processes associated with obtaining them ■ Sustainable		

[a] Knowledge worker: An individual whose main capital is knowledge and has an emphasis on nonroutine problem solving that requires a combination of convergent, divergent, and creative thinking.
Data from Reinhardt, W., Schmidt, B., Sloep, P., & Drachsler, H. (2011). Knowledge worker roles and actions: Results of two empirical studies. *Knowledge and Process Management, 18*(3), 150–174. http://dx.doi.org/10.1002/kpm.378

because his or her work is based on knowledge capital and includes nonroutine problem solving and creative thinking (Reinhardt, Schmidt, Sloep, & Drachsler, 2011).

First, the leader role is accountable for creating the organizational context for value creation—a context that provides the support necessary to ensure that appropriate decisions and actions are undertaken along with adequate resources for the work and desired outcomes. Like all roles, the leader bases decisions on evidence and the importance of creating new evidence where none is available. The leader is aware of the confluence and consonance of interactions among external environmental forces and internal relational, operational, and behavioral responses to an ever-changing set of circumstances (Frandkov, 1999). Members of an evidentiary community reflect attitudes, competencies, and specific role behaviors to support the transformed organization.

The role of leadership in this movement is self-evident. Because leaders have the predominant role in creating the context and providing the supports necessary to ensure that appropriate decisions and actions are undertaken, resourcing and applying structure to these new models are obligations of the leader role. Performing this role effectively requires clarity of the conceptual role, personal knowledge, leadership principles, collaboration, synthesis, knowledge management, and mentoring. Aware and informed healthcare leaders stay abreast of the changing conditions and context for the application of clinical service. Through deliberation and dialogue at the strategic and tactical levels of the organization, these managers facilitate the planning and construction of designs for creating infrastructure and processes that would support point-of-service, evidence-based data integration and translation of its utility into clinical practice.

The manager represents the contemporary application of the theory and research of the action of complex systems and the translation and use of that understanding in decisions and actions in the workplace. For the manager, just as for the clinician, the development of the infrastructure reflects the application of complexity theory and complex adaptive systems to the work relationships, behaviors, and structures constantly operating to influence clinical practice and outcomes. The manager recognizes the action of complexity and the value of establishing the evolving role factors, including new roles responding to the current circumstances and the activities unfolding within them.

The manager's requisite abilities related to scanning, predictive capacity, and adaptation now come to bear as a critical skill set in the creation of the structures and processes in support of contemporary evidence-based initiatives (Hesselbein, 2002). Indeed, managers represent in their own practice and performance the use of evidentiary strategies and tactics in advising decisions and taking actions related to resource use, demonstrated in their own management of human, fiscal, material, support, and systems accountabilities. The role played by strong, evidence-committed management leaders is enhanced by their willingness to both model and mentor evidentiary dynamics as the appropriate contemporary framework within which all work relationships and clinical performance unfold. Caregivers are accountable for the performance of patient care interventions and the achievement of clinical outcomes using the latest evidence-based interventions. In particular, caregivers are owners of their nontransferable capital and capacity of the application of their work. Their knowledge is mobile and portable—their knowledge goes with them wherever they go.

After the role descriptions are clear for the leader, manager, and direct care giver, the associated accountabilities are identified. These distinctions are necessarily driven from evidence rather than experience and intuition. **TABLE 6-3** provides an overview of requisite knowledge, skills, and abilities for innovation thinking. **TABLE 6-4** lists essential competencies for this innovation work.

TABLE 6-3 Innovation Knowledge, Skills, and Abilities Assessment

Knowledge—a body of information applied directly to the performance of a function.

Skill—an observable competence to perform a learning psychomotor act.

Ability—competence to perform an observable behavior that results in an observable product.

		Meets	Exceeds	Exceptional
	KNOWLEDGE			
1	Understands the role that nursing/discipline has in clarifying the meaning of innovation			
2	Self-confidence and self-knowledge about innovation			
3	Understands complex change/innovation theories			
4	Recognizes and differentiates change, management, and innovation			
5	Understands the significance of information management and its relationship to innovation			
6	Cross-disciplinary knowledge; aware of how strategic partnerships can facilitate innovation			
7	Synthesizes knowledge of innovation from educational and experiential opportunities			
8	Disruptive change and its impact on organizational norms			
9	Principles and value of empowerment			
10	Has high regard for the value of innovation			
11	Has a clear vision for innovation			

		Meets	Exceeds	Exceptional
	SKILLS			
1	Communicates the value of innovation			
2	Is optimistic about the future and the unknown			
3	Creates the conditions for innovation to occur			
4	Creates a culture of innovation			
5	Positive open attitude toward change			
6	Fosters a culture of inquiry where employees are free to inquire and challenge the status quo			
7	Rewards and recognizes innovation work			
8	Able to assess the feasibility of an opportunity			
9	Experiments			
10	Tests ideas with others			
11	Emphasizes big-picture thinking			
12	Recognizes new patterns and insights			
13	Engages in deep-dive experiences to foster creativity			
14	Synthesizes ideas from different fields			
15	Uses boundary spanning thinking			
16	Empowers others to be as innovative as they can be			
17	Collaborates with nursing research and process improvement to define strategies for testing ideas			

(continues)

TABLE 6-3 Innovation Knowledge, Skills, and Abilities Assessment *(continued)*			
	Meets	**Exceeds**	**Exceptional**
18	Fosters high interprofessional and team collaboration			
19	Implements unit-level teams of practice councils			
20	Builds and uses networks			
21	Embraces failure as a learning opportunity			
22	Makes risky decisions			
23	Asks the best questions			
24	Breaks open entrenched and intractable problems			
25	Supports positive deviance behaviors for innovation			
ABILITIES				
1	Integrates evidence, new knowledge, and research findings into practice and contributes to the *advancement of clinical practice*			
2	Evaluates and demonstrates *individual growth* in clinical practice with attention to guidelines, standards, regulations, and quality indicators			
3	Participates in *elevating the quality of care and/or the environment of care* while ensuring safety and the appropriate use of resources			
4	Competent in translating innovation to operations			
5	Ensures the availability of financial resources for innovative work			

		Meets	Exceeds	Exceptional
6	Implements roles to address the new work identified by innovation			
7	Translates innovation into operations and includes requirements for process changes, role modifications, staffing and resource needs			

TABLE 6-4 Performance Evaluation: Innovation Competency Statements

	Innovation Competency Statement	Leader	Staff Nurse	Both	Neither
	GENERAL				
1	Integrates evidence, new knowledge, and research findings into practice and contributes to the *advancement of clinical practice*				
2	Evaluates and demonstrates *individual growth* in clinical practice with attention to guidelines, standards, regulations, and quality indicators				
3	Participates in *elevating the quality of care and/or the environment of care* while ensuring safety and the appropriate use of resources				
4	Competent in translating innovation to operations				
5	Ensures the availability of financial resources for innovative work				
6	Implements roles to address the new work identified by innovation				
7	Hires employees who value creativity and innovation				

(continues)

TABLE 6-4 Performance Evaluation: Innovation Competency Statements *(continued)*

	Innovation Competency Statement	Leader	Staff Nurse	Both	Neither
	KNOWLEDGE				
8	Self-confidence and self-knowlege				
9	Uses knowledge and experiences in the process of innovation				
10	Recognizes and differentiates change management and innovation				
11	Understands the significance of information management and its relationship to innovation.				
12	Cross-disciplinary knowledge				
	CREATIVITY				
13	Communicates the value of innovation				
14	Is optimistic about the future and the unknown				
15	Creates the conditions for innovation to occur				
16	Creates a culture of innovation				
17	Has high regard for the value of innovation				
18	Has a clear vision for innovation				
	RECOGNITION OF OPPORTUITIES				
19	Positive, open attitude toward change				

	Innovation Competency Statement	Leader	Staff Nurse	Both	Neither
20	Embraces disruptive change				
21	Fosters a culture of inquiry where employees are free to inquire and challenge the status quo				
22	Rewards and recognizes innovation				
23	Assesses the feasibility of an opportunity				
	DESIGN THINKING/ EXPERIMENTATION				
24	Translates innovation into operations				
25	Experiments				
26	Tests ideas with others				
27	Emphasizes big-picture thinking				
28	Recognizes new patterns and insights				
29	Engages in deep-dive experiences to foster creativity				
30	Synthesizes ideas from different fields				
31	Uses boundary spanning thinking				
	COLLABORATION				
32	Empowers others to be as innovative as they can be				
33	Collaborates with nursing research and process improvement to define strategies for testing ideas				

(continues)

	Innovation Competency Statement	**Leader**	**Staff Nurse**	**Both**	**Neither**
	TABLE 6-4 Performance Evaluation: Innovation Competency Statements *(continued)*				
34	Fosters high interprofessional and team collaboration				
35	Implements unit-level teams of practice councils				
36	Builds and uses networks				
	EMBRACING FAILURE				
37	Embraces failure as a learning opportunity				
38	Makes risky decisions				
39	Asks the best questions				
40	Breaks open entrenched and intractable problems				
41	Supports positive deviance behaviors for innovation				
42	Considers outside-the-box thinking				

▶ Role Accountability, Responsibility, and Knowledge Ownership

Each of the described roles have associated behaviors to support a complex system in which evidence and innovation are inexorably interwoven and reflect clear expectations for professional accountability, responsibility, and the management of knowledge.

Accountability

In knowledge work environments such as hospitals and healthcare systems, the notion of accountability takes on special meaning. Knowledge workers own the means of their own capital, and this means is now as significant as any other sources of capital and human-intensive organizations (Reinhardt et al., 2011; Sveiby, 1997). Knowledge workers have an individually driven sense of ownership with regard to their knowledge and its demonstration in the applications of work (Hooker &

Csikszentmihalvi, 2003). Embedded in this understanding of knowledge work ownership are the mobility and portability of that knowledge because the knowledge worker carries the knowledge wherever he or she operates in the system. This flexibility is another important consideration with regard to accountability. Knowledge workers do not transfer the locus of control for their accountability to institutions, organizations, or others outside their knowledge work community. Accountability for the performance and achievement of outcomes rests exclusively and solely with each role. Accountability for creation of the context of accountability rests with the leader. Accountability for facilitating and designing the infrastructure for practice rests with the manager.

This notion of ownership in relationship to accountability is critical to the professional knowledge worker; it also informs the management of these workers. As such, ownership for the work of practice does not transfer to the management role, and managers cannot be held accountable for the outcomes of practice owned by the caregivers whose capacity and competence are essential to both achieving and sustaining outcomes (Porter-O'Grady, 2000). Because ownership is invested in each role, if the desired outcomes are to be achieved, management's role is to create an organization and systems context that facilitates, supports, and encourages the ownership and expression of accountability (Albrecht, 2003).

In short, the accountability of management differs in important ways from the accountability of the direct care provider. The effectiveness of work and the achievement of outcomes belongs to the knowledge worker caregiver; the creation of context that frames and supports the work and accountability of staff is the source of accountability for management (Dotlich & Cairo, 2002). The outcome of the knowledge worker management role is the same as that of the knowledge worker staff: effective patient care that leads to positive clinical outcomes. However, accountability for achieving those ends is significantly different in a management role compared to the knowledge worker staff role. The activities associated with one are differentiated from the activities associated with the other. Yet both roles are necessary to create the dynamic—the intersection—necessary to sustain performance outcomes.

DISCUSSION

Accountability is a concept often bandied about and misinterpreted. After there is understanding that accountability requires the licensed person to perform interventions as indicated for the patient, there are often challenges from others to modify practice. Consider the following situation:

You are instructed to discontinue protective isolation by the chief executive officer (CEO) because the patient's family has a high profile and does not want to be bothered. Using the principles of accountability, how would you handle this? Can the clinician take directions about patient care from the CEO?

Management accountability relates to the quality and integrity of the direction, infrastructure of systems, and the degree of integrity of their relationship with the work and performance outcomes of the knowledge worker stakeholders. In partnership with knowledge workers, the organization's leaders aggregate the efforts of systems and people in a mosaic of intersection and performance that networks strategy, infrastructure, resources, and knowledge work in the configuration (a dance, if you will) of consonance and contribution that advances both the clinical outcomes for patients and the organizational viability of the system (Pidd, 2004).

Managers represent in their own practice and performance the use of evidentiary strategies and tactics in advising decisions and taking actions related to resource use, demonstrated in their own management of human, fiscal, material, support, and systems accountabilities. The role played by strong, evidence-committed management leaders is enhanced by their willingness to both model and mentor evidentiary dynamics as the appropriate contemporary framework within which all work relationships and clinical performance unfold. As the new context based on complexity emerges within the three foundational roles and accountability expectations, there are four competencies or attitudes that are also essential behaviors within each of these roles.

Competencies

There are four essential competencies or attitudes for all members of the organization: inquisitive, vulnerable, inclusive, and proactive. **TABLE 6-5** presents the core content of each competency and role expectation for the leader, manager, and direct caregiver. These are often challenging to identify objectively; however, the results of these competencies are evident in the increasingly successful outcomes of the organization at the individual, organization, and community levels.

TABLE 6-5 Evidentiary Competencies: Basics for Advancing New Work in Complex Organizations

Competency	Core Content	Role: Leader, Manager, Caregiver
Inquisitive	Innovation knowledge Self-knowledge; personal management; self-care	Knowledge system manager Data manager Role knowledge
Vulnerable/ courageous	Courageous Challenges practice and assumptions for increased understanding and improvement Open to new ideas	Experimenter and tester of new ideas
Inclusive	Relationship builder	Facilitator of individuals and teams to achieve value; coach, mentor, collaborate Diversity facilitator; conflict embracer/engager Technology versus humanness
Proactive	Synthesizer; strategist	Critical strategist and value creator; business case creator

Inquisitive

Successful individuals are continually inquisitive about the nature of the work, the factors affecting and the evidence supporting current work, and new ideas that are being introduced. In particular, individuals demonstrate a high regard for and value creativity, have an openness to new ideas, are comfortable in challenging assumptions, and can see conflict as diversity. As agents of change, these individuals are continually enhancing their knowledge of innovation and change content, tools, processes, and challenges. Knowing the science and art of innovation is essential.

There are numerous descriptions and definitions of innovation (**BOX 6-2**) that guide the work of innovation leaders. As knowledge in innovation leadership emerges, more descriptions will be presented. The skeptic often dismisses innovation with the belief that nothing new ever really occurs; rather, it is only new combinations and iterations of existing products and processes that occur. This approach may be an example of a delaying tactic and does little to address the need for the organization to be contemporary in its work. Becoming tangled in the conceptual precision discussion may serve only to delay meaningful discussion and attention to the future.

Individuals are also inquisitive about their own personal skill sets. Self-knowledge and competence with innovation and change further assist individuals. A clear understanding of one's personal strengths and limitations as they relate to the evidentiary dynamic is essential to create the business case for developing new ideas.

BOX 6-2 Change and Innovation: Common Descriptions

- The implementation of new or altered products, services, processes, systems, organizational structures, or business models as a means of improving one or more domains of healthcare quality (AHRQ Health Care Innovations Exchange, n.d.)
- Anything that creates new resources, processes, or values or improves a company's existing resources, processes, or values (Christenson, Anthony, & Roth, 2004)
- The power to redefine the industry; the effort to create purposeful focused change in an enterprise's economic or social potential (Drucker, 1985)
- The conversation of knowledge and ideas into a benefit that may be for commercial use or for the public good; the benefit may be new or improved products, processes, or values (Christenson et al., 2004)
- The power to redefine the industry; the effort to create purposeful, focused change in an enterprise's economic or social potential (Drucker, 1985)
- A new patterning of our experiences of being together as new meaning emerges from ordinary, everyday work conversations (Fonseca, 2002)
- The first practical, concerted implementation of an idea done in a way that brings broad-based, extrinsic recognition to an individual or organization (Plsek, 1997)
- A historic and irreversible change in the way of doing things; creative destruction (Schumpeter, 1943)
- Emergent continuity and transformation of patterns of human interactions understood as ongoing ordinary complex responsive processes of human relating in local situations in the living present (Stacey, 2007)
- Innovation is something new, or perceived as new by the population experiencing the innovation, that has the potential to drive change and redefine health care's economic and/or social potential (Weberg, 2010)
- Fresh thinking that leads to value creation (Vaitheeswaran, 2007)

Assessments of decision making, communication, and conflict resolution styles are foundational areas of focus in self-knowledge assessment. The Myers & Briggs (http://www.myersbriggs.org) and DiSC (https://www.discprofile.com/what-is-disc/overview/) assessments are examples of helpful assessment tools for individuals. Although individuals often overemphasize self-assessments to learn about styles, strengths, and limitations, the label or category into which the individual falls should never be the primary focal point. Rather, the information about styles is intended to provide insight into an overall set of behaviors and does not reflect all activities. The ability to understand others and collaborate with multiple styles in multidisciplinary teams are essential competencies.

Individuals also assess their information processing and thinking systems styles as a means to excel. The relationship between emotions and intellectual content is important in understanding not only one's personal style but also the abilities of others. Consideration is also given to understanding rational and experiential information processing styles (Cerni, Curtis, & Colmar, 2008). Rational processing is analytical, intentional, logical, and slower, whereas experiential information processing is holistic, automatic, associative, and faster. Necessarily, both modes of processing are required to be effective. Areas of strength and areas of development opportunities guide professional development and growth.

Self-care is another area the individual focuses on as part of the self-knowledge assessment. The individual's sense of self is well developed along with the importance of maintaining high levels of performance and wellness. The work in an evidentiary organization is demanding and unrelenting, requiring individuals to be healthy, energetic, and resilient. There is often a need for a little bit of narcissism— self-care is essential for energy renewal for the innovation leader. Taking time to balance work with one's personal life is essential to sustain high levels of performance and productivity.

Vulnerability

The second competency is about vulnerability—being open and comfortable with uncertainty and being comfortable with the limitations of one's knowledge (Whitehurst, 2015). Vulnerable individuals are comfortable with the fact that one can never know everything and that this perpetual incompleteness is a fundamental trait of all individuals. The essential work is connecting and creating meaningful relationships with others who have different areas of expertise.

Courage is an element of vulnerability in that the individual is willing to discuss sacred cows and challenge long-standing practices and dare to eliminate obsolete healthcare dogma and not be afraid of criticism or ridicule that might result. This courage also guides the innovation leader in facilitating effective and difficult dialogue. When things are not going well, the individual examines and evaluates the situation and facilitates the appropriate course correction quickly. This course correction emphasizes learning from experience without ascribing blame to anyone.

Inclusive

The third competency is about being inclusive of multiple individuals and points of view. As a collaborator, individuals demonstrate a high-level competence in listening, encouraging feedback, and conflict utilization. Differing perspectives and values are not seen as conflicts to be resolved or mediated but rather as expressions of diversity. Many obstacles are encountered along the innovation continuum. Individuals, equipment, resources, and time can be the sources of conflict among team members. The innovation leader perceives conflicts as opportunities to learn more about the issues and to gain insight into the values and beliefs of others. The leader avoids efforts to neutralize or minimize the differing opinions until more information is gained. Necessarily, the innovation leader is a master change facilitator and is able to use conflict as an opportunity to gain further insight of pertinent issues.

For individuals in this type of organization, effective collaboration is about moving from a group of assembled individuals to a team of highly interactive, participative, goal-oriented individuals. Individuals thrive in multidisciplinary teams—the fundamental unit in the organization. The individual is always considered incomplete because one can never know all there is to know. Working alone or in single-discipline dialogue is inefficient and ineffective. Transdisciplinary dialogue is the norm to address issues of complexity and innovation. The innovation leader is patient, tolerant, and interested in a diverse discussion to facilitate teamwork. Innovation leaders seek out those known for strong opinions, the ability to challenge others, taking risks, and thinking creatively. In addition, the goal of being inclusive is about learning from others to find common ground while avoiding the rubber stamps of prattled conversation. Principles of appreciative inquiry guide interactions.

Teams often include disparate disciplines, such as clinicians, engineers, computer specialists, designers, and representatives from several generations and ethnic cultures. Courageous individuals are role models in the activities of challenging traditional norms and practices, and confronting each other when resistance is evident. As team members, they encourage comments on others' ideas; withholding feedback is considered counterproductive to the entire process. The goal is for sharing feedback to be a core rather than an optional behavior.

Within each role of leader, manager, and caregiver, the attitude of inclusiveness begets facilitation, coaching, and mentoring. Individuals facilitate the development of innovation principles and strategies among colleagues, adult learning, and the importance of system change. Further, individuals work to empower the creative genius in others. Creative genius is that part of each individual that has a possibilities-oriented, can-do attitude and way of being that communicates to everyone that anything is possible; it is about being full of excitement, energy, and ideas (McGlade & Pek, 2008).

These contextual attributes are realized in the dynamic evidentiary organization in which communication is encouraged and permission is not required to collaborate with others across departments and levels in the organization. There is a spirit of candor and a free flow of information without fear of criticism or reprisal. The reality is that some individuals have information at different times, and sharing ideas informally can increase the organization's capacity to solve problems and meet challenges. The goal is to use information to support optimal organizational performance; it is not to gossip or engage in one-upmanship competitions.

The behaviors of all individuals should reflect communication in an unrestricted manner, interest in new ideas, and willingness to challenge long-held assumptions. This open culture requires tolerance for the possibility of error and a climate in which errors can be discussed freely and the underlying causes investigated and corrected quickly (Whittingham, 2003). The successful culture is one in which leaders are competent across organizational operations, transformations, and innovations.

These competencies assume a high level of trust among individuals in the organization. As the culture evolves, greater trust is earned with much effort and consistency of behaviors. The culture is truly brought to life by the organization's leaders as they role-model their competencies. To be sure, this is an iterative process of cultural evolution and development of leader expertise.

Proactive

The fourth competency is about being proactive, about thinking into the future. Individuals want to be actively planning for a better future. The leader moves from reliance on historical knowledge to imagining, intuiting, inspiring, and reflecting the present as the means to the future (Scharmer & Kaufer, 2000).

The proactive individual demonstrates competence as a synthesizer and strategist and thrives with the rapid and continuous introduction of new ideas, processes, technology, and equipment. Managing and gathering large amounts of data to elicit evidentiary adequacy, value, and potential outcomes further exemplify performance. Information is quickly synthesized from multiple sources to create a comprehensive set of next steps for advancement using the wisdom of all team members and combined into a critical mass of expertise. New ideas are introduced after careful analysis using a business case for innovation. Individuals formulate key data into formal documents to identify the value of new work, the level of current evidence, and its clear relationship to the mission and vision of the organization.

From this proactive, evidence-building approach, creation of the business case becomes powerful. A business case or the rationale for expenditure of resources under certain circumstances is essential to support appropriate resource allocations (Burns, 2005). The elements of a strong business case for innovation include the following:

- A description of the new product or service
- The intended purpose or goal of the innovation
- Projection of costs specific to accomplish the innovation
- Costs excluded from the proposal and rationale for exclusion
- Projected benefits and rationale for valuing of benefits
- A timeline for the project from initiation to benefits realization
- Anticipated profit or loss
- Expected nonfinancial benefits
- Anticipated risks and plans to mediate risks
- Overall summary of both short-term and long-term value to the organization and community (Invest Northern Ireland, n.d.)

Within these major categories of the innovation business case, information specific to anticipated productivity changes, reductions in cost, market share, patient quality outcomes, new partnerships, and risks for not moving forward, such as losing market share, productivity loss, employee turnover, and profit margin reduction, must be included. Further, information that identifies how the new work could differentiate the organization from competitors, benefit multiple constituencies in the organization, and extend the life of the organization as a value-producing entity is an important element of this business case (Merrifield, Calhoun, & Stevens, 2008).

Building the strategic business case for new and untested ideas requires a modified approach from preparing a traditional business plan because of the unknown outcome of the innovation and the inadequacy of operational tools for innovation. Creating a sustainable budget or projection for an innovation requires knowledge about the past, which may be completely irrelevant, and estimations about the future that include cost of materials, technology, and human resources, and expected revenues. Christensen, Kaufman, and Shih (2008) identified the challenges in creating the business case as the lack of good financial tools to understand the market, build brands, find customers, select employees, organize teams, and develop strategies to advance the work. Specifically, when an organization relies on traditional discounted cash flow and net present value to evaluate investment opportunities, the real returns and benefits are often underestimated. Consideration of fixed and sunk costs using traditional models creates an unfair advantage on challengers and inhibits incumbent firms that attempt to respond. Finally, the emphasis on earnings per share as the primary metric for success diverts resources from investments whose payoff occurs at a much later date. According to Christensen and colleagues (2008), although these tools are good for operations, they create a systematic bias against innovation. It is challenging but not impossible to create the case for new work processes and products given the need for improvements in patient safety and quality outcomes. These four competencies are essential areas for growth and development of contemporary healthcare workers as they continue to develop high-level professional accountability. In addition, each role in the evidentiary organization must be able to access and manage the appropriate data for specific role accountabilities.

▶ Evidence-Driven Decision Making and Analysis: Managing Data and More Data

In an evidentiary dynamic organization, management of data by all three roles is critical. To be sure, all organizations are awash with data. It is not so much the collection of data that is important but rather the ability to use those data, analyze them, and make decisions and take action based on what the analysis reveals (Chakravarthy, 2003; Garvin & Roberto, 2001; Porter-O'Grady & Afable, 2003). Without question, in today's information-driven business world, the ability to manage data and use it appropriately is a fundamental management skill set. This love for and attachment to data, including the management of data and the analysis of its impacts, is a central prerequisite and an essential tool in the armamentarium of the good leader (Davenport, 2006). Attachment to data means having competence for gathering, aggregating, translating, interpreting, and applying it in a way that is meaningful and makes a difference in the lives of those who will use the data. It is important to note that knowledge is the lifeblood of innovative and complex organizations. Leaders then help to translate data into knowledge that will assist members of the organization. Data-driven decision making means more than simply relating to the data. It means establishing an intense relationship with data processes so that the structure of data becomes both a facilitating factor and a seamless integration. The data-driven process supports real-time communication and information, and the application of data entails real-time informing, guiding, and solution seeking at the point of decision and action (Ball, 2000; Oostendorp, 2003). Consider three questions posed by Allworth, Wessel, and Levie (2015):

1. What is the job to be done?
2. In a perfect world, what information would help you complete that job?
3. If you had this information, what inside your organization would need to change?

Of real importance is the ability to make this strong attachment or connection to data and analysis a part of the fundamental work experience for each individual in the organization. Translating data management into a real attachment to the use of data by knowledge workers is a formidable undertaking. Nevertheless, if the connection can be made between the value of work and the extent to which it is informed by data-driven decision making and evaluated by data-clarified measures, then leaders can begin to establish an attachment between the use of data and evidence, and the clinical decisions made and actions taken at the point of service. To accomplish this goal, such processes must be seamlessly integrated into the recording, collection, and assessment of information, and directly connected to the decision processes whose value and accuracy depend on both the veracity and the utility of the knowledge produced in real time by such data processes (Goad, 2002). The fluidity, portability, and mobility of data systems and processes as they are incorporated into knowledge worker activity are the keys to accelerating their viability as tools for both informing decisions and evaluating actions. Competent managers now view this approach not as a new way of doing business but rather as the *only* way to think and do the work effectively.

To create a meaningful attachment or connection to data and the analytics related to creating relevance from it will require that both practitioners and information systems experts and developers focus on the utility of such systems from the users' perspective (Hildreth & Kimble, 2004). To date, much data have been collected in health care, yet much of those data are neither relevant nor valuable to individuals at the point of service, where the ability to establish the evidence of clinical viability is compromised without this input. The heavy, complex, and overwhelming systems for collecting and managing data simply make them untenable in the work life of the knowledge worker, especially given the myriad clinical pressures constraining his or her time. Continuing emphasis on the development of portability through the use of mobile data devices, remote data access, and handheld devices is essential to creating ease-of-use conditions that satisfy the point-of-service user who needs ready access to critical and real-time data. It is the obligation of managers, in their role of creating and enabling context for evidentiary practices, to make sure that such data processes are both available and useful. If the point-of-service utility of data management systems does not advance, the currently great distance between truly effective evidence-based processes and clinical practices will be sustained over a long period of time (Geisler, Krabbendam, & Schuring, 2003).

Building effective analytics calls for organizations to recalibrate the way in which they collect and integrate data. In hospitals, for example, financial, flow, patient, and clinical performance data should not be looked at as separable elements. Instead, they should be viewed as representing distinct components of essentially the same data set. Each of these elements of data affects the others, thereby providing multiple sources of related information for guiding decision making and action (Locsin, 2001). From a purely business perspective, clinical requirements generated from patient assessment have a direct and immediate impact on financial considerations; they influence how hospitals will get paid for those activities because they invariably fall both under and outside the auspices of third-party payers. This, in turn, has a direct impact on both the patient and the organization—one that can be ignored only at the peril of both. Evidence-based management requires knowing the value of these interfaces, recognizing how the implications of the data may affect both the business and the practices of the organization, and subsequently taking the requisite actions necessary to positively problem-solve (Jurewicz & Cutler, 2003). Laying the foundation for analytics as a process for linking and integrating the business of care with the practice of care is essential to generate practitioner-centered values that directly relate to the patients that practitioners serve, the decisions they make, and the positive outcomes they attempt to achieve. It is especially important in the transformation to a higher level of digital processes and resources that health-care work remain a human-relational process that enhances health and well-being and not a robotic process that eliminates the need for human contact, understanding of social situations, and the individual persona. Thoughts on the human–technology interface should be considered in the creation of a data management infrastructure.

▶ Technology and Human Integration

The interface between humans and technology is now of great concern and interest to both patients and healthcare workers. There is great interest in new devices and software that is coupled with concern for health care becoming too impersonal or robotic. Algorithms are emerging to support decision making in new and creative ways (Frick, 2015); however, human judgment must still be the cornerstone for patient care. As new technologies are introduced into the marketplace, individuals are inundated with new devices and software applications believed to enhance the value of healthcare services. Decision making for the addition of software or devices necessarily follows an evidentiary process. Evidence that the additional technology will provide additional value to the organization is often not readily available, in spite of overwhelming enthusiasm about the additional technology from an emotional perspective. The creation of human-centered technologies has assisted many health populations in monitoring diseases such as diabetes and hypertension, patient safety alerts, and stress management sensors. Robots are now entering health care to do many standardized tasks, and some even have artificial intelligence capacity. An essential consideration in choosing technology in a complex organization is how to retain a balance of humanness in a highly technological world. Individuals in highly technological environments must work hard to avoid total reliance on technology and, at the same time, envision a better future.

▶ Overcoming Dogma and Belief

Increasing one's capacity can only be done with the addition of more hours—or with the elimination of nonvalued work. No matter how intensely one wishes to do more with less, that is not possible. It is about doing only work that results in value for the user of the healthcare system. To be sure, the process of eliminating non-value-added work is often blocked by historical dogma and beliefs. Past practice, historical precedent, dogma, belief, and ideology serve to create a contextual framework that informs action. Professions—most notably, nursing and medicine—have long historical attachments to process in the memories, mythologies, fantasies, and stories that create an idealization of practice and a disconnect from fact and reality (Anderson & Willson, 2008). For example, the traditional attachment to policy and procedure now represents a significant impediment to building evidence-based systems and infrastructure. Policy and procedure are anathema to evidentiary processes representing a mental model and organizational framework that operate with constructs demonstrating a polar difference from the ones that now represent the fluidity of information management and clinical decision making (Birch, 2007; Oostendorp, 2003). Reliance on policy and procedural constructs represents an understanding of practice as being part of a fixed operational and clinical system. Policy and procedural constructs demonstrate a belief that change is external, incremental, and situational—none of which, as we now know, holds true. Individuals now must purposefully give consideration to elimination of existing work that might be duplicative, outmoded, or nonvalue producing. Eliminating duplicative or unnecessary work is one of the more difficult tasks for the team. Too often, emotional attachment or personal interest in tasks becomes the primary rationale for retaining duplicative or ineffective processes. At some point the team needs to work together to collaboratively abandon those processes. Failing to eliminate dogmatic practices and unnecessary work obstructs or negates the new work as it becomes burdensome and perceived as an add-on.

▶ Caveat: Beware of Motivation Strategies

There is one final thought about the work in creating and assessing one's infrastructure for evidence and innovation (**BOX 6-3**). If the forces of motivation were understood and the research related to those forces were incorporated into management capacity, managers might spend more of their resources and energy on creating the conditions of alignment (Barry, Murcko, & Brubaker, 2002; Fottler, Ford, & Heaton, 2002). Aligning individual motivations with organizational goals has a much longer history of well-researched validation than do efforts at employee motivation (Gottlieb, 2003; Lencioni, 2002). Creating both the infrastructure and the expectation of alignment of individual behaviors with organizational goals requires a particular set of skills, including ownership, engagement, investment, and strong-linked and integrated efforts at performance evaluation and course correction (Malloch & Porter-O'Grady, 2006). Good evidence suggests that efforts in this arena have a direct payoff in terms of accomplishment and outcomes. No such body of evidence has been uncovered for organizational efforts at employee motivation.

BOX 6-3 Evidence-Based Motivation: Truth

You cannot motivate anyone to do anything! People are already motivated. However, their motivation may not be aligned with group goals. The role of the leader is to create this alignment, not to motivate people.

🔍 *CASE EXAMPLE*

John Stanton, RN, MBA, is the critical care director for a small healthcare organization in the Midwest. He has reviewed the national driving forces for healthcare reform and believes he has a good understanding of them. He believes changes are needed in his organization, and he is unsure where to start to determine what needs to be changed and where innovation would be needed. John is also uncertain about the innovation competencies of his team members. He believes all the key stakeholders should be involved in this assessment. He would like to have a list of questions to begin the discussion. He formulated the following list to present to the team to begin the process.

Using the valued outcomes diagram as a focal point, John planned to ask individuals to share their perceptions of the level of understanding for each of these concepts:

- Personal knowledge:
  - What does complexity mean to you as a caregiver?
  - Share an innovation experience that you believe was successful.
  - How is your role unique as a member of this unit?
  - What interventions that you do are directly linked to patient improvement?
  - What measures do you think are important to evaluate the quality of your care?
- System perceptions:
  - How ready do you believe the organization is for the full implementation of the Patient Protection and Affordable Care Act?
  - What would our unit need to do to provide 100% fully integrated continuum care?
  - Which care processes or interventions that are provided in our unit result in value to the patient?
  - Which care processes do not result in value and could be considered for elimination?

John is hopeful that if he can understand the current level of team member understanding about the drivers for change, the members' unique role contributions, and the nature of value-based health care, he will be able to develop a plan to make evidence-driven improvements and identify opportunities for innovation in his unit.

Questions
1. Do you think John is on the right track?
2. What will be the obstacles to this process?
3. What suggestions would you make to John?

🔍 *CASE EXAMPLE*

Leaders are continually steeped in complexity and change. Several competencies are essential for survival in the contemporary healthcare organization. After reading this chapter, Melissa Rogers, chief nursing executive of a large Southwest healthcare system, believed a leadership development program focusing on complexity was needed for her leaders. Melissa also reviewed additional leadership literature and believed most leaders were transactional in nature. She engaged the shared governance council to share her ideas.

(continues)

🔍 *CASE EXAMPLE*   *(continued)*

The goals of this process included the following:

1. Gain an increased understanding of the basic attributes of complexity science to create a common foundation for all leaders.
2. Develop scenarios that reflect the reality of complexity attributes in routing practice to demonstrate the pragmatic value of learning about complexity and the potential impact of outcomes.
3. Describe the differences between complexity leadership and transactional leadership to further illustrate how leadership behaviors could be more facilitative and less directive as a means to increase team engagement.

The council then created and implemented a yearlong formal plan to engage leaders in learning new behaviors. The plan included didactic online sessions for each leader and monthly team sessions in which complexity leadership scenarios were discussed.

To evaluate the impact of this work, Melissa believed there would be changes in nurse satisfaction and patient engagement. Using your facility satisfaction surveys for both nurses and patients, what specific items do you believe should improve? Can you link the improvement to a specific complexity principle? For example, is an improvement in staff perception of involvement related to a better understanding of the attribute of interrelatedness?

▶ Summary

Changes in communication modalities, new work flow processes, multivariate evaluation measurement variables, innovative outcome expectations, and the quest for clear and visible value are undeniable for organizations. These evolutions reflect the new realities of space, time, structure, and substance. Effective organizational cultures must now support a more pronounced evidentiary work dynamic that fully integrates the contents and interrelationships of the evidence–innovation continuum. This will necessarily result in more effective operations and the continual creation, evaluation, and introduction of new and better ideas.

References

Agency for Healthcare Innovations Exchange. https://innovations.ahrq.gov/

Albrecht, K. (2003). *The power of minds at work: Organizational intelligence in action.* New York, NY: AMACOM.

Allworth, J., Wessel, M., & Levie, A. (2015). 3 questions to get the most out of your company's data. Retrieved from https://hbr.org/2015/01/3-questions-to-get-the-most-out-of-your-companys-data

Anderson, J., & Willson, P. (2008). Clinical decision support systems in nursing: Synthesis of the science for evidence-based practice. *CIN: Computers, Informatics, Nursing, 26*(3), 151–158.

Ang, Y., & Yin, S. (2008). *Intelligent complex adaptive systems.* Chicago, IL: IGI.

Ball, M. J. (2000). *Nursing informatics: Where caring and technology meet* (3rd ed.) New York, NY: Springer.

Barnsteiner, J., Disch, J., & Walton, M. K. (2014). *Person and family centered care.* Indianapolis, IN: Sigma Theta Tau International.

Barry, R., Murcko, A., & Brubaker, C. (2002). *The Six Sigma book for healthcare.* Chicago, IL: Health Administration Press.

Bennis, W., Goleman, D., & Biederman, W. (2008, Fall). Creating a transparent culture. *Leader to Leader,* 21–27.

Birch, D. (2007). *Digital identity management.* Los Angeles, CA: Gower.

Blum, M. (2006). *Continuity, quantum, continuum, and dialectic: The foundational logics of Western historical thinking.* Chicago, IL: Peter Lang.

Boradkar, P. (2010). Transdisciplinary design in the classroom. In T. Porter-O'Grady & K. Malloch (Eds.), *Innovation leadership: Creating the landscape of health care* (pp. 109–133). Sudbury, MA: Jones & Bartlett Learning.

Burns, L. R. (Ed.). (2005). *The business of healthcare innovation.* New York, NY: Cambridge University Press.

Castells, M. (1998). *The information age: Economy, society and culture* (Vol. III). Malden, MA: Blackwell.

Cerni, T., Curtis, G. J., & Colmar, S. H. (2008). Information processing and leadership styles: Constructive thinking and transformational leadership. *Journal of Leadership Studies, 2*(1), 60–73.

Chakravarthy, B. (2003). *Strategy process: Shaping the contours of the field.* Malden, MA: Blackwell.

Christensen, C. M., Anthony, S. P., & Roth, E. A. (2004). *Seeing what's next: Using theories of innovation to predict industry change.* Boston, MA: Harvard Business School Press.

Christensen, C. M., Kaufman, S. P., & Shih, W. C. (2008). Innovation killers: How financial tools destroy your capacity to do new things. *Harvard Business Review, 86*(1), 98–105.

Columbia University. (2017, November 28). *Global leadership in the 21st century at the Columbia University World Leaders Forum.* Retrieved from https://www.youtube.com/watch?v=-dFk7rBeulk

Davenport, T. H., & Harris, J. (2017). *Competing on analytics: The New Science of Winning* (rev. ed.). Boston, MA: Harvard Business Review Press.

Dotlich, D. L., & Cairo, P. C. (2002). *Unnatural leadership: Going against intuition and experience to develop ten new leadership instincts.* San Francisco, CA: Jossey-Bass.

Drucker, P. F. (1985, May/June). The discipline of innovation. *Harvard Business Review, 63,* 67–72

Drucker, P. F. (2001). *The essential Drucker: Selections from the management works of Peter F. Drucker.* New York, NY: HarperBusiness.

Drucker, P., & Stone, N. (1998). *On the profession of management.* Boston, MA: Harvard Business School.

Endsley, S. (2010). Innovation in action: A practical system for getting results. In T. Porter-O'Grady & K. Malloch (Eds.), *Innovation leadership: Creating the landscape of health care* (pp. 59–86). Sudbury, MA: Jones & Bartlett Learning.

Fonseca, J. (2002). *Complexity and innovation in organizations.* London, UK: Routledge.

Fottler, M., Ford, R., & Heaton, C. (2002). *Achieving service excellence.* Chicago, IL: Health Administration Press.

Frandkov, A. (1999). *Nonlinear and adaptive control of complex systems.* New York, NY: Springer.

Freshwater, D., & Rolfe, G. (2004). *Deconstructing evidence based practice.* New York, NY: Routledge.

Frick, W. (2015). Here's why people trust human judgment over algorithms. *Harvard Business Review.* Retrieved from https://hbr.org/2015/02/heres-why-people-trust-human-judgment-over-algorithms

Garvin, D., & Roberto, M. (2001). What you don't know about making decisions. *Harvard Business Review, 79*(9), 108–118.

Geiger-Brown, J., Rogers, V. E., Trinkoff, A. M., Kane, R. L., Bausell, R. B., & Scharf, S. M. (2012). Sleep, sleepiness, fatigue, and performance of 12-hour-shift nurses. *Chronobiology International, 29*(2), 211–219. http://dx.doi.org/10.3109/07420528.2011.645752

Geisler, E., Krabbendam, K., & Schuring, R. (2003). *Technology, health care, and management in the hospital of the future.* Westport, CT: Praeger.

Giacco, A. F. (2003). *Maverick management: Strategies for success.* Newark, NJ: University of Delaware Press.

Goad, T. W. (2002). *Information literacy and workplace performance.* Westport, CT: Quorum Books.

Gottlieb, M. R. (2003). *Managing group process.* Westport, CT: Praeger.

Hesselbein, F. (2002). *Hesselbein on leadership.* San Francisco, CA: Jossey Bass.

Hildreth, P. M., & Kimble, C. (2004). *Knowledge networks: Innovation through communities of practice.* Hershey, PA: Idea Group.

Hooker, C., & Csikszentmihalvi, M. (2003). Rethinking the motivation and structuring of knowledge work. In C. Pearce & J. Conger (Eds.), *Shared leadership: Reframing the hows and whys of leadership* (pp. 217–233). Thousand Oaks, CA: Sage.

Invest Northern Island. (n.d.). Use innovation to start or grow your business. Retrieved from https://www.nibusinessinfo.co.uk/innovationgrowth

Jurewicz, L., & Cutler, T. (2003). *High tech, high touch: Library customer service through technology.* Chicago, IL: American Library Association.

Kelly, T. (2005). *Ten faces of innovation.* New York, NY: Doubleday.

Lencioni, P. (2002). *The five dysfunctions of a team.* San Francisco, CA: Jossey Bass.

Locsin, R. C. (2001). *Advancing technology, caring, and nursing.* Westport, CT: Auburn House.

Malloch, K., & Porter-O'Grady, T. (1999). Partnership economics: Nursing's challenge in a quantum age. *Nursing Economics, 17*(6), 299–307.

Malloch, K., & Porter-O'Grady, T. (2006). *Introduction to evidence-based practice in nursing and health care.* Sudbury, MA: Jones & Bartlett Publishers.

Martin, D. J. (2014). Literature review: Nurse fatigue related to shift length. *Missouri State Board of Nursing Newsletter, 16*(1), 7. Retrieved from http://pr.mo.gov/boards/nursing/publications/newsletters/ 2014-02-01.pdf

McDaniel, C. (2004). *Organizational ethics: Research and ethical environments.* Burlington, VT: Ashgate.

McGlade, J., & Pek, A. (2008, Summer). Spark your creative genius. *Leader to Leader,* 1–15.

McNamara, O. (2002). *Becoming an evidence based practitioner: A framework for teacher–researchers.* New York, NY: Routledge/Falmer.

McSherry, R., Simmons, M., & Abbott, P. (2002). *Evidence informed nursing: A guide for clinical nurses.* New York, NY: Routledge.

Merrifield, R., Calhoun, J., & Stevens, D. (2008). The next revolution in productivity. *Harvard Business Review, 86*(6), 73–80.

Miller, J., & Scott, P. (2007). *Complex adaptive systems: An introduction to computational models of social life.* Princeton, NJ: Princeton University Press.

Mintzberg, H. (1990). The manager's job: Folklore and fact. *Harvard Business Review, 48*(2), 163–176.

Morrison, K. (2007). *Complexity leadership.* Charlotte, NC: Information Age.

Murphy, E., Ruch, S., Pepicello, J., & Murphy, M. (1997). Managing an increasingly complex system. *Nursing Management, 28*(10), 33–38.

Oliver, R. W. (2004). *What is transparency?* New York, NY: McGraw-Hill.

Oostendorp, H. V. (2003). *Cognition in a digital world.* Mahwah, NJ: Lawrence Erlbaum.

Pidd, M. (2004). *Systems modeling: Theory and practice.* Hoboken, NJ: John Wiley & Sons.

Plsek, P. E. (1997). *Creativity, innovation and quality.* Milwaukee, WI: ASQ Quality Press.

Porter-O'Grady, T. (2000). Interdisciplinary shared governance: A partnership model for high performance in a managed care environment. *Seminars for Nurse Managers, 8*(3), 158–169.

Porter-O'Grady, T., & Afable, R. (2003). The technology of partnership. *Health Progress, 84*(3), 41–52.

Price, T. L. (2006). *Understanding ethical failures in leadership.* New York, NY: Cambridge University Press.

Reinhardt, W., Schmidt, B., Sloep, P., & Drachsler, H. (2011). Knowledge worker roles and actions—results of two empirical studies. *Knowledge and Process Management, 18*(3), 150–174. http://dx.doi.org/10.1002/kpm.378

Rogers, A. E. (2002). Sleep deprivation and the ED night shift. *Journal of Emergency Nursing, 28,* 1–2.

Rouse, W. (2007). Complex engineered, organizational and natural systems: Issues underlying the complexity of systems and fundamental research needed to address these issues. *Systems Engineering, 10*(3), 260–271.

Scharmer, O., & Kaufer, K. (2000). Universities as the birthplace for the entrepreneuring human being. Retrieved from http://www.ottoscharmer.com/docs/articles/2000_Uni21us.pdf

Shan, Y., & Ang, Y. (2008). *Applications of complex adaptive systems.* Hershey, PA: IGI.

Shumpeter, J. (1943). *Capitalism, socialism, and democracy.* New York, NY: Harper.

Smith, P. (2004). *Shaping the facts: Evidence based nursing and health care.* New York, NY: Churchill Livingstone.

Solomons, N. M. (2016). *A relational view of hospital and post-acute staff communication and adherence to evidence-based transitional care* (Unpublished dissertation). Arizona State University, Phoenix, AZ.

Solow, D., & Szmerekovsky, J. (2006). The role of leadership: What management science can give back to the study of complex systems. *Emergence: Complexity and Organizations, 8*(4), 52–60.

Stacey, R. (2007). *Complexity and the experience of leading organizations.* New York, NY: Routledge.

Stimpfel, A. W., Lake, E. T., Barton, S., Gorman, K. C., & Aiken, L. H. (2013). How differing shift lengths relate to quality outcomes in pediatrics. *Journal of Nursing Administration, 43*(2), 95–100.

Suh, N. P. (2005). *Complexity: Theory and applications.* New York, NY: Oxford University Press.

Sveiby, K. (1997). *The new organizational wealth.* San Francisco, CA: Berrett-Koehler.

Tourish, D., & Hargie, O. (2004). *Key issues in organizational communication.* New York, NY: Routledge.

Trompenaars, A., & Hampden-Turner, C. (2002). *21 leaders for the 21st century: How innovative leaders manage in the digital age.* New York, NY: McGraw-Hill.

Vaitheeswaran, V. (2007, October 11). *A survey of innovation: A discussion with Vijay Vaitheeswaran of* The Economist [Audio podcast]. Retrieved from http://www.economist.com/node/9934754

Wager, K., Wickham, F., & Glaser, J. (2005). *Managing healthcare information systems: A practical approach for healthcare executives.* San Francisco, CA: Jossey-Bass.

Watkins, S. (2004). 21st-century corporate governance: The growing pressure on the board toward a corporate solution. In R. P. Gandossy & J. A. Sonnefeld (Eds.), *Leadership and governance from the inside out* (pp. 27–36). New York, NY: John Wiley & Sons.

Weberg, D. (2010). Transformational leadership and staff retention: An evidence review with implications for healthcare systems. *Nursing Administration Quarterly, 34*(3), 246–258.

Whitehurst, J. (2015). Be a leader who can admit mistakes. Retrieved from https://hbr.org/2015/06/be-a-leader-who-can-admit-mistakes

Whittingham, R. B. (2003). *The blame machine: Why human error causes accidents.* Boston, MA: Elsevier.

Wolper, L. F. (2004). *Health care administration: Planning, implementing, and managing organized delivery systems* (4th ed.). Sudbury, MA: Jones & Bartlett Publishers.

Yin, S., & Ang, Y. (2008). *Applications of complex adaptive systems.* Chicago, IL: IGI.

Zimmerman, B., Lindberg, C., & Plsek, P. (1998). *Edgeware.* Irving, TX: VHA.

CHAPTER 7

Shifting Workforce Paradigms: From Quantity to Value-Driven Staffing Using Evidence and Innovation

Kathy Malloch and Tim Porter-O'Grady

The enterprise that does not innovate inevitably ages and declines. And in a period of rapid change such as the present . . . the decline will be fast.

— **Peter Drucker**

CHAPTER OBJECTIVES

Upon completion of this chapter, the reader will be able to:

1. Examine the driving forces and current challenges requiring change in health care.
2. Develop insights into an innovative healthcare value model as the infrastructure to improve nurse staffing adequacy.
3. Assess the clinical productivity model as a strategy to integrate disciplines across the continuum.

▶ Introduction

Since this chapter was written, the persistent issues about nurse satisfaction with staffing continue. Little has been updated in research publications related to nurse staffing models, which leaves us with the principles for evidence-driven value-based staffing as presented in this chapter. This work is about the processes to address the goal of appropriate staffing that results in minimal adverse outcomes to our patients and caregivers. As an innovator, each of us needs to explore the negative issues of staffing and ponder what new and creative solutions are needed. Or perhaps staffing is routinely adjusted and managed at the facility level, and the problem is not as critical as we once believed. If not, there is another approach that is worth considering and would require a significant disruption in our healthcare organizations. Sharmer (2017) worked at Massachusetts Institute of Technology to address the global issue of climate change, which in many perspectives may be similar to addressing adequate staffing in healthcare facilities. Consider the discussion on shifting social fields and reflect if there is a possibility to apply this approach along with the content in this chapter to continue our journey.

Discussion: Five Conditions for Shifting Social Fields

Participants are identified from diverse backgrounds, positions, and accountabilities with a desire to create profound individual and institutional innovation and change. Participants remain in their existing jobs and meet in small coaching circles over 15 months' time. Expert facilitators come from global finance, data-driven science, mindful systems change, systems dynamics, and experiential learning environments. Participants are asked to identify:

1.   What year would there be improvement?
2.   What year would measurable improvements be recognized?
3.   What are the projected financial contributions for all participants?

From this work over the course of 15 months, participants realized it was difficult to change practices as they recommended doing the same thing in their first problem-solving session. Dysfunctional posturing occurred regularly as silos were reinforced before a more global solution could be embraced.

Participants and expert facilitations recognized five conditions for social change or the center of gravity in a system to change:

1.   A container for stakeholders for innovative interactions—a safe space for change.
2.   Science or data from which to move past everyone's favored opinion.
3.   Dialogue to close the feedback loop between collective action and awareness, or rather make the system see itself for what it is.
4.   Visualization and perception of the issue from an aesthetic perspective, specifically, the viewable impact of the problem.
5.   Facilitation that holds the transformative space ever-present and avoids back sliding.

Thought for consideration: Is there an innovative, more global approach to addressing the persistent, unresolved problem of nurse staffing?

Background

Providing adequate caregivers and staff support for patient needs is foundational for effective healthcare organizations, clinics, and home care settings to be able to achieve valued outcomes. This work is complex and clearly affected by emerging evidence, new technology, innovative ideas, and the existing organizational culture in which care is provided. In this chapter the driving forces requiring change, the new opportunities that support innovations in healthcare delivery, challenges and obstacles to progress, and a value-based approach for more effective care from an evidentiary perspective, as well as the anticipated outcomes from this value-driven model, are presented. The content of this chapter focuses on available evidence as the foundational content for effective work and identifies gaps in knowledge or the absence of evidence as opportunities for innovation and innovative strategies. Challenges in advancing this work should be viewed not as obstacles but rather as opportunities to tap into the infinite wisdom of healthcare colleagues and move forward with energy and enthusiasm in changing health care for the better. The interactive dynamic of evidence and innovation provides a purposeful framework from which to view this work.

The key to success is for you to make a habit throughout your life of doing the things you fear.

—Vincent Van Gogh

▶ Driving Forces for Change and Innovation in Staffing

There are numerous drivers and incentives to improve not only the management of nurse staffing but also the overall quality of the healthcare experiences that are nearly always affected by the quality of nurse staffing. Several regulatory and accrediting agency drivers that are facilitating significant change in the way health care is delivered include the Centers for Medicare and Medicaid Services (CMS), the Health and Medicine Division (HMD), and the Institute for Healthcare Improvement (IHI).

The CMS road map for value-based purchasing (CMS, n.d.) and the Medicare Modernization Act and the Deficit Reduction Act have shifted the government from a passive payer of services to an active purchaser of higher-quality, affordable care. The overall intent of these regulations is to promote efficiency in resource use while providing high-quality care in settings such as hospitals, home health, nursing homes, and medical homes. Nursing is a significant part of resource allocations and necessarily must embrace more effective, evidence-driven ways of providing care.

CMS has also advocated for and legislated improvements in care coordination, alignment of financial incentives with outcomes, adoption of electronic health records, e-prescribing, increases in the percentage of population-based payment, and joint team accountability for outcomes (CMS, 2015; Welton, 2010). The meaningful use initiative now requires increasing levels of electronic documentation.

The IHI identified the Triple Aim of simultaneously improving population health, improving the patient experience of care, and reducing costs per capita as the expectation for transformed healthcare systems (2012). The Triple Aim has become an organizing framework for the U.S. National Quality Strategy. Improvements in nurse staffing and resource use are essential in supporting the Triple Aim.

▶ New Opportunities

In addition to the driving forces, there are several advances that provide opportunities to improve the healthcare system. These include an increased evidentiary focus, technology advances, and increasing consumerism focusing on value.

Evidentiary Focus

Much attention has been given to staffing based on evidence or research that has tested and validated practices. A critical mass of research supporting the presence of registered nurses in hospitals is now recognized. Nurses educated at the baccalaureate level also have a positive impact or decrease patient mortality (Aiken, Clark, Cheung, Sloane, & Silber, 2003; Aiken, Clark, Sloane, Sochalski, & Silber, 2002; American Nurses Association, 2017; Buerhaus, Donelan, Ulrich, Norman, DesRoches, & Dittus 2007; Kane, Shamliyan, Mueller, Duval, & Wilt, 2007; Lang, Hodge, & Olson, 2004; Needleman, Buerhaus, Mattke, Stewart, & Zelevinsky, 2002; Needleman, Buerhaus, Pankratz, Leibson, Stevens, & Harris, 2011; Savitz, Jones, & Bernard, 2005; Tourangeau, Cranley, & Jeffs, 2006; Upenieks, Akhavan, Kotlerman, Esser, & Ngo, 2007; White, 2006). Further, new science specific to healthcare organizations in the Magnet Recognition Program shows better patient outcomes on mortality measures and significantly better outcomes compared to non-Magnet hospitals (Friese, Xia, Chaferi, Birkmeyer, & Banerjee, 2015).

New science for staffing specific to clinical specialties, skill mix, environmental influences, and the linkage of staffing models to clinical outcomes is being developed and published regularly (Malloch, 2015; Needleman et al., 2011). In addition to new staffing science is evidence for HMD interprofessional practice (IPP). IPP has an impact on patient safety, provider and patient satisfaction, quality of care, community health outcomes, and cost savings, as well as a direct impact on the relationship among interprofessional education (IPE) and patient, population, and system outcomes (Institute of Medicine, 2015).

Value research is also emerging. The Agency for Healthcare Research and Quality (AHRQ) has advanced value research, which focuses on finding a way to achieve greater value in health care with cost and waste reductions while maintaining or improving quality (AHRQ, 2015)

Technology Advancements

Advances in technology continue to emerge for both patient care delivery and the management of information. With the introduction of the electronic health record, platforms for the management of large data sets are now available as well as the introduction of standardized clinical language. The standardized language further supports data comparisons across settings and enables providers to coordinate and collaborate more easily on patient care, which can improve healthcare outcomes and enable providers to achieve performance standards (CMS, n.d.).

Consumerism

Finally, users of the healthcare system are more involved than ever. Person- and family-centered care is now the expectation (Barnsteiner, Disch, & Walton, 2014), whereby persons are empowered, actively participate, and are informed of all costs and the anticipated value of services. Both provider and healthcare organization performance metrics, as well as Hospital Consumer Assessment of Healthcare Providers and Systems (HCAHPS) scores, are published regularly. Consumers also access staffing data for healthcare facilities on a routine basis. The importance and utility of a personal health record continues to increase. Users of the healthcare system want their information consolidated into one file and readily accessible when needed. User ownership and management of one's personal health record is now an expectation of increasing numbers of patients. These opportunities, along with other driving forces, continue to support the case for value-based health care, of which staffing is an integral part.

Embedded within each of these initiatives are issues and concerns about the availability and productivity of nursing resources. As previously noted, the work of changing current systems and practices is complex and requires courage, persistence, and evidence to shift the current trajectory. While there is supporting evidence for this journey, there are also obstacles and challenges that must be reckoned with. The obstacles or challenges to this work are discussed in the next section.

▶ Challenges and Obstacles to Change

There are many challenges and obstacles within the healthcare system that make it difficult to move forward with improvements to the healthcare system. Despite the clear and convincing theoretical rationale for system change, it is often ignored. These obstacles to making the needed transformation happen cannot be dismissed or taken lightly. Creating a new healthcare model requires support, passion, evidence, and resources. For many healthcare leaders, the process involved in making a significant system change is far too complex to embrace. Many leaders will struggle with any modification of the current system under the misguided notion that the system is functional and provides the appropriate information to make decisions supportive of quality patient care outcomes. In this section, several of these challenges will be discussed. The control and influence of the existing powerful organizational infrastructures over nursing resource allocation, coupled with the inability of nursing to articulate its specific work and outcomes achieved within the existing productivity framework, the environment of health care, and the determination of productivity using a single metric are imposing obstacles that many may find difficult to challenge.

Historically, services are provided and documented by siloed or individual disciplines and then pasted together into a summative document without identified connections among the individuals contributing to patient care. Most healthcare organizational cultures are steeped in traditions that support the silo mentality and stability of operations.

The historical adequacy of the overarching position of medicine and its specific measures of procedural-based coding and billing have precluded the need for more accurate clinical productivity measures for nursing that are quantifiable, credible, and useful. Unfortunately, the development of appropriate measures for nursing work tend to garner attention only during times of a nursing shortage and nursing dissatisfaction.

Organizations today may struggle to control costs through cost reductions associated with the poorly defined work of nursing, yet the need for competently educated practitioners remains significant. Despite the increases in nursing education and the increasing complexity of nursing work, clarity in the work of nursing and appropriate workforce measures have not emerged to achieve the desired recognition of the value of nursing work in the marketplace. Because it is poorly defined and described, nursing work is difficult to measure and evaluate, which too often results in uncertain patient outcomes. When attempts are made to decrease or increase nursing resources for work that is poorly defined, the effects of these measures on patient outcomes is uncertain as well. While it is believed that less nursing care results in poor patient outcomes, such conclusions are not universally supported. The lack of evidence identifying the specific interventions of nursing and their implications for patient outcomes must be addressed. Tallying simple hours of care, without delineating the actual work performed, will not produce data that can be confidently correlated to patient outcomes, whether those outcomes are positive or negative. Describing the work of nursing from an evidence-based perspective is the first step in the process; the second step, integrating these principles into practice, is evolutionary and ongoing.

Inconsistent Identification of the Work of Nursing

Not all work of nursing is visible and measurable; intuition, caring behaviors, and trust are essential in the provision of care and yet are not readily captured in traditional knowledge worker models or productivity systems. The tangible work of nursing is more easily measured than intangible work. While the work of nursing is defined in each state's nurse practice act and professional standards of the American Nurses Association (ANA), each organization has created unique models and frameworks to guide the practice of nursing. Most frequently, the frameworks are based on body system checklists and assessments. Few organizations focus on nursing care interventions on the basis of practice acts or professional standards.

Another challenge is the work that nurses actually do during their work time. A high percentage of time is spent on activities not related to direct patient care. In a Hill-Rom study of acute care organizations, approximately 85% of nurses' time was spent on direct and indirect activities that did not move the patient along the care path (Lanser, 2001). Murphy (2003) reported that wasteful work—including excessive documentation requirements; inefficient shift-to-shift or departmental reports; and searching for colleagues, supplies, and equipment—consumed 35% of hospital employees' time. More recently, the Advisory Board Company identified that nurses spend 25% of their time on indirect patient care (2012).

Another aspect of this challenge is that nurses find it quite difficult to give up any of their current nursing work because all work is believed to be valuable and appropriate. Non-value-added work includes both direct and indirect nursing work and work resulting from system inefficiencies. The following examples identify tasks that do not provide value to patient outcomes:

- Provision of patient education to patients who are historically noncompliant: It is unrealistic to expect that an 80-year-old diabetic patient will become enlightened and change his or her behaviors in an acute care setting. Extensive reviews and presentation of information in these situations serve only to complete checklists and provide inappropriate feelings of accomplishment. Brief, meaningful encounters with known noncompliant patients are necessary to check for new interest; however, this is more effective in post-acute-care settings. In the value equation, unrealistic interventions render the equation out of balance given the lack of outcomes and overuse of scarce resources associated with these efforts.

- Frequency of vital signs: When a patient has consistent and stable vital signs, is it necessary to repeat these measures every 4 hours, especially when caregivers are present who can monitor the patient?
- Telemetry monitoring: Is all telemetry monitoring value based? Is the intervention of telemetry monitoring linked to improvements in the patient's status, and is it an effective use of available resources? Or is telemetry monitoring used for routine patient oversight?
- Searching for equipment and supplies: Does this task promote the patient's movement along the healing continuum?
- Passing out meal trays: Is this the best use of a nurse's time? Should someone from another division or support staff handle this task?
- Searching for other providers and colleagues: Is this an appropriate task for nurses?
- Replenishing procedure carts and monitoring levels in supply rooms: Do these activities directly affect the patient?
- Searching for information and reference manuals: Can this task be managed differently?

Lack of Linkage Between Nurse Actions and Patient Outcomes

The next challenge is not only the lack of linkage between nurse work and patient outcomes but also the inconsistent use of linkage evidence that is available. The evidence supporting a relationship among caregiver performance, patient outcomes, and financial performance is strong (Aiken et al., 2003; Aiken, Smith, & Lake, 1994; Blegen & Vaughn, 1998; Cho, Ketefian, Barkauskas, & Smith, 2003; McCue, Mark, & Harless, 2003). Evidence supporting the relationships among variables in the organizational structure and patient outcomes has also been identified. Unfortunately, the intervening specific work processes that produce those outcomes have not been clearly articulated nor are they embedded in the analysis of these relationships.

The challenge in identifying truly valued work is coupled with the reality that evidence is lacking to support some interventions that may, indeed, positively affect patient outcomes. The historic lack of connection between the economic viability of the organization and its effects on the satisfaction and performance of its nursing resource is an untenable factor in the future consideration of the viability of healthcare organizations. The failure to clearly tie practice elements and activities to specifically defined outcomes makes it exceptionally difficult to identify any unique and specified value for nursing practice. Nurses cannot claim value on one hand and provide little definitive evidence of that value on the other hand.

Too many nurses ignore the need to balance clinical performance against resource availability and quality outcomes. Because of the history of nursing and its predominant focus on clinical process rather than specific identification with clinical outcome, many nurses have become addicted to process (Hughes & American Nurses Association, 1958). For many nurses, the process has become ritual, routine, and intellectually mindless. Further, experience itself has become a mantra, even though in most cases experience tends to be a limitation; the more experience one has, the more one is inculcated in the values that experience provides (Smith, 2002). *Competent* practice is *changing* practice. As technology enhancements and innovations continually challenge the foundations of clinical practice, it is the very fluidity, flexibility, and mobility of clinical practice that ensures its continuing viability and efficacy. This blind dependence and valuing of experience over innovation and education must be overcome if meaningful value is to be found and defined (Corey, 2001).

Inconsistent Time Allocations for Nursing Work

There is precious little data about how much time is required for nursing interventions and the recognition of the optimal provider to do this work. The greatest stumbling block for quantification of nursing work is the lack of consensus about the appropriate measurement technique, such as motion and time studies, historical use of nurses' time, and comprehensive assignment analysis methods (Malloch, 2015).

Calculation of time requirements for patient care needs requires more granularity than previously considered. Time considerations for the additional handoff requirements of admissions, discharges, and transfers have been identified and continue to be studied using electronic records. Time for nurse surveillance and nursing care that encompasses oversight of the patient without a specific intervention has also been calculated and linked to adverse patient outcomes when not provided.

Limited Productivity Measurement and Evaluation

The current metric of hours per patient day identifies how long it took for the care to be delivered but not what was done; it is an incomplete representation of the work of nursing that does not incorporate structural and environmental considerations in productivity measures. Relative value unit (RVU) measures attempt to recognize the degree of patient care variation based on a median unit, but they are limited by the description of the value of 1.0 unit. The limited accuracy and completeness of describing 1.0 RVU continues to be problematic because descriptors for all categories of the core work of nursing are not included in this system.

Measurements that are limited to comparisons of total hours worked per patient day and projected budgeted hours can only provide a limited perspective of value. Such comparisons provide no information specific to the level of patient acuity, provision of appropriate interventions, achievement of clinical outcomes, and absence of adverse outcomes—all of which require a framework for productivity measurement based on principles that integrate values of effectiveness, utility, and cost.

Knowing which outcomes resulted from which work performed by which category of caregiver is critical if the profession is to effectively articulate its value and contribution to the health of individuals. Understanding the important relationships among specific work processes and integrating them into the productivity measurement systems of organizations will require new knowledge, new mental models, and commitment to staffing on the basis of evidence or trend data created from best practices.

Unfortunately, this approach and limited analysis have been used in most organizations to measure nurse productivity and to make decisions specific to the allocation of staffing resources. The hours used are typically compared to patient units of service without considering the actual output, which is an essential component of a productivity measure. These traditional productivity measures of hours used per patient day represent a limited analysis and do not reflect the notion of theoretical productivity, which calls for the greatest output for the least input (Drucker, 1990).

Nonsupportive Physical Environment

Pinkerton and Rivers (2001) identified 64 variables that affect nurse staffing needs, including variables specific to interdepartmental interactions, intradepartmental interactions, the care environment, professional competency, physicians, and the external environment. Physical environments are a critical element of the care dynamic itself, not only for patients, but also for providers. Unfortunately, there is wide variability in the use of evidence in the creation and sustaining of current healthcare environments. The building, structural format, color, inclusion of nature, and peaceful aesthetics help create a viable milieu to work within (Ulrich, Quan, Zimring, Joseph, & Choudhary, 2004).

Poorly designed work spaces, heavy equipment, the absence of patient lift equipment, and the lack of noise control have negative impacts on both patients and caregivers. Further, the conditions of stress embedded in clinical work have a tremendous impact on retention and turnover in clinical practice. Nurse fatigue and burnout have been identified as major stressors for both nurses and patients (Geiger-Brown et al., 2012; Martin, 2014; Stimpfel, Lake, Barton, Gorman, & Aiken, 2013).

Mixture of Technology and Minimal Interoperability/ Lack of Actionable Data

The use of multiple applications for clinical documentation and management information requires users to sign in and sign out of multiple applications during their work time. The inefficiencies of isolated applications render the information fragmented and leaves the aggregation of data to the user to obtain meaningful information for clinical decisions. Further, within applications, caregivers are required to review multiple other areas of documentation to determine the status of the patient condition.

Evidence Lacking in Staffing and Assignment Processes

The nurse–patient assignment process has also lacked an evidentiary foundation; namely, matching required hours of patient care to the appropriately competent caregiver. The simplicity of ratio calculations for nurse–patient assignments has overshadowed the benefits (including greater accuracy) that might be realized with the use of multiple data values. Overcoming the deeply entrenched tradition of ratio or grid-based staffing models to create evidence-based processes that recognize and address the daily variations of patient care needs and staff availability requires courage and commitment to the creation of a better system. The obvious simplicity of these historical calculations is antithetical to the real goal of quality patient care. To overcome this resistance, increasing numbers of organizations are selecting computerized database management systems to provide more sophisticated, more complex, and timely data that can be used to develop the next generation of productivity measurements. The reality is that it is difficult to use resources effectively without such systems and evaluations.

Lack of Standardized Language

In attempting to arrive at the truth, I have applied everywhere for information, but in scarcely an instance have I been able to obtain hospital records fit for any purposes of comparisons.

—Florence Nightingale

At one point, the ANA approved 13 standardized languages that support nursing practice, 10 of which are considered languages specific to nursing care (Rutherford, 2008). The use of multiple descriptions for similar concepts is confusing and difficult to automate. Information in healthcare records must be searchable, shared, and synthesized as needed (Warren, 2012). The use of standardized healthcare language requires that the interventions of nursing must be specified and described with sufficient clarity so another researcher or practitioner can replicate the action. Standardized language comprises terminology and communication styles that can be used in all settings by all clinicians, is grounded in clinical practice and research, is functionally appropriate for computerized clinical documentation systems that need to simplify the exchange, and makes it easier to manage and integrate clinical data into the electronic health record. The language must allow for the measurement of patient, family, and community healthcare interventions and outcomes (Moorhead, Johnson, & Maas, 2004).

Although this next section focuses on the work of nursing, it is imperative for all professional and support providers to recognize the current limitations in determining their value and create similar linkages among services and valued outcomes. The proposed innovative model is designed to serve as a framework for the conceptualization of the interrelationships of organizational elements.

A pile of rocks ceases to be a rock pile when somebody contemplates it with the idea of a cathedral in mind.

—Antoine de Saint-Exupéry

▶ The Value Approach: An Innovative Model to Advance Staffing Adequacy

At long last, the rules are changing! Value is now the driver for healthcare work as identified earlier in this chapter. It is now back to the future as healthcare leaders work to achieve the expected value outcomes from an evidentiary paradigm. Considering both the challenges and the opportunities in health care, leaders are well positioned to advance the value model. In this section, the basic components of a healthcare staffing value model are presented (**FIGURE 7-1**). These components

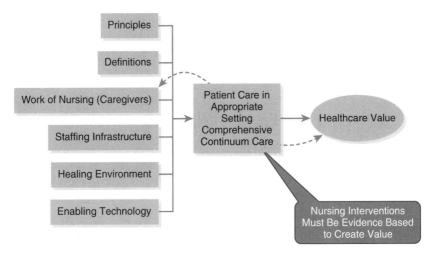

FIGURE 7-1 Healthcare value model mind map: Basic components.

include principles for an evidentiary value model, a description of healthcare value, description and measurement of nursing work using a clinical productivity model, and anticipated outcomes from a value-driven system.

Principles in a Value Model

Foundational principles to guide the development of this innovative model are presented. Principles for designing this model are more effective in a complex and ever-changing world than specific procedures and algorithms. Principles should be longer lasting, and procedures and algorithms change rapidly. The principles include the following:

- Person- and family-focused care is provided within the context of each patient's life position
- Coordinated team efforts are essential for and by providers and patients
- Objective and measurable outcomes are associated with each intervention or strategy
- Providers are selected based on cost and outcomes; the goal is the highest quality and the lowest cost optimizing the full scope of practice for each role
- The environment is supportive of patients and caregivers
- The most current evidence is integrated into this work

Value Definitions

Although there are many definitions of value and value-based health care, the following are simple and reflective of the desired outcome:

- Value is considered as patient health outcomes per dollar spent; value is the only goal that can unite the interests of all system participants. It will require fundamental restructuring of healthcare delivery, not incremental improvements (Porter, 2012).

- Value-based care means safe, appropriate, and effective care with enduring results at a reasonable cost; it means using evidence-based medicine and proven treatments and techniques that take into account the patient's wishes and preferences (Dartmouth-Hitchcock, 2015).

▶ Clarifying the Work of Nursing

The challenge is to create a value-driven model based on evidence for nursing work that includes all valued nursing care, its economic component, and the intangible work that nurses bring to the bedside (Welton, 2011). There are three types of nursing work: objective and observable interventions, intangible interventions or absence factors, and overlapping interventions. All must be included in a staffing productivity model.

The work of nursing is about providing appropriate goal-oriented services rather than providing as many services as possible regardless of the cost and outcomes. Value choices for care, rather than rich choices (choices for care that are nice but not linked to the outcome, such as back rubs twice a day or bed baths for ambulatory patients), that take into account fiscal implications; appropriateness of nursing care specific to outcomes; and goodness of fit, service quality, and patient impact are needed. The process of quantifying and enumerating the work of nursing must be embraced if we are to develop valid and reliable information and systems to guide nurse staffing. This effort will in turn provide credibility within the financial sectors of health care.

To identify value, there also needs to be objective and measurable elements that can be related to outcomes using standardized language to embed in current measurement structures and electronic databases. The description also requires recognition and integration of a societal mandate for nursing, the professional scope of practice, and the economic realities of the marketplace (ANA, 2003). A qualitative, descriptive overview of the work of nursing must include more than just tasks that are easily observed and quantified, such as procedures and administration of medications.

Quantifying the work of nursing using a standardized approach to patient intensity is the foundation for a valid and reliable patient intensity needs system, another important element of an evidence-based workforce management system (ANA, 2008). The patient intensity level used by an organization must reflect the major clinical intervention categories applicable to all clinical specialties. At a minimum, categories specific to the technical work of nursing, monitoring activities, interdisciplinary coordination, communication, and leadership must be represented. Examples of interventions within those categories include patient assessment, medication administration, intravenous access and line management, pain management, safety or restraint management, and interpretation of vital signs.

In addition to these categories, the following must be included:

- Monitoring progress and oversight of patient conditions
- Management of information, namely, knowing not only what to communicate but also to whom and when to communicate
- Patient and family education as well as information management among members of the caregiver team

- Creating and modifying plans of care in a timely manner based on patient conditions
- Leadership behaviors specific to the delegation and supervision of work processes of other staff and precepting new nurses
- Continuum care coordination, namely, coordination of the work of all disciplines caring for the patient

It is clear that to ensure effective resource management, workforce systems must be transformed into evidence-based systems and reflect a prevailing and sustaining reality (ANA, 2012). Optimum nursing care, according to Welton (2011), represents a balance between the intensity and quality of the delivered nursing care, including costs, safety, and outcomes of that care.

Continuum Care Coordination

The work of care coordination has been moved among clinical roles and typically focuses on utilization management or the amount of resources or dollars that are available for a patient. Historical goals have been to avoid overuse of resources at the expense of patient achievement of desired goals. The proposed value model requires the registered nurse to assume the care coordination role across the continuum for several reasons. The nurse is located at the intersection of the provision of all healthcare services. It is the nurse's role to coordinate, integrate, and facilitate all the clinical functions related to the delivery of patient care. Nurses are deeply entrenched in daily processes of relationship management with all patient care team members (e.g., physicians, nurses, managers, allied health personnel, and unlicensed assistive personnel). Experience and collective wisdom emerge from team members who work together effectively. It is vital to recognize nursing's central role, however, as nurses integrate all the work of other disciplines with regard to a patient's progress along the healing continuum. This realization is the key to the clinical success of the entire health organization (While et al., 2004). However, empirical evidence of the critical value of *intersection management*—that is, interdisciplinary coordination—is needed.

Continuum care coordination is a much-needed service for patients within the value model. As previously noted, it has been difficult to determine and quantify the value of those activities that are predominantly focused on coordinating and integrating processes. Because this type of coordination and integration accounts for the majority of professional nursing activity (in terms of value), it is clearly important to provide a financial definition for it (Rubin, Plovnick, & Fry, 1975). Although nursing must clearly delineate its own specific functions and activities, the importance attached to those functions and activities is not gained unilaterally.

Fulfilling the role of care coordination clearly places the nurse in a critical position with regard to the financial and service viability of the organization. In addition, elements of high levels of quality in the delivery of clinical service are influenced and often coordinated by nursing professionals. Nurses are the eyes of all other providers; in this eyes-and-ears role, nurses evaluate the patient's condition, response, and progress in a timely fashion. Therefore, in a high-level interface, nurses have a direct and powerful impact on the clinical and service viability of the organization. Through this direct relationship, nurses control the financial variables that ultimately affect the economic viability of the organization as a whole (Finkler & Graf, 2001).

Missed Nursing Care

Missed nursing care must also be considered. Examination of nursing from the opposite side of the outcome—namely, from the time before nursing occurred or in the absence of nursing as it is now known—is both illustrative and enlightening to assist in the description of nursing. When nursing is absent, it is not merely medications that are not administered and dressings that are not changed; much more occurs. What is lost is subtle at first and then overwhelmingly thunderous. Patients are not monitored regularly for condition changes; failure to rescue is common, and emergency codes occur; condition changes are not communicated to physicians; care is not coordinated; patient knowledge is not improved; and measures of preventable conditions, such as pressure ulcers, urinary tract infections, pneumonia, and length of stay, all increase—these are the intangible interventions that need to be described and included as nurse work. Kalish (2014) has identified nine elements of regularly missed care: ambulation, turning, delayed or missed feedings, patient teaching, discharge planning, emotional support, hygiene, intake and output documentation, and surveillance. Failing to fully account for the work of nursing and to be sure that there is not missed care will compromise the integrity of the value model.

DISCUSSION

Nurses in your department believe there is much nursing care that is missed. What is available in your current systems to determine what has not been done? How would you propose to determine if discharge planning has been missed? Or if hygiene has been missed and how often it has been missed? After you quantify this information, how can you use the clinical productivity model to ensure that the care will not be missed in the future? Finally, how were patient outcomes affected in light of missed care?

Overlapping Patient Care

The nature of nursing practice should be closely examined to better understand the boundaries of nursing; that is, boundaries that overlap with other disciplines and boundaries that are unique to the nursing profession. The work of care coordination, assessment, planning, and identified procedures should be retained by nurses, and activities of daily living, vital sign monitoring in many situations, and administration of routine medications should be delegated and shared with appropriate disciplines, such as paramedics, nursing assistants, and licensed practical nurses (Pittman & Forrest, 2015; Rheaume & Belliveau, 2015).

Some of the work performed by nurses can be performed by other disciplines or support staff. Nursing will have an especially difficult time in meeting the obligations of discipline-specific definitions if it continues to perform these tasks without further evaluation and efforts to ensure the highest quality of care at the lowest cost. Examples of overlapping interventions include vital sign monitoring, activities of daily living, and medication administration in selected settings. The challenges for nursing derive from its historical commitment to the process and its lack of a clearly defined relationship to clinical outcomes. The more valuable activity for nursing in undertaking this process will be to assess the time commitments related to coordinating, integrating, and facilitating the clinical work of all the disciplines, then assign a specific value to that time and effort. Important to this process, which will put nursing farther along the road to adoption of an evidence-based format, is attention to the following factors:

- Establishing a clear value for the support functions of managing supplies and equipment for nurse work.
- Enumerating the type and character of coordinative and integrative activities that are fundamental to the role of the nurse.
- Specifically identifying particular clinical practice standards and professional performance characteristics against which value can be established so the outcomes indicated by them can be more clearly defined.
- Creating a method (formula) for determining costs and value related specifically to the clinical and coordinative activities undertaken at the point of service that reflect the standard of practice identified there.

The elimination of non-value-added work also provides more time for nurses to give comfort to and talk with patients, develop and update plans of care, and provide patient and family education—all types of work that are typically foregone when time is scarce.

Creating Linkages Between Work and Value for the Patient

After the work of nursing is described, its linkage to patient outcomes and available resources must be established. A specifically defined tie among clinical tasks, best practices, and the payment formats within which they are financed is an essential element of the value model. The value equation in which clinical practice, performance outcomes, and the available payment structure are examined serves as a template to assess the overall value of the nursing work (Malloch & Porter-O'Grady, 1999). Desirable outcomes of nursing interventions include achievement of clinical goals, improvement in the ability to manage one's own health, and a safe environment as measured by the absence of adverse outcomes. Examples of outcomes specific to nursing that affect not only the patient but also the conditions that influence a patient's health include the following:

- Increased ability to provide self-care
- Improved mobility
- Improved stress management and coping skills
- Improved knowledge of clinical condition
- Improved knowledge of healthy behaviors specific to nutrition and mobility
- Improved parenting skills
- Community health and well-being
- Improved knowledge of behaviors for safety specific to health care

The purpose of quantification of caregiver work is to develop information to extend the current productivity system that identifies the direct link among the evidence-based work of caregivers, value-based outcomes, and payment. Necessarily, this effort requires quantification of the specific work and the link or relationship of the work to the achievement of desired value-based outcomes. The health status of the patient must be affected positively to justify the resource expenditure.

DISCUSSION

Achieving value in healthcare organizations begins at the unit or shift level. Using the value equation, resources will result in the desired clinical outcome for the patient, a group of nurses in a Magnet organization decided to see if their pain management service resulted in value for the patients. Nurses were aware that the revenue for this unit exceeded budget targets, and the hours for nurse staffing were within the budgeted allocation. As the team discussed this process of value analysis, they realized that patient feedback specific to sustainable pain relief was not a metric considered in evaluating the program.

- What is your reaction to this scenario?
- What changes do you think are necessary to determine the value of this program to patients?
- If the revenue and hours of nursing care were over budget and the patients experienced significant relief from their pain, what would be the next steps in your assessment of the pain clinic?
- Are there other areas of patient care in which this analysis would be similar?

To clearly delineate nursing value, it is crucial to utilize the prevailing methodology, which uses payment factors as a part of value determination. The most obvious unit of value is the Diagnosis-Related Group (DRG), the predominant value unit that is used for payment in healthcare organizations. No matter which approach is ultimately identified and used, it must be consistent, be reducible to financial value, integrate and link the contributions of the healthcare disciplines, and be useful as an evaluative and comparative mechanism. In addition, it should provide an opportunity to evaluate the criteria, performance, and impact of medical practice.

Finally, there are several tools to examine the value of nursing in addition to clinical outcomes. These analyses can further document the value of nursing care. Each method is based on specific goals (Stone, Curran, & Bakken, 2002); these tools include the following:

- Financial metric of cost minimization: Costs are compared among alternatives only; equal effects are assumed; no outcomes are measured
- Value metric of cost effectiveness: Consequences are measured in the same units among alternatives; outcomes are measured using ratios such as expenditures/outcome or dollars/life years gained
- Value metric of cost utility: Effects include both quantity and quality measures; measures are dollars or quality of life years gained
- Financial metric of cost benefit: Effects are measured as a single dollar measure; measures are in dollars gained
- Value metric of cost consequences: Costs and effects are listed separately; effects among alternatives may have different measures; expenditures and a separate list of outcomes are measured

Each of these evaluation methods offers a different lens through which to view the work of nursing. Ultimately, a combination of several methods is likely to better represent nursing work based on the intended goals and resources.

Supporting Effective Staffing Infrastructure Elements

To achieve staffing adequacy, specific organizational infrastructure elements are needed. The first is appropriate caregiver resources, that is, competent caregivers and support staff to meet identified patient care needs. The staffing infrastructure also includes a scheduling system, patient needs system, and time and attendance systems that are preferably interconnected and interoperative so that staffing adequacy can be obtained. The following elements are essential components within an effective staffing system:

- Nursing time required to perform identified care (Malloch, 2015)
- Appropriate skill and competence of each caregiver, addressing the overlapping of selected interventions by different disciplines
- Performance standards, including levels of expectations for clinical competence, differentiation among provider levels, and clearly delineated performance expectations for specific patient populations or DRGs
- Nurse–patient assignment criteria and a staffing adjustment process that addresses changes in patient conditions and needs
- Understanding of environmental factors affecting staffing and the cost factors associated with delivery of care
- Available resources (supplies, equipment, medication, etc.) for each patient

Supportive Environment

There are several considerations for the environment of care. First is a culture with supportive leadership embracing engagement, openness, and valuing of the clinical provider as a key aspect of creating an appropriate supporting structure. A host of considerations must be taken into account in regard to the physical work environment and its impact on risk and safety from both providers' and patients' perspectives. These issues also exert a powerful effect on the cost of providing service and the ability to create an environment that establishes a marketable relationship between the organization and those whom it serves. Much evidence supports the existence of a close relationship between environmental issues of safety and clinical error rates. As a consequence, fiscal and service leaders should make a clear distinction of the costs associated with these environmental and structural factors. Also, these factors should be incorporated into any data analysis related to productivity and work value determinations.

The Center for Health Design's Pebble Project model addresses issues including the desirability of the environment for the patient; the market value of a healing environment to the community; and the fiscal impact of reducing length of stay, care intensity, and patient need. According to this model, creating a physical environment that facilitates healing is as important as other influences on cost (Berry et al., 2004).

Environmental considerations are critical in establishing evidence of the environment's influence on clinical practice as well as economics and health service costs. In building an evidentiary value model, the following issues and relationships should be considered:

- Identification of specific healing, comfort, and patient satisfaction considerations related to the physical environment and structural context for care
- Delineation of the structural and organizational (delivery system) considerations affecting clinical practice and specific elements of work flow

- Enumeration of the impact of physical plant, environment, and structures on provider attitudes, satisfaction, and turnover rates
- Determination of the impact of environment and structure on issues of clinical error, patient safety, and circumstances of care
- Incorporation of structural and environmental considerations in productivity measures and formulas associated with appropriate resource use and service time values

Enabling Information Technology Platform for Data Management

The development of a data management system that collects, sorts, and provides reports in an easy-to-access format is essential in an evidentiary model. Using an evidence-based framework to determine optimal productivity, patient–staff ratios, clinical assignments, provider categories, and relationships to patient outcomes is now fundamental in efforts to accurately determine value and its effects on quality and cost (Harrington & Estes, 2004). Indeed, the accuracy of the financial data pertaining to the clinical relationship between patient and provider is now an essential construct of appropriate, meaningful, and sustainable delivery of clinical services. Failing to include these environmental and structural considerations in the determination of productivity and clinical care not only contributes to a lack of cost control but also facilitates the inappropriate and possibly expensive use of unevaluated human resources.

A new productivity metric is needed that reflects the complex work involved in the practice of nursing. This new metric would replace the traditional comparison of hours worked to hours budgeted. Metrics that reflect the output of care compared to the input of providers and are adjusted for environmental factors provide a more accurate representation of nursing productivity.

An integrated data infrastructure in which nursing practice is included according to the context of both clinical quality and financial enumerators is necessary for monitoring and evaluating the value model. Integrated data systems that link services, costs, and outcomes add the nurse–patient assignment to electronic operational databases to allow specific identification of which nurse cared for which patients. Moving in this direction will significantly change how we view nursing performance (Welton, 2010). The financial success of system participants does not equal patient success; rather, it is the aggregated cost the patient is responsible for, such as deductibles and non-covered items. It is important to be transparent and identify costs around the full cycle of care for the patient's medical condition rather than charges billed or collected (Porter, 2012).

The purpose of creating a new clinical productivity model is not to more accurately represent the work of nursing as we now know it but rather to create a new mindset that moves leaders from expecting adequate numbers of nurses to focusing on achieving adequate patient care outcomes within the existing healthcare structure and resources. Three strategies are essential in the creation of a more contemporary model:

- Embedding the new measures within existing systems
- Evaluating performance in an aggregated model
- Managing the variance or system feedback to ensure system sustainability

From an evidence-based practice perspective, it may be more helpful to clearly articulate nursing's value within an economic framework to join all interdisciplinary activities under the rubric of an integrated clinical standard of practice. It is this linkage and integration among the disciplines that will create the composite framework for value determination. The evidence of impact on patient outcome, the viability of clinical processes, and the cost framework that supports clinical practice can be more clearly elucidated when the disciplines speak the same language and use a common framework. Until that time, however, focusing on effective nursing workforce management and creating an integrated structure for valuing that work will be critical first steps toward valuing nursing practice, establishing its relationship to financial and payment concerns, and providing a baseline with which nursing resource value can be connected across the interdisciplinary healthcare network.

An integrated data set connects the financial, accounting, and budgeting processes of the organization to workforce management and resource allocation within the context of specific clinical protocols or DRGs. Developing, refining, and maintaining a clinical resource information infrastructure for real-time data related to acuity, patient demand, resource allocation, clinical standards or protocols, structural and environmental considerations, and a continuous and effective reporting mechanism requires an evolutionary process in which longtime disparate processes can be strategically linked.

An integrated data management system also supports the work of addressing the challenges of change and innovation. Improvements that focus on the elimination of non-value-added work and increasing productivity include computerized electronic health records, technology for communication, pocket reference guides, personal digital assistants, and pocket-sized hand sanitizer packets.

Variance Management: A Daily Dynamic

Daily data assessments of critical variables specific to clinical and financial targets are important not only to understand the current state but also to make course corrections if needed.

The most significant information produced from any system relates to variances, that is, the differences between the desired outcome and the actual outcome. Seldom is there a perfect match between what is desired and what actually results. The resulting variance between time for patient care needs and time provided by staffing resources reflects the reality of balancing the workforce processes with the inherent expectations for reducing, eliminating, or managing these differences. It is this variance that provides the data from which to manage, monitor, and improve system performance. Merely counting and documenting the desired and actual outcomes does not provide any value for the system in outcome management. Instead, ensuring the accountability of the articulation and reporting of variance management is the essential unifying link in the process. Efforts to produce high levels of quality without devoting adequate human or financial resources to support those efforts is irrational and doomed to eliminate (destroy) the system. Effective evaluation processes lay the foundation for safe and timely management of the variance between what is desired and what actually (**BOX 7-1**).

Leaders are continually challenged to consider variations in the known natural clinical variances of disease; levels of severity; patients' responses to treatment; variability in work flow due to random arrivals of patients; and inherent variability

---

BOX 7-1 Key Variance Assessment Questions

1. How many shifts are within, under, or over targeted staffing?
2. How many nurse–patient assignments were within capacity? Over? Under?
3. How do these results compare with target performance goals?
4. How many adverse patient outcomes occurred when targets were not met?

DISCUSSION

As the nurse manager on a unit, you would like staff nurses to become familiar with variance management for their own shift. What guidelines would you establish for determining when a variance is over or under target? How would you assist the nurses in determining if patient care is or will be negatively affected? Is this about using evidence that is available, or being innovative and creating a new strategy for variance management?

---

of clinicians in regard to their knowledge, critical thinking, prioritizing, and communication skills. According to Long (2002), the goal is to eliminate artificial variance—that is, clinical errors, medication errors, lack of knowledge, inappropriate scheduling, and scheduling based on staff needs rather than patient needs. Leaders should focus on further managing the natural variation or the uncertain occurrence of care needs by patients, both predicted and unpredicted, and the inherent professional differences in ability that will always exist.

System variances result in high and low levels of workload, characterized by frequent internal diversions of patients to other units, backups in the postanesthesia care unit, external diversions from the emergency department, staff overload, and increased length of stay as a consequence of system gridlock. When a system variance is identified, the following management practices are indicated:

- Delineate protocols and link their required interventions to desired outcomes.
- Create a framework to examine performance standards.
- Define the linkage among interventions, best practice, and payment formats.
- Continue to monitor, evaluate, and adjust for gaps in desired linkages needed for value (cost–service–quality).

A staffing variance occurs when there is a difference between the identified patient care needs and the resources available to meet those needs. Given that there will always be discrepancies between needs and available staff, and given that nurses will continue to accept responsibility for providing safe, competent care, the development of strategies to manage this type of variance is essential. When a staffing variance is identified and efforts to obtain additional staff are exhausted, consider the following 10 strategies:

1. Take a teamwork approach: Commit to working as a team to address the gap. Planned variance management from a team perspective is proactive and minimizes stress. In contrast, individual variance management is impulsive, reactive, and highly stressful.
2. Prioritize: Identify specific patient care issues that require immediate attention and those that can be safely left until later in the shift or for the next shift.

3. Manage decision making: As a team, determine how work will be organized or reorganized, then assign work for the shift based on the type of staff available and patient needs. Decide which aspects of care can be eliminated or safely assigned to others.

4. Delegate and supervise: Delegate work to the appropriate caregivers and supervise accordingly to ensure that the work is being performed as required.

5. Control work flow to the unit: Reroute admissions if possible and appropriate.

6. Communicate: Arrange for a short midshift report to assess how well all team members are managing the workforce and reassign and reprioritize tasks as needed. Communicate how breaks and lunches will be organized.

7. Plan: After the team is organized, have each team member do a quick walkabout to assess those clients identified as high priority.

8. Evaluate: If circumstances require modification of a patient's plan of care, inform the patient about these changes and provide clear, factual information about the care the patient can expect.

9. Document: Complete a variance report that identifies the specific patient care concerns. Clearly describe the safety concerns. Provide examples of care that could not be completed or situations in which the timing of prescribed interventions was delayed.

10. Communicate: Share the variance management data with stakeholders and develop plans to minimize future gaps.

Variations from target staffing can also be calculated on a shift-by-shift basis. These data provide an overview of staffing patterns and opportunities to sustain or adjust current practices. In a large study by Needleman and colleagues, 15.9% of all shifts were 8 hours or more (8-hour shifts) below targeted staffing requirements. Both below targeted staffing and high turnover were associated with increased levels of mortality (Malloch, 2015; Needleman et al., 2011). Organizations will necessarily establish target performance levels and determine if 15.9% is acceptable.

New Units of Service: Comprehensive Continuum Approach

The historical inadequacy of summative task workforce calculations can be improved upon by using an aggregated or comprehensive workforce unit approach to measure patient care; the latter approach better represents the essence of the work of not only nursing but also all other caregiver work.

New models that embrace and reflect the reality of nursing patient care services, focusing on the holistic and dynamic human condition with associated scientific, societal, and economic factors, will improve the ability of leaders to manage resources from an evidence-based perspective. A model that views and measures the work of patient care as an aggregated whole rather than as a series of disconnected tasks better represents the work of caregivers in a much simpler way. An extension of the nursing patient classification system to include all disciplines providing care further enhances the robustness of a clinical productivity system. The ideal workforce management system is one in which the unit of service is multidisciplinary and patient specific for a defined period of time. All disciplines providing services are integrated and considered as a multidisciplinary comprehensive unit of care. The work of each discipline can be identified on the basis of interventions and associated contributions to patient outcomes. This unit of care represents the integrated, interwoven contributions of associated disciplines, such as hospitalists, physical therapy, respiratory therapy, and social services.

This new model also must integrate the achievement of clinical outcomes resulting from the services provided, the number of hours of care for the service, and the level of provider required to achieve these outcomes. Further, the effects of this integration are reflected in the patient care value equation in which resources, outcomes, and value are examined and evaluated, forming the philosophical foundation for a new, aggregated productivity model.

The purpose of modifying current processes and measures is not to devalue the historical clinical productivity measurement but rather to extend the existing productivity system to quantify the relationship among patient care services, value, and payment, and to adjust for those variables that influence the work of nursing. To be sure, this work may prove challenging. Reengineering anything is a risk that requires knowledge of not only the desired state of improvement but also the failures that one desires to correct. Successes provide confidence that something right is occurring but not necessarily *why* it is right. Failures provide unquestionable proof that we have done something wrong. Creating new measurement models for healthcare clinical labor productivity requires knowledge of the best features of effective existing processes and failures that have negatively influenced outcomes.

As we move though the productivity enhancement journey, it is important to remember that 100% productivity requires homogeneity—namely, patients with the same disease, patients arriving at the same rate, providers equal in their ability to provide patient care, and families with the same level of knowledge and understanding. In other words, 100% productivity is a mythical, ideal state that does not exist in clinical settings. The most reasonable approach for operational decision making is longitudinal monitoring of productivity by organizational units combined with indicators of patient care quality (Advisory Board Company, 2014; O'Brien-Pallas et al., 2004). This care must be described, documented, and measured using a standardized patient classification system to support decisions that will support safe patient care. O'Brien-Pallas and colleagues (2004) identified 85% as the optimal nursing unit productivity, with 93% as the maximum productivity because 7% of the shift is made up of mandatory breaks.

▶ Anticipated Outcomes from a Value-Driven System

Making changes and improvements in healthcare staffing to create an optimal value model will evolve over time. Using an evidentiary approach strengthens the quality and reliability of decisions and further illuminates opportunities for innovation. Using a value model framework is intended to improve not only allocation and matching of staff resources to patient needs but also clinical outcomes through coordinated care, more affordable care, the availability of actionable data, and data to identify gaps in processes and opportunities to reduce those gaps. **FIGURE 7-2** provides an overview of the component details of the value model.

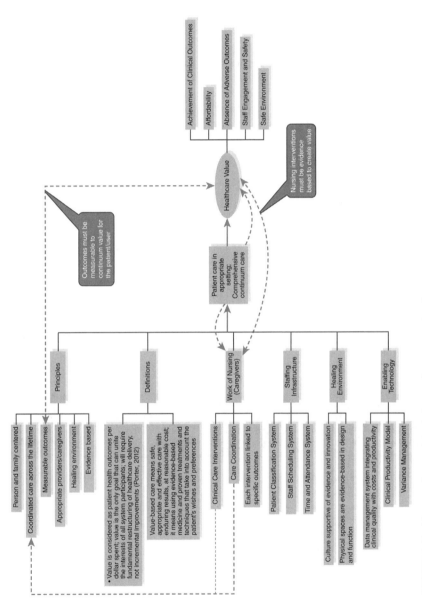

FIGURE 7-2 Healthcare value model mind map: Component details.

All care providers must now be cognizant of the relationship among what they do, what it costs, and what is achieved as a result of having done it. In an evidence-based value format, managerial decisions must reflect a balancing of the value equation—namely, the tension among service, resources, and outcomes (Malloch & Porter-O'Grady, 1999). This three-legged stool upon which clinical and performance viabilities are based becomes unbalanced when any one of the value factors is emphasized in a way that sacrifices its relationship to the other factors. Untenable and uncontrolled emphasis on providing service without consideration to issues of resource utilization creates an imbalance that ultimately diminishes service sustainability. Equally important, a focus on producing high levels of quality without efforts to develop the human or financial resources necessary to obtain and sustain that quality creates an imbalance. An uncontrolled and overriding focus on managing costs ultimately limits and threatens the organization's ability to provide adequate service or to ensure the high quality of that service. Again, the imbalance inherent in these situations is obvious.

The economic and financial sustainability of the organization depends on finding a continuous and dynamic balance among the three elements of the value equation and keeping them in accord. To achieve this goal, productivity measurement must transcend its current constraints and evolve into a multifaceted model that reflects the complexity of the work of nursing. This level of understanding is much different from the simple and limited cost–benefit evaluation that compares work hours to budgeted units of service. Imagine the long-term impact that reactive cuts to the nursing resource create during an economic downturn and the turnaround toll that is later exacted when these reduced numbers increase both risks and costs, alter the organization's market position, and raise recruitment and salary costs to untenable levels. Cutting out the core of a business does more than just alter the current balance sheet; it ultimately damages the sustainability of the business itself and positions it on a negative trajectory from which it may never fully recover.

🔍 CASE EXAMPLE: CARE COORDINATION ASSESSMENT

Cynthia Walker, RN, MSN, has recently been promoted to chief operating officer. One of her executive responsibilities is to ensure that there is an appropriate infrastructure for care coordination across the patient life span. She has a good understanding of the work and intended outcomes of this initiative; however, she is not certain how to assess current staffing for care coordination across the continuum life span. She would like to know the current status of care coordination. She believes the following information is needed:

- Identify those involved in handoffs, care planning, discharge planning, home health, and nonacute care placements.
- Identify and review existing policies and protocols for handoffs, care coordination, case management, and discharge planning processes. Identify the level of available evidence to support these policies and protocols.
- Interview 10 patients who use the organization's services and have chronic disease conditions, and ask them about their perceptions of care coordination across their life span.

- Interview 10 wellness users who access organizational services for regular health support and wellness maintenance about their perceptions.
- Review available metrics specific to care coordination processes.

Questions

1. Will this information be adequate to achieve Cynthia's desired goals?
2. Is additional information needed?
3. Is some of the information unnecessary?
4. What would be the next steps in this process after the assessment is completed?
5. What innovations are needed to facilitate the required changes?

CASE EXAMPLE: STAFFING ADEQUACY

Sheila Baumgarten, PhD, RN, has been the director of the medical product line for 20 years. She is also a nurse informaticist and would like to see more use of software for clinical and management analyses. She is responsible for both acute care and post-acute care services, including clinical, diagnostic facilities, and home health services. She has long been challenged by the limited utility of the financial productivity model. She recognizes that some of the resistance of executives has been due to the lack of software applications to collect and sort essential data elements for more comprehensive analysis of multiple data points.

The organization recently purchased the ideal software to create a comprehensive clinical productivity system. The nurse executive of the system asked Sheila to lead a team to develop the optimal clinical productivity system. She is excited and also cautious about how to do this work effectively using the current evidence for practice and outcomes and how to be innovative in designing a robust model to address the current challenges. She has decided to start small and selected DRG 89, simple pneumonia and pleurisy, to begin this work.

Sheila identified key stakeholders to collaborate with and create the desired model. The following information has been identified by the group as necessary to create a clinical productivity system:

- Inputs:
  - Number of patients with DRG 89 for the past 12 months
  - Hours of care provided to each patient by registered nurses (RNs) and nursing assistants (NAs)
  - Intensity projected needs for patient care (patient acuity) in hours
  - Budgeted hours of care for each patient
- Outcomes:
  - Actual length of stay (average)
  - Target length of stay (average)
  - Cost of care (average per patient)
  - Hospital Consumer Assessment of Healthcare Providers and Systems (HCAHPS) scores for patients (average)
  - Patient satisfaction with clinical outcomes
  - Number of falls, medication errors, and pressure ulcers

The following information was readily available:

- 200 patients with diagnosis DRG 89
- RNs provided an average of 47 hours to each patient (data extracted from patient acuity system and staffing information)

(continues)

🔍 *CASE EXAMPLE: STAFFING ADEQUACY*

(continued)

- NAs provided an average of 14 hours to each patient
- Patient intensity hours from the acuity system averaged 65 hours for each patient
- Budgeted RN and NA hours for each patient averaged a total of 68 hours for the RN and NA
- Patient satisfaction is 10% lower than the target performance goal
- Patient falls with injury increased by 10%
- No change in pressure ulcers or medication errors

Questions

1. As a team, consider these data and what they mean.
2. Is this data adequate for a new clinical productivity system?
3. What actions would you take, knowing that the hours used were below both the acuity and budgeted hours?

References

Advisory Board Company. (2012). Survey: Nurses spend 25% of shift on indirect patient care. Retrieved from https://www.advisory.com/daily-briefing/2012/02/02/nurses

Advisory Board Company. (2014). Nursing productivity benchmark generator. Retrieved from https://www.advisory.com/technology/workforce-compass/members/tools/nursing-productivity-benchmark-generator http://www.ahrq.gov/cpi/portfolios/value/index.html

Agency for Healthcare Quality and Research (2015). 2015 National Healthcare Quality and Disparities Report and 5th Anniversary Update on the National Quality Strategy. Retrieved from https://innovations.ahrq.gov/qualitytools/2015-national-healthcare-quality-and-disparities-report-and-5th-anniversary-update

Aiken, L. H., Clark, S. P., Cheung, R. B., Sloane, D. M., & Silber, J. H. (2003). Education levels of hospital nurses and patient mortality. *Journal of the American Medical Association, 290*(12), 1–8.

Aiken, L. H., Clark, S. P., Sloane, D. M., Sochalski, J., & Silber, J. H. (2002). Hospital nurse staffing and patient mortality, nurse burnout, and job dissatisfaction. *Journal of the American Medical Association, 288*(16), 1987–1993.

Aiken, L. H., Smith, H. L., & Lake, E. T. (1994). Lower Medicare mortality among a set of hospitals known for good nursing care. *Medical Care, 32*(8), 771–787.

American Nurses Association. (2003). *Nursing's social policy statement* (2nd ed.). Washington, DC: Author.

American Nurses Association. (2008). Safe staffing saves lives. Retrieved from http://www.nursingworld.org/HomepageCategory/Announcements/Safe-Staffing-Saves-Lives.html

American Nurses Association. (2012). *Principles of nurse staffing* (2nd ed.). Silver Spring, MD: Author. Retrieved from http://www.nursingworld.org/MainMenuCategories/ThePracticeofProfessionalNursing /NursingStandards/ANAPrinciples/ANAsPrinciplesofNurseStaffing.pdf

American Nurses Association. (March 2017). Safe staffing literature. Retrieved from: https://www.nursingworld.org/~49ebbb/globalassets/practiceandpolicy/work-environment/nurse-staffing/safe-staffing-literature-review.pdf.

Barnsteiner, J., Disch, J., & Walton, M. K. (2014). *Person and family centered care*. Indianapolis, IN: Sigma Theta Tau International.

Berry, L., Parker, D., Coile, R., Hamilton, D. K., O'Neill, D., & Sadler, B. (2004). *Can better buildings improve care and increase your financial returns?* Chicago, IL: Frontiers of Health Services Management.

Blegen, M. A., & Vaughn, T. (1998). A multisite study of nurse staffing and patient occurrences. *Nursing Economic$, 16*(4), 196–203.

Buerhaus, P. I., Donelan, K., Ulrich, B. T., Norman, L., DesRoches, C., & Dittus, R. (2007). Impact of the nurse shortage on hospital patient care: Comparative perspectives. *Health Affairs, 26*(3), 853–862.

Centers for Medicare and Medicaid Services. (n.d.). Roadmap for implementing value driven healthcare in the traditional Medicare fee-for-service program. Retrieved from http://www.cms .gov/Medicare/Quality-Initiatives-Patient-Assessment-Instruments/QualityInitiativesGenInfo /downloads/vbproadmap_oea_1-16_508.pdf

Centers for Medicare and Medicaid Services. (2015). Better care, smarter spending, healthier people: Improving our health care delivery system. Retrieved from http://www.cms.gov/Newsroom /MediaReleaseDatabase /Fact-sheets/2015-Fact-sheets-items/2015-01-26.html

Cho, S. H., Ketefian, S., Barkauskas, V. H., & Smith, D. G. (2003). The effect of nurse staffing on adverse events, morbidity, mortality, and medical costs. *Nursing Research, 52*(2), 71–79.

Corey, M. (2001). *Groups: Process and practice.* London, UK: Wadsworth.

Dartmouth-Hitchcock. (2015). What is value-based care? Retrieved from http://www.dartmouth -hitchcock.org/about_dh/what_is_value_based_care.html

Drucker, P. (1990). *Managing the nonprofit organization.* New York, NY: HarperCollins.

Finkler, S., & Graf, C. (2001). *Budgeting concepts for nurse managers.* New York, NY: W. B. Saunders.

Friese, C. R., Xia, R., Chaferi, A., Birkmeyer, J. D., & Banerjee, M. (2015). Hospitals in "Magnet" program show better patient outcomes on mortality measures compared to non "Magnet" hospitals. *Health Affairs, 34*(6), 986–992.

Geiger-Brown, J., Rogers, V. E., Trinkoff, A. M., Kane, R. L., Bausell, R. B., & Scharf, S. M. (2012). Sleep, sleepiness, fatigue, and performance of 12-hour-shift nurses. *Chronobiology International, 29*(2), 211–219.

Harrington, C., & Estes, C. L. (2004). *Health policy: Crisis and reform in the U.S. health care delivery system* (4th ed.). Sudbury, MA: Jones & Bartlett Publishers.

Hughes, E. C., & American Nurses Association. (1958). *Twenty thousand nurses tell their story: A report on studies of nursing functions sponsored by the American Nurses Association.* Philadelphia, PA: Lippincott.

Institute for Healthcare Improvement. (2012). A guide to measuring the Triple Aim: Population health, experience of care, and per capita cost. Retrieved from http://www.ihi.org/resources /Pages/IHIWhitePapers /AGuidetoMeasuringTripleAim.aspx

Institute of Medicine. (2015). Measuring the impact of interprofessional education (IPE) on collaborative practice and patient outcomes. Retrieved from https://www.iom.edu/Reports/2015 /Impact-of-IPE.aspx

Kalisch, B. J. (2014). Missed nursing care: A qualitative study. *Journal of Nursing Care Quality, 21*(4), 306–313.

Kane, R. L., Shamliyan, T. A., Mueller, C., Duval, S., & Wilt, T. J. (2007). The association of registered nurse staffing levels and patient outcomes: Systematic review and meta-analysis. *Medical Care, 45*(12), 1195–1204.

Lang, T. A., Hodge, M., & Olson, V. (2004). Nurse–patient ratios: A systematic review on the effects of nurse staffing on patient, nurse employee and hospital outcomes. *Journal of Nursing Administration, 34*(7–8), 326–337.

Lanser, E. G. (2001). Leveraging your nursing resources. *Healthcare Executive, 80*(10), 50–51.

Long, M. C. (2002). *Translating the principles of variability management into reality: One physician's perspective.* Boston, MA: Boston University, School of Management, Executive Learning.

Malloch, K. (2015). Measurement of nursing's complex health care work: Evolution of the science for determining the required staffing for safe and effective patient care. *Nursing Economic$, 33*(1), 20–25.

Malloch, K., & Porter-O'Grady, T. (1999). Partnership economics: Nursing's challenge in a quantum age. *Nursing Economic$, 17*(6), 299–307.

Martin, D. (2014). Literature review: Nurse fatigue related to shift length. *Arizona State Board of Nursing Regulatory Journal, 9*(3), 4–5.

McCue, M., Mark, B. A., & Harless, D. W. (2003). Nurse staffing, quality, and financial performance. *Journal of Health Care Finance, 29*(4), 54–76.

Moorhead, S., Johnson, M., & Maas, M. (2004). *Nursing outcomes classification (NOC)* (3rd ed.). St. Louis, MO: C. V. Mosby.

Murphy, M. (2003). *Research brief: Eliminating wasteful work in hospitals improves margin, quality, and culture.* Washington, DC: Murphy Leadership Institute.

Needleman, J., Buerhaus, P., Mattke, S., Stewart, M., & Zelevinsky, K. (2002). Nurse staffing levels and the quality of care in hospitals. *New England Journal of Medicine, 346*(22), 1715–1722.

Needleman, J., Buerhaus, P., Pankratz, S., Leibson, C. L., Stevens, M. S., & Harris, M. (2011). Nurse staffing and inpatient hospital mortality. *New England Journal of Medicine, 364*, 1037–1045.

O'Brien-Pallas, L., Thomson, D., Hall, L. M., Pink, G., Kerr, M., Wang, S. . . . Meyer, R. (2004). Evidence based standards for measuring nurse staffing and performance. Retrieved from http://www.researchgate.net/publication/228738285_Evidence-based_Standards_for_Measuring_Nurse_Staffing_and_Performance.

Pinkerton, S., & Rivers, R. (2001). Factors influencing staffing needs. *Nursing Economic$, 19*(5), 236–237.

Pittman, P., & Forrest, E. (2015). The changing roles of registered nurses in Pioneer ACOs. *Nursing Outlook, 63*(5), 554–565. Retrieved from http://www.nursingoutlook.org/article/S0029-6554(15)00179-7/references

Porter, M. E. (2012). *Value-based health care delivery.* Presentation at HBS Healthcare Initiative & Healthcare Club, March 7, 2012.

Rheaume, A., & Belliveau, E. (2015). The changing boundaries of nursing: A qualitative study of the transition to a new nursing care delivery model. *Journal of Clinical Nursing, 24*(17–18), 229–2537.

Rubin, I. M., Plovnick, M. S., & Fry, R. E. (1975). *Improving the coordination of care: A program for health team development.* Cambridge, MA: Ballinger.

Rutherford, M. (2008). Standardized nursing language: What does it mean for nursing practice? *OJIN: The Online Journal of Issues in Nursing.* Retrieved from http://www.nursingworld.org/MainMenuCategories/ThePracticeofProfessionalNursing/Health-IT/Standardized NursingLanguage.html

Savitz, L. A., Jones, C. B., & Bernard, S. (2005). Quality indicators sensitive to nurse staffing in acute care settings. In K. Henriksen, J. B. Battles, E. S. Marks, & D. Lewin (Eds.), *Advances in patient safety: From research to implementation* (pp. 375–385). Rockville, MD: Agency for Healthcare Research and Quality.

Sharmer, O. (2017). 5 conditions for shifting social fields. Retrieved from https://www.huffingtonpost.com/otto-scharmer/five-conditions-for-sifti_b_5943120.html

Smith, J. (2002). Analysis of differences in entry-level RN practice by educational preparation. *Journal of Nursing Education, 41*(11), 491–495.

Stimpfel, A. W., Lake, E. T., Barton, S. Gorman, K. C., & Aiken, L. H. (2013). How differing shift lengths relate to quality outcomes in pediatrics. *Journal of Nursing Administration, 43*(2), 95–100.

Stone, P. W., Curran, C. R., & Bakken, S. (2002). Economic evidence for evidence based practice. *Journal of Nursing Scholarship, 34*(3), 277–282.

Tourangeau, A. E., Cranley, L. A., & Jeffs, L. (2006). Impact of nursing on hospital patient mortality: A focused review and related policy implications. *Quality and Safety in Health Care, 15*(1), 4–8.

Ulrich, R., Quan, X., Zimring, C., Joseph, A., & Choudhary, R. (2004). *The role of the physical environment in the hospital of the 21st century: A once in a lifetime opportunity.* Concord, CA: Center for Health Design.

Upenieks, V. V., Akhavan, J., Kotlerman, J., Esser, J., & Ngo, M. J. (2007). Value added care: A new way of assessing nursing staffing ratios and workload variability. *Journal of Nursing Administration, 37*(5), 243–252.

Warren, J. (2012). Importance of standardized terminology in healthcare information systems. Retrieved from http://www.aacn.nche.edu/qsen-informatics/2012-workshop/presentations/warren/Importance-of-Standardized-Terminology-Warren.pdf

Welton, J. M. (2010). Response to nurse staffing and quality of care with direct measurement of inpatient staffing. *Medical Care, 48*(100), 940.

Welton, J. M. (2011). Value based nursing care. *Journal of Nursing Administration, 40*(10), 399–401.

While, A., Forbes, A., Ullman, R., Lewis, S., Mathes, L., & Grifiths, P. (2004). Good practices that address continuity during transition from child to adult care: Synthesis of the evidence. *Childcare Health and Development, 30*(5), 439–452.

White, K. M. (2006). Policy spotlight: Staffing plans and ratios. *Nursing Management, 37*(4), 18–22, 24.

CHAPTER 8

Failure and Resilience: Driving Sustainable Innovation

Tim Porter-O'Grady

Genius is 1% inspiration and 99% perspiration.

—**Thomas Edison**

CHAPTER OBJECTIVES

Upon completion of this chapter, the reader will be able to:

1. Examine the elements and characteristics of failure in the innovation process, and appreciate its contribution to sustainable innovation.
2. Identify the recovery strategies related to managing failure on the trajectory toward successful innovation and its implementation.
3. Use particular strategies and processes directed to managing the landscape of failure and utilizing failure as an incremental measure for success.

▶ Understanding Failure

In the early stages of the space shuttle program, in what was later called the *Challenger* incident, a rocket carrying astronauts into space blew up in midair. The Rogers Commission report explored the decision-making processes leading up to the accident and concluded that there was a serious flaw in the process that led to the disastrous launch of the shuttle on January 28, 1986. The report found that management practices were at odds with many of the system needs, and failure to communicate with all parts of the system led to a breakdown in understanding and communication, both of which were identified as major contributors to the cause of the accident (U.S. Congress, Senate Committee on Commerce, Science, and Transportation, Subcommittee on Science, Technology, and Space, 1986).

The report of the Nuclear Regulatory Commission's assessment of the Three Mile Island disaster also found a failure in communication and misunderstanding with regard to processes and procedures, and the level of mutual understanding among leaders and the system related to those processes, policies, and procedures (Sills, Wolf, & Shelanski, 1982).

Both of these disasters reflected common, ordinary failures in operating processes that can be replicated in many organizations and systems around the world. Failures such as these occur daily in organizations in every place on the globe in ways that reflect errors arising out of routine activities.

Enormous numbers of activities are undertaken in routine and ritualistic ways every single day in every workplace in the world. These ritualistic and repetitive activities are often quickly noted, briefly addressed, then placed in the historical dustbins of the organization, long forgotten while anticipating and addressing the next opportunity with all the potential error of previous initiatives. Error and failure are central to the human experience. Failure is a requisite on everyone's journey through life, learning, and adaptation. Without failure there is simply no measure for success (Bennis, Sample, & Asghar, 2015). Within this context, success can be said to be the appropriate aggregation of sufficient error. Failure can serve as both a stimulus and a deficit, depending on how it is perceived and addressed. Regardless of perception, the action of error can be a productive and important part of all or any of the elements of innovation. Innovation depends on failure and error as its way of both discerning and delineating the stage of the innovation process and what works and what does not work (**FIGURE 8-1**). Without this demarcation, there is no way to ascertain progress, or lack of it, toward the creation of the new, the different, and the previously unconceived (Akintoye, Goulding, & Zawdie, 2012). As James Joyce suggested, "Mistakes are the portals of discovery" (Cleary, 2014). Innovators stimulate reflection and recalibration, suggesting new tweaks or approaches or ways of undertaking an issue or finding a solution to a problem. The millions of silly and even monumental errors that one will confront on the journey to innovation serve as the highway to the seminal or more significant failures that provide the demarcation between the major movements or processes, and their challenges, on the journey to producing an innovative outcome.

Most of the time errors and failures are essential constituents of the journey of innovation. The landscape and processes associated with successful innovation require embracing error and failure and incorporating them into the operational mechanics and processes associated with successful innovation dynamics. Good leadership of innovation counts on the utility of failure and uses it as a part of the measurement mechanism essential to determine the viability and validity of decisions, choices, and processes associated with the positive movement toward successful innovation.

▶ The Truth about Failure

Innovation research consistently shows that most systems, organizations, and innovation processes are not terribly comfortable with accommodating embedded failure (Anderson & Costa, 2010). Most leaders are uncomfortable with failure because

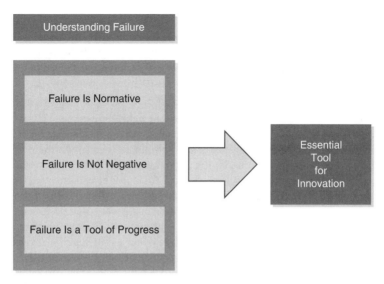

FIGURE 8-1 Understanding failure.

it is often seen as a reflection of one's competence, capacity, success, or lack of it. Historically, failure was used as a template to assess whether companies or individuals were successful in their undertakings and efforts. Failure, of course, was deemed unacceptable. This attitude created a perception about failure that alienated it as a legitimate part of organizational dynamics and clearly defined it as a deficit when assessing leadership behavior. In short, organizations and their leaders abhor failure. The emotional response and reaction to the presence of failure is so palpable in leaders that any mention of failure as a value generates a sense of incongruence, contradiction, and disbelief. In the history of leadership, there is only horror and negative reaction to the remotest suggestion that error and failure contain anything of value.

At a personal level, the deep pain associated with the negative notion of failure leaves a lasting imprint on both mind and experience. Because the negative impulses create much more reactive pain and depth of feeling than do pleasure and success, failure is deeply remembered and recalled often with only the darkest of images. The intensity of these memories creates a painful psychodynamic relationship to the concept of failure and error that any belief that they could be used as a positive force and an essential measure of success simply strains individual credulity. Therefore, from every place in the organization, from personal to collective experience, the notion of error and failure as a positive dynamic creates such cognitive dissonance that it is virtually impossible to overcome and creates an organizational psychology that makes embracing failure inconceivable and unlikely. Simply, learning to love failure violates every notion we have of organizational and professional integrity.

The conceptual and actual vision of failure is experienced as a bitter pill that, at best, is taken as bad-tasting medicine and, at worst, considered a terminal event. Therefore, organizationally and personally, failure is seen as something to be avoided at all costs, whether in our thoughts or in our deeds. Any notion of incorporating it into our legitimate operating processes or using it as a measure of progress goes far beyond the realm of possibility and creates a cognitive and organizational noise that makes it impossible to explore error and failure with any level of objectivity or intentional examination in a way that can make it useful and viable as a learning tool.

There are five basic scenarios or circumstances within which organizations and leaders approach the notion of failure that are negative and nonproductive but are common and consistent with contemporary management practices:

1. The organization completely rejects mistakes as legitimate. In this case, the organization finds mistakes completely unacceptable, rejects them, and does everything possible to eliminate them, hide them, ignore them, sweep them under the rug, or simply let them fall into oblivion. The organization has no mechanism for engaging or addressing error or failure, and undermines its capacity to create the milieu that provides the opposite: a perception of success, good choices, and positive attribution for all its processes and accomplishments. The failure-evading organization creates a leadership climate that is only superficially positive and reacts strongly to failure in any of its forms.

2. The organization can acknowledge error and failure but works diligently to hide and cover both. In this scenario, leaders in the organization recognize that error and failure do occur but consider them, at their foundation, exceptions, unusual circumstances, and unacceptable. Because they do occur, it is important in these systems to identify errors, not to give them value but to find where the blame needs to be placed to isolate each error, eliminate it, or punish it so it will not again raise its ugly head. In these organizations and management cultures, error and failure are to be feared, and those who are associated with either are to be shunned and/or punished in a way that leaves a message to the organization and its people that error occurs, but it is unacceptable, and failure is not a strategy that leads to rewards or positive relationships in the organization.

3. The organization recognizes that error occurs and that it occurs regularly, and it can turn up at any time and any place in the organization. Still, in this organization, error and failure remain unacceptable—anomalies to which leaders must object. If an error is found, it is to be analyzed and studied deeply to find out its characteristics and genesis, why it arose, what it means, what went wrong, and how to eliminate it from the processes and functions of the organization going forward so it will not have an opportunity to arise again. In this case, error is seen as a necessary and present deficit that, if studied carefully and deeply, can be managed and eliminated from processes in a way that minimizes it and, hopefully, over time, diminishes or eliminates it. Here again, error and failure are seen as deficits, but if studied appropriately, they can be acknowledged as part of identifying the root cause in an effort to diminish or eliminate both and replace them with positive and successful processes that reduce the chance of error or failure arising again.

4. Error and failure are recognized as parts of any process of implementation and are present in unrecognized forms in every design and project. Here again, error and failure are seen as deficits, uncontrolled outliers or variances that invariably rise to the surface because of the normative imperfection of planning, strategizing, or acting on an

initiative or undertaking. Error or failure in this case will always arise and must be accommodated and expected as one of the normal vagaries of any human undertaking. Still, the accommodation of an error is not the engagement of it. In this scenario, failure is still visualized as an arc of unaccepted variants that must be accommodated because it invariably appears, not because it is a tool of measure that may indicate specific viable and valuable data regarding effective process and decision making. Here again, the accommodation of the organization leads to an effort to reduce the impact of error and failure and to manage it in a way that reduces its risk and negative influence. If not for the error or failure, the situation is seen as an otherwise positive and successful process.

5. A standard of behavior in many organizations is the consideration that there are some people in the organization that are either personally committed to the failure of a project or do not actively embrace it, ultimately leading to its failure. Here again, failure and error are seen as deficits, in this case, personal and intentional ones, where stakeholders do not invest or commit to the strategy or undertaking of the organization in a sufficiently robust way to ensure that an innovation or initiative will be successful and sustainable. This lack of engagement and embracing the strategic imperative or design trajectory of the organization causes or creates error and failure, thus affecting the organization's viability and measures of success. In this case, it is believed that if the leaders in the organization can obtain sufficient engagement and embracing of a project or initiative by all the affected stakeholders, they can diminish the potential for failure and accelerate the potential for success. Here, the notion of error and failure is invested in the insight regarding whether individual commitments or participation operates at a sufficient level of intensity to minimize the chance for failure and maximize the opportunity for success. The belief of leadership in this scenario is that engaging and embracing the initiative or activity is positive. The risks of error and failure are minimized because of the offsetting energy of the collective commitment, ownership, and engagement of stakeholders in the work of the initiative or innovation. In this perception, it is believed that this full sense of engagement and empowerment creates a critical mass that inherently diminishes or eliminates the potential for error and failure in the organization (von Held, 2012). And, of course, it does not.

DISCUSSION

How has your organization historically approached the issue of failure? How has it affected your attitude toward failure as a member of that organization?

These five examples demonstrate how fear of error or failure becomes entrenched and embedded in the organization's culture. This occurs in a way that facilitates and expands individual fear, uncertainty, and downright opposition to the presence of error and failure in the dynamic processes of the organization. These sentiments create an operating milieu where the positive role of failure is significantly diminished. In truth, the chances of accelerating the potential for failure are enhanced simply because the organization fails to recognize failure as an elemental and positive force on the trajectory of good design, implementation, and outcome.

▶ Prediction and Failure

It appears that the survival rates of natural organisms and companies are about the same. This complexity phenomenon was studied by Paul Ormerod, who found that the trajectory of the extinction rate of species over time matches the extinction rate of companies when measured over the same period of time. No matter the intensity of the effort, most companies tend to fail over the long term (Ormerod, 2010). As pointed out in Tim Harford's best-selling book *Adapt* (2012), the long-term success of companies and their ability to survive extinction had nothing to do with their degree of success in strategic planning. Although some companies, like Shell and General Electric, have survived over the decades, the vast majority of companies did not. Therefore, we should be suspicious of any predictions of long-term success for companies, ventures, or initiatives in our current age.

This same data, with regard to the predictability of the survival of companies, applies to almost every other prediction you can make. The predictions of so-called experts appear to produce no more accurate certainty than the prediction of the life trajectory of a company. Nobody cannot safely predict whether anything will succeed or fail. This understanding drives the notion that failure is deeply embedded in all dynamics and endeavors at every level of nature and human enterprise. Our efforts cannot protect us from the vagaries of failure and uncertainty, nor are we able to predict and anticipate sufficiently to prevent or control failure. The real issue is to demonstrate resilience in the face of inevitable and inherent failure, and to successfully manage the realistic eventuality of failures in the course of our experiential journey.

▶ Structural Failure: An Impediment to Innovation

Among others, there are two deterministic characteristics that have a direct impact on failure management: structural failure and intentional (design) failure (Kale, 2015). Of the two, structural failure is the most dangerous because it impedes the mechanics of innovation and operates in opposition to the activities necessary to stimulate innovation. Structural failure is deeply embedded in the traditional hierarchical design of most organizations and companies, and it operates in a way that opposes the dynamics essential to facilitate and stimulate the innovation process (Davila & Epstein, 2014).

Structural innovation is a metaphor for organizational hierarchy. The more rigid the organizational hierarchy, the less likely it is that it can make room for innovation. Hierarchy acts against innovation insofar as it is structured to support strategic, operational, and functional alignment within the narrow parameters of planning and acting. These structural impediments facilitate failure before any definitive action can be taken leading to any measurable level of innovation. Structural impediments embedded in the hierarchy create such a narrow locus of control and such rigid process protocols that the potential for innovation, with all the vagaries necessary to support it, makes it impossible for innovation to succeed. The notion that the entire organization is driven structurally solely through its strategic trajectory and its associated processes strangles any potential for innovation before it even arises.

The creativity, discourse, openness, and collateral character of the innovative environment simply has no room to thrive in a rigid hierarchy, and therefore all the elements that would contribute to the potential for innovation are skewed or missing. Almost all healthcare organizations are designed in a way that provides a structural impediment to the potential for innovation. The only work-around is the construction of some unique forum, compartment, department, or institute that demonstrates a vehicle to get around the existing rigid parameters in a way that supports the innovation dynamic. In other words, when rigid structures and processes define the organization, innovation is either compartmentalized into a specific team, or innovation exists in the shadows, waiting to be found and stopped.

As a result, there is precious little evidence in these kinds of organizations of the action of innovation. Their structural framework does much to contribute to the long-term sensitivity of the organization to the negative vagaries of change to which organizational leadership has precious few resources to respond. The convergence of these negative forces works in concert to contribute to the decline or demise of a system (**FIGURE 8-2**).

Structural failure results from an infrastructure that does not allow for the possibility of trial and error and the quirks associated with the multidirectional and multilevel processes inherent in the innovation dynamic. Without a direct relationship to the strategic imperatives and permission from the structured management leadership or the functional mechanisms that support the operation of the bureaucracy, innovation simply has no place to grow. The constraints and rigidities of a clearly defined hierarchical infrastructure represent the supposition that failure and errors are simply unacceptable. This strong insulation from the risks and possibilities of experimentation and failure shields leaders from the potential that is entangled in accommodating failure and instead offers the stability and organizational

FIGURE 8-2 Structural failure.

rigidity that often cloisters its leaders from change and keeps the organization from anticipating, predicting, and creating its own future.

Sustainable innovation is never driven from the top of an organization and is therefore anathema to a hierarchical decision-making framework because innovation is stimulated and sustained the closer it generates and operates from the point of service or productivity that energizes and sustains it. The more involvement and interaction of stakeholders and the looser the rigidities of control and organizational permission giving, the more likely an environment for thriving innovation can be created. Structural rigidities are the enemy of innovation and create both an attitude and a disposition toward the essential elements of innovation, including failure, that create a context that makes it impossible for innovation to operate.

🔍 CASE EXAMPLE: FAILURE

The Blue Ridge National Health System has a long and storied history of success as a major health provider for a multistate region. It has been well noted for its high-quality, excellent physicians; wonderful nursing care; and its clinical model that has been identified as one of the best in the nation. This health system has always been identified as a unique provider, constantly out front in all measures of care and quality. In the past, its clinical model has been touted as one of the best in the country and has been broadly covered by every television network in America.

Rebecca Brown, RN, DNP, has recently been appointed as the new chief executive officer of this very successful health system. She was hired because of her major success in another health system across the country and had been identified as a strong up-and-coming, young administrator capable of providing strong and innovative leadership. When Becky arrived, she found an organization that was traditional, conservative, proud of its accomplishments, and firmly standing on its laurels. She also found many structures and systems that were highly entrenched, many medical and departmental silos, highly compartmentalized patient care services, high cost per unit of service, and leaders with a history and experience of protecting their turf from threat or encroachment.

In addition, the medical system is beginning to experience challenges from competitors who are slowly chipping away at its clinical model and patient population, and are busy innovating new kinds of care delivery systems driven by the demands of building a value-based service network. Many of its competitors are decentralizing health care, emphasizing ambulatory care, and growing community-based services. On the other hand, the Blue Ridge National Health System is highly institutional, with many buildings on a fixed site, a number of related clinics, and very little dispersed community presence. Becky also noticed that there is not much community outreach, representation, or involvement in the strategic or tactical health decisions of the community. Furthermore, much of the decisions are controlled by a handful of powerful physicians with little engagement of other disciplines and the staff at the point of service. Becky identified that what she is confronting is a structural failure in the health system, and she saw that she had much work ahead of her to create a culture of innovation and engagement, which is essential to the health system's future success.

Discussion

We clearly see here an organization with a long history of success. The organization has embraced its success as its permanent identity in a way that ultimately insulates it from the realities and vagaries of a new, different, challenging, transforming, and relevant system prepared to create its future organization. Many of the structures in place are clearly unsustainable, requiring that leadership undertake a full 180-degree shift in strategy, culture, design, behavior, and impact.

Questions

In a team of four to seven members, discuss Becky's role and emerging priorities that will help the system confront its structural impediments to innovation (failures to innovate).

1. What makes this health system structurally unable to engage in impending and necessary innovation?
2. How does an organization's history act to position it to fail in responding to overwhelming indicators of the need for change and innovation?
3. What specific challenges must Becky confront as she assesses the organization's capacity to change its structures to support innovation at the strategic (governance), operational (senior leadership), functional (departmental and unit), and individual (professionals and employees) levels of the organization?
4. As you consider Becky's role, what would be the initial steps or activities you would suggest she take to begin the process of removing the structural impediments to innovation in the health system?
5. How will the organization need to be different, and what will be the new leadership roles that will exemplify the organization's capacity to embrace innovation and engage the staff in transforming the health system?

It is important to note that hierarchical structures are currently threatened by the emergence of complexity science in organizational contexts and the implications of network realities. The leadership of predominantly relational systems and the intersections that describe how these networks operate has served to change the very dynamics of leadership and the organization of work (Ledema, Verma, Wutzke, Lyones, & McCaughan, 2017). In health care, the emergence of value-grounded processes and the move from volume-based models to value algorithms has served to shake the organizational landscape, flatten hierarchies, and empower decisions and actions operating at the point of service (Wilson, Gole, Bharat, & Jitendra, 1916). This move to more point-of-service configurations and the requirement for decisions and actions generating from these places has rewritten the script for health services and has driven systems to confront their vertically controlled organizational designs. In the face of the need for entrepreneurial, evidence-grounded, and just-in-time decision and action models, leaders now have no choice but to test and experiment with new models of organizing work and structuring for innovation. The demands of collective wisdom and team-based action in the exercise of integrated clinical activity across the continuum require more local leadership, planning, and decision making to ensure clinical relevance and efficacy. All these emerging circumstances serve to create the conditions where it is less of an option to maintain rigid hierarchies in the face of growing demand for nimble, mobile, just-in-time clinical decisions and actions, all within a digital infrastructure. The hierarchy in a well-matrixed and -networked organization does not seek to maintain its formal control of the work, but rather the hierarchy provides guiderails, energy channels, and catalysts for innovation. The structure in an innovative organization helps innovation thrive. The structure challenges innovation at the edge of chaos, helping to maintain information feedback loops associated with success and failure, ensuring that the organization can evolve and thrive.

▶ Intentional Failure: Essential Facilitator of Innovation

Intentional failure is simply a metaphor for a context or environment that is, by design, supportive of the dynamics and processes associated with sustainable creativity leading to useful innovation (Bolman & Deal, 2013; Guzzini & Iacobucci, 2017). Intent implies a level of understanding regarding the structural facilitators and requisites necessary to advance the elements and products of innovation. Innovation demands a high degree of interaction, relationship, communication, experimentation, and trial and error. An environment that facilitates all the characteristics and processes supporting these dynamics is the essential underpinning leaders provide to support sustainable innovation. Intentional failure implies that the organizational constructs have been carefully thought out and that the relationship between sufficient organizational structure and the work of innovation has been just as carefully constructed and operationalized in a way that ensures the presence of the structural underpinnings supportive of innovation (Hoque & Baer, 2014).

Intentional failure suggests a level of understanding of the role failure plays in innovation (Tawfik, Rong, & Choi, 2015). In this understanding of failure, leaders recognize the central and essential value of the role it plays in the innovation trajectory and in the assessment of progress and the determination of success. The recognition is that through experimentation, trial and error, and the incorporation of the risks associated with failure, the innovator and innovative system can actually innovate (Talukder, 2014). Within the paradigm of intentional failure, leaders can construct and use the tools of assessment and progress evaluation to better determine what is and what is not working. Clear to the leaders in intentional failure is the recognition that the delineation of both progress and failure serve an equal role in explaining and measuring the elements of progress in determining what is and what is not working (Kumar & Kumar, 2016). In this case, innovation leadership embraces failure in equal measure to other indicators of progress, recognizing that all of them are important determinants of points of reference on the innovation trajectory. Furthermore, the judgment of failure is no different from the judgment of progress. Each serves as an objective measure of movement and provides a specific demarcation of the development and progress of any innovation. With dispassionate approaches and objective yet definitive tools, innovation leadership can harness the measures of failure as an evaluation of progress and, from it, strengthen choices, change them, and/or adjust the trajectory in any way that can facilitate the potential for positive outcome or impact (**FIGURE 8-3**).

▶ Harnessing Failure as a Strategy of Success

Understanding the role of failures in innovation is to understand the dynamics of innovation. Failure through the lens of innovation is an operational element, as much

FIGURE 8-3 Intentional failure.

a part of the processes of innovation as any other element. The purpose and work of failure is directed to the following:

- Failure is a tool and component of trial and error in which measurement of progress is essential. Error (thus, failure) is a metric that serves to identify where one is in the process of design or implementation. Failure tells the innovator where he or she is in the process and where the trajectory leads or does not lead. Knowing where not to go or what not to do in the innovation dynamic is equally important to knowing what is affirmed or validated in the innovation trajectory.

- Failure serves as a data point, a source of information, a point of reference that helps the innovator know where he or she is in relationship to other activities associated with the innovation process. Success in innovation can be said to be the sufficient aggregation of appropriate error. This acknowledges that the role of aggregated failure is helping to ascertain the demarcations of progress and the sum of the activities necessary to determine success.

- Failure serves to help identify the critical points of change in a trajectory or direction. A failure becomes seminal when it indicates the need for a major reconceptualization or reconfiguration of the innovation process. While innovation is a process, it is not a straight line. Points of failure lead to moments of revolution that may require new thinking or processing and thus completely revamp the dynamics in a way that leads to new thinking or a new direction.

- Failure serves as a vehicle for disruption in a way that may actually cause a stop in a process or create conditions that may completely alter the path of an innovation. The disruption is usually significant enough to invalidate the current trajectory or work and is a cause for shift or change so significant that it can be said that it is essentially not the same process. In these cases, the products of innovation may become different and the disruption may be so complete that the product of innovation may be entirely different from that originally conceived.

- Failure may indicate a problem with conception or with the frame for thinking about an innovation. Failure may actually challenge, even invalidate, a method of conceiving or thinking about an invention or innovation. Indeed, the opportunity to turn the corner on an innovation may actually be embedded in transforming how one thinks about what is being created or altering images of

FIGURE 8-4 Failure as a positive tool for innovation success.

process and product such that this challenge may serve as the very catalyst for positively moving forward on a stalled or ineffective strategy or tactic in the innovation dynamic.

■ Finally, failure may act to invalidate the value and the process of a particular innovation effort. The significance of the failure may be such that the innovation itself is invalidated, making further progress on it purposeless. In this case, failure serves to inform the innovator of the complete nonviability of the innovation or demonstrate that conditions have eclipsed the value or relevance of the innovation in a way that ultimately stops it in its tracks. The positive take on this traumatic realization is that further expenditure of time, energy, and resources are halted, and those efforts can be transferred to other initiatives or innovations.

In each of these cases, failure is a positive tool for the innovation leader (**FIGURE 8-4**). It serves as a strong metric at every point in the innovation process that relays important data regarding progress and the movement toward success. Free of negative emotion and stigma, it serves as simply another tool, a metric for determining progress, priority, or change.

▶ Trial and Error: Partnering Failure and Innovation

All innovation uses mechanisms of trial and error. Different from an improvement that advances something that already exists, innovation is primarily the creation of something that does not exist. Innovation mostly begins with an idea. However, an idea is not an innovation. An innovation is always the product of the work of translating an idea into action or a product. Keep in mind that in any health system or organization, an innovation must ultimately add value in a way that affects care, service, outcome, or price; the innovation is itself the product.

Because design is the discipline or the work of innovation and is essentially a process of creation, the ultimate product of innovation is usually not fully known.

The innovation process is filled with the elements of discernment, discourse, and discovery. Through the collective wisdom and processes of the stakeholders of the innovation, it slowly unfolds and takes shape. That shape forms as a result of small tests, experimentation, and trails along its trajectory. Deeply rooted in this process are all the indicators of progress and failure, each doing its part in validating and moving the innovation process along. Tests of utility lead to further refinement or enhancements or abandonment—shifts or changes in the innovation course. Accomplishment and success validate process; failure stimulates redesign or change. Trial and error contain equal measures of both. The veteran innovator knows that there will be a good measure of both success and failure, and each will do its part to inform the process of innovation and help make the necessary responses to keep the innovation process on track.

Failure also serves to mature the innovator and deepen his or her discernment and reflective process. Many an innovator has suggested that the most important and definitive moments in the innovation process were driven out of a spectacular failure that was so precise and devastating that it caused a dramatic demand for reflection and rethinking. In the time following a failure, new synapses, connections, and ideas are often generated in a way that serves as a tipping point such that the whole innovation hinged on the work done after failure. Indeed, for many an innovator, failure was the catalyst that served as the incubator that ultimately redefined the innovation and served to spark a new genesis along its trajectory toward realization and success.

DISCUSSION

How safe is it in your organization to experiment, test, and explore new approaches or different methods of solving a problem, influencing patient care, or advancing the patient experience? What are the boundaries or barriers that keep you from using trial and error as a tool for innovating practice?

Failure acts as a discipline in the dynamic of innovation. Failure is often the sobering point in the process that salts the excitement of ideation and creativity with the reality and sobriety of truth or reality, countering the realm of fantasy that fuels the dreams and hopes that stoke the energy and spirit of the innovation process. Creativity takes the innovator to the heights of possibility; failure provides the sobering foundation that supplies the stark truth about progress and the substance of the innovation in a way that helps inform the reality of the journey. In short, failure is a vital tool in assessing progress and informing the innovator about the realities and potentials of the innovation process itself.

▶ Failure as a Tool Set for Effective Change

When failure is recognized in its role as a part of all the elements and processes of the innovation dynamic, the leader's attention shifts from failure as error to failure as a tool for advancing the innovation process. The degree of utility and vitality brought to the use of failure in the dynamic of innovation determines the veracity and the effectiveness of adaptation, adjustment, or a radical change in course. The use of the tool of failure calls the leader to understand the mechanisms associated with it and to bring intentionality to the use of failure as a normative management strategy. Some of the issues related to the utility of failure are as follows:

- Identify the potential for failure early: If failure is to prove useful, the leader must first have dealt with personal attitudes and dispositions toward the notion of failure. Structuring failure as a normative component of the innovation process seems inherently counterintuitive. Each individual's developmental history informs the attitude toward failure by virtue of how failure was both perceived and handled in the individual's own life journey. Most of us have seen failure either as a challenge, at the minimum, or a devastating occurrence, at the maximum. On either end of a continuum, failure is identified as personal, having both an intimate and a relational impact.

  These personal notions related to perceptions of failure inform the mental model the innovator and the innovation leader bring to their roles. The positive and contributing characteristics of failure operate successfully only after having recognized that the occurrence of failure is a normative circumstance deeply embedded inside the innovation journey. It is important to surrender attachment to the past notions and sentiments regarding failure and equally important to recognize it more objectively as a positive tool set that helps assess points of reference, positive metrics, and potential decisions affecting the innovation process.

  As the leader moves more confidently into an objective assessment mental model with regard to the innovation process and embedded error, the utility and value of failure become increasingly obvious. In this more objective framework, the only values that count in managing failure are early identification and early engagement. Much like conflict, the ability to respond positively to the failure in process, approach, strategy, or effort depends on the earliest possible identification and engagement. The sooner an emergent failure is recognized by the innovation leader and the earlier this leader predicts both the content and impact of the failure of effort, focus, strategy, or process, the easier it is to adjust and recalibrate in addressing their implications. The more positive the notion and attitude toward the dynamic associated with failure in the innovation process, the more alert the leader is for the potential contribution and value that emergent failure provides in informing and managing the innovation process.

- Failure is an indicator of the veracity of the idea: Many ideas engender excitement and enthusiasm in people who generate them and those who are affiliated with them. Often, this excitement and enthusiasm helps inform the conceptual frame of reference with regard to the value and potential of the idea going forward. While this enthusiasm is essential to generate the energy necessary to stay the course in the innovation process, it is also a trap. This conceptual trap serves to create the conditions where the energy is the driver leading to sidelining some of the basic tenets of logic, rationality, measurement, value, and sustainability.

  Besides its association with creativity, openness, and free association, innovation is also a discipline. It has stages with definitive activity identified within them and specific measures and mechanisms that test the innovation potential and viability (LaRusso, Spurrier, & Farrugia, 2015). Good innovation leaders recognize that if the products of innovation are to be achieved, faithfulness to this process will be critical to success. While the enthusiasm associated with the generation of ideas and the subsequent innovation process is important in keeping it going, the more rational and dispassionate phases of the innovation dynamic provide the more rigid and systematic template and tools essential to move it to successful completion. Failure of an element, component, stage, phase, or notion associated with the innovation serves as a point of measurement where the innovation leader can undertake some objective assessment of the meaning and value of any particular failure and its impact on subsequent decisions and actions related to the innovation. In this case, failure sometimes reflects the lack of veracity or relevance of the innovative idea and causes the leadership and innovation team to reflect and to discern the appropriateness of the originating idea and the substance of innovation going forward, should that be a rational decision (Weberg, 2017).

Equally as possible is the determination that the innovation idea is not viable, relevant, or doable. Knowing when to stop an innovation or the innovation process to reevaluate the value equation is a key leadership behavior that is equally as important as fostering the innovation. Whether or not it is viable should be the product of these more rational processes that subject the innovation in the moment of failure to a more rigorous, rational, and focused assessment using objective metrics that inform and effectively advise correct decision making related to the innovation.

- Value failure for its role in destructive creativity: The leader's assessment of potential or impending failure does not necessarily need to lead to the consideration of the innovation as a terminal event. Failure serves a range of purposes. While one of them is certainly an indicator of the viability of the innovation, there are other factors associated with a particular failure that do the opposite. Sometimes failure is simply delivering the message regarding either choices made or the trajectory of the innovation. Examination of the failure can lead the innovation leader to reflection regarding strategies or processes chosen and their effectiveness in leading to the intended innovation or outcome.

Sometimes the failure merely calls attention to errors in strategy, process, trajectory, or individual actions. In this case, a reexamination of any or all of these factors and their impact on the lack of positive progress can call the leader to reconfiguration or recalibration of decision, effort, trajectory, or priorities. Having made the necessary course correction, the innovation leader may thereafter create conditions where better convergence around successful innovation processes emerge and, for the next stage or phase, the more successful progress can be noted. Here, failure serves simply as a demarcation for measurement, a moment of reflection, and an opportunity for the innovation team to reconfigure its efforts in a way that better addresses issues leading to the moment of failure and helps the team push past that moment with renewed insight, tools, and tactics that better align with the innovation's trajectory.

- Failure is a tool for redefining the innovation: When an innovation process or the trajectory of innovation is clearly not working and the options for success following the planned trajectory are limited or nonexistent, this failure, again, may not necessarily lead to a termination of an innovation. In complex adaptive processes, often what might appear as a terminal event may actually be the ground floor of a more emergent circumstance leading to an innovation or change not previously conceived or visualized in the originating innovation process.

Often, out of the ashes of a clearly failed innovation process are born the seeds of a new innovation. This new innovation is often better, more viable, and potentially more significant than the failed innovation out of whose ashes it emerged. Indeed, in the innovation dynamic, the death of an innovation may cause the innovators to turn a corner, look sideways, dig deeper, and clear the conceptual decks in a way that makes space for a different conception and a much more viable trajectory leading to something not previously conceived but that now demonstrates a value for which there was simply no vision while pursuing the previous innovation process that unwittingly led to its conception and generation. Here again, the circumstance is a reminder to the innovation leader that in the innovation dynamic, closing the door to a failed effort does not end the work of innovation; often it simply changes its course. Faithfulness to the discipline of innovation helps create the conditions where destruction, deconstruction, and termination can actually serve as a rich medium out of which new and more viable innovation emerges.

- Failure acts as the catalyst for evaluation of the effectiveness of the innovation process: Failure in the pursuit of a particular innovation may actually have nothing to do with the innovation. Often the failure in the innovation is a symptom rather than effect. Such a failure calls the innovation leader to review the dynamics and processes associated with the discipline of innovation. Through review of the stages and phases of the innovation process and the resources and mechanisms supporting it, the innovation leader often finds points of challenge that lead to an understanding of brokenness and failure in the process itself.

Because innovation is both a dynamic and a process, the failure to achieve the desired outcome may have more to do with inadequacy in the process than in the potential veracity and value of the innovation. Here again, when failure is recognized as normative and serves as an objective tool of assessment or evaluation, information of significance regarding the dynamic is obtained. This information can then yield more effective or aligned elements or processes supporting the innovation trajectory. A regular and focused examination of the characteristics and elements of the innovation process and its appropriate support structures helps innovation leaders to further refine the process in ways that make it more predictable, dependable, and trustworthy. Although each innovation has its own developmental characteristics, all innovation has a common frame of reference within which the foundational set of processes and parameters routinely operate to support and facilitate the innovation dynamic.

Flaws in the process, missing elements, irregular flow, and limits on effective evaluation all converge to create conditions that negatively affect the discipline and processes of innovation. For the innovation leader, the best predictors of flaws in the innovation process are the degrees of repetition in the occurrence of patterns of failure over time. Failing to address these or lack of awareness of their operation can often cause the leader to focus on the innovation rather than on the mechanisms that advance it. More often than not, the failure lies in the mechanics of innovation, not the idea driving it.

Failure as Value	Failure as Deficit
• Objective	• Subjective
• Assessment	• Unsafe
• Measurement	• Terminal
• Influence Direction	• Negative
• Set Trajectory	• Destructive

FIGURE 8-5 Failure as value versus failure as deficit.

Objectively managed, failure is clearly a viable and useful tool in refining and advancing any innovation toward success. However, it takes a manager or leader with an adjusted attitude and insight toward failure to use these objective tools to successfully traverse the landscape of innovation. Careful and serious use of the tools of the discipline of innovation help facilitate and enhance the dynamic of innovation. This more balanced and realistic insight about the processes of innovation and its effectiveness grounds the leadership of innovation and increases the likelihood of its successful movement through all stages of development (**FIGURE 8-5**).

▶ Minimizing the Potential for Unnecessary Failure

Although it is clear in this chapter that we have emphasized the fact that failure is a fundamental—a necessary—element of the innovation process, it is important to suggest that not all failure is necessary. Sometimes failure occurs because of inappropriate decision making, inadequate processes, or poorly constructed innovation support structures. Each of these failures is conditional, meaning it can be addressed and managed, and when it is fixed, it no longer acts as an impediment affecting the innovation process. Keep in mind, however, that correcting structural flaws in the innovation process does not necessarily diminish the potential emergence of other errors and failures inside the innovation dynamic. Operational flaws are separate circumstances and create different conditions. Structural errors embedded in the process can always have a strongly negative impact on the innovation process and therefore on the innovation itself. Errors of this type operate in a different way from operational error and failure that more simply reflect problems with the processes of innovation.

Innovative organizations are just as intensely human as any other organizations. Essentially, this means that the potential for mistakes, misjudgments, poor planning, bad choices, and uninformed decisions and actions can be just as apparent in the innovative organization as they are in any other system. With an awareness of this reality, the leader recognizes that he or she is constantly assessing the environment for their presence and evaluating, learning, adjusting, and correcting systems to keep them on course and to support effective innovation processes.

Leaders of innovation can exhibit several behaviors to help minimize unnecessary failure:

- Be bold: Voicing concerns about the alignment, trajectory, and evolution of the innovation is part of the process. Laissez-faire leadership in innovation can lead to value-negative outcomes. The inaction of team members in the innovation dialogue about value, process, and alignment can lead the innovation to lose adaptability and stagnate or cause the innovation to spin into more chaos. Leaders of innovation must both speak up and facilitate speaking up.
- Bridge structural errors: As discussed, many organizations have structural and cultural foundations that can minimize or inhibit innovation. Leaders of innovation can work to bridge these structural gaps through building strong networks of conspirators, external contacts, and linkages to fellow innovators. The network of agents will always be stronger than any hierarchal force. Building a network of innovation is key to minimizing unnecessary error caused by rigid structures and culture.
- Focus on the outcome: Although it is easy to become fixated on the process of innovation (brainstorming, ideation, prototyping, etc.), leaders of innovation must equally focus on the outcomes the innovation will achieve. Many times the innovation morphs and shifts through the process, and teams can lose sight of what they are trying to accomplish. Keeping the vision of the outcome visible to the team will help maintain alignment of the process and minimize errors associated with wasted time, unnecessary iterations, and lack of focus.

▶ Innovation for Value

Perhaps one of the most significant shifts in recent history in health care is the current move from a volume-driven system to one based on value. Currently, the most significant contextual failure that innovation leaders will need to contend with is that related to the move from volume to value. Almost any innovation that emerges today needs to represent the emergence of value-based realities driving much of the strategic work of organizations. No innovation will have any sustainable meaning or even succeed over the long term in its implementation from idea to product if it does not in some way anticipate, facilitate, or advance the engagement of value. The entire arena of health services must now reflect value drivers in a way that now fulfills the obligations of the Triple Aim.

As mentioned previously, innovation should relate to organizational purpose and strategic imperative. Although there is a challenge in the contest between the unique characteristics of an innovation and the opportunity it provides to undertake something that is new and/or different, the innovation still needs to reflect the major purposes of the organization. In health care, regardless of the changes that are occurring, any innovation that seeks to thrive in the healthcare environment in some way or another needs to advance the service, quality, or price interests of the healthcare organization. A sound element of the discipline of innovation is the assurance that innovation undertakings, regardless of their creativity, somehow directly relate to advancing the healthcare enterprise. In this case, it is the role of the innovation structure to provide that framework, the discipline, if you will, that keeps the generation of resources supporting any innovation undertaken within the framework of the value of the organization. Failing to do so robs the organization of its resources and its capacity to exercise good judgment and action in a way that advances its purposes and value. The following are some critical factors influencing the success of innovation:

- Innovation and strategic relevance: There are all kinds of innovations that are important, meaningful, valuable, creative, and relevant. To the innovation leader, none of them matters if all these elements do not in some way lead to advancing the interests, viability, and sustainability of the organization within the context of its purpose and the service it provides. In health care, supporting innovation activities need to demonstrate how they uniquely contribute to advancing the interests of the organization and provide a foundation for the quid pro quo essential to advancing a thriving health service environment. The significant failure to do so relates specifically to the nonalignment of the innovation efforts with the purposes and roles of the health institution and the efforts necessary to advance the health of those it serves.

    The failure to align strategy and innovation at the systems level creates a critical condition for the organization with its larger environment. Health systems are directed within the contemporary value equation to advance the health of the communities within which they live and operate. Essential to this exercise is the appropriate and careful use of organizational, financial, and human capital in ways that serve that essential purpose (Owens & Fernandez, 2014). In the value equation, evidence of having done so is delineated by the organization's capacity and success in advancing metrics that demonstrate a high level of user satisfaction, strong performance on quality metrics, and competitive pricing of the services and products of the health system. The innovation priorities of the organization that advances performance in these arenas of value measures indicate strong alignment among the priorities and activities of the organization and its strategic positioning for success.

- Failure and inadequate resourcing for value: Perhaps the most significant anticipated and predicted failure in the innovation process is the lack of organizational and financial support for innovation activities. Often what occurs in organizations regarding innovation is the provision of a great deal of verbal and personal support with no structural and financial infrastructure to sustain it. For many leaders, innovation is the generation of ideas and thus never lifts off toward a structure for change. As a result, organizations are inundated with ideas related to technological, process, and product innovation with precious little progress toward producing something that matters or makes a difference for the health system.

    Innovation projects or processes that are inadequately funded generally die on the vine. These innovations have no way to develop or thrive simply because the most obvious indicator of support—financial resources—is either inadequate or missing. Making appropriate resources available for innovation is the most concrete proof of the organizational support for that innovation. Leaders indicate significant value for any undertaking through the medium of the number of dollars devoted to move the innovation toward product or impact. Lacking that, no amount of verbal and personal support for the work of innovation will ever move the innovation anywhere near the fulfillment of its potential.

- Failure of an adequate infrastructure to support the discipline or process of innovation: As clearly identified throughout this text, innovation is specifically defined as an enumerated process with identifiable elements, stages, and metrics that elucidate its properties. In the popular press and in the imaginations of some leaders, innovation is often seen as a series of loosely defined, highly variable, often unstructured dynamics and processes that relate more to idea management than to any definitive and disciplined process that could ultimately produce a product or create an impact on the life of the organization. However, more often than not, nothing could be further from the truth.

Innovation, like any process of production, has elements and stages through which it grows that are necessary for its implementation. Ultimately, an innovation must produce something: either a change or a product. None of this can occur without the capacity to do what is necessary to produce something. Structures related to idea management, knowledge generation, product refinement and development, experimentation and small tests of change, integration of effort, resource management, intellectual property and legal issues, production, evaluation, marketing, and so forth, are embedded within the processes and functions essential to the long-term viability and ultimate success of the proposed innovation.

With all of these components and stages essential to the success of an innovation, it comes as no surprise that few innovations make it anywhere near completion. If organizations are to be successful in managing their innovation processes, the essential tools, infrastructure, metrics, resources, and processes must be carefully constructed and aligned to ensure that all appropriate and necessary efforts converge to positively facilitate the innovation toward successful completion. This essential infrastructure provides both the frame and the glue that enables innovators and associates on the positive trajectory to access supports necessary to accelerate the opportunity to succeed. Failure to build this essential infrastructure is a failure to equip both the innovator and the innovative process with virtually everything they will need to thrive within the process and to move positively and successfully toward fulfilling the potential of the innovation. It is important to remember that even with the right set of factors energizing the innovation, failure still may occur. For example, even the most successful venture capital firms have about a 10% success rate in funding innovative start-ups.

- Failure of relevance: Leaders have an obligation to the organizations they lead to make sure that the activities and priorities of the organization best represent three critical elements: (1) the driving characteristics and demands of the larger environment within which the organization lives and operates, (2) the trajectory of the organization is traveling in a way that best demonstrates its response to the environmental and contextual demands within which it lives, and (3) the appropriate decisions and actions that represent the best response to the demands of the environment and the requisites of the trajectory.

Any organization that seeks to thrive must attend to its capacity to be relevant. Relevance represents the characteristics and activities of individuals, groups, or organizations in a way that best exemplifies the broader social, political, technological, and economic forces converging to influence their capacity to thrive. Leaders must demonstrate the essential skills that help them forget inevitable and emerging shifts in reality brought by each of these forces and the impact of those shifts on the decisions and actions of the organization in a way that is timely and appropriate. This predictive and adaptive capacity is a fundamental skill set of leadership within the context of innovation; it is no longer

FIGURE 8-6 Two major leadership capacities.

optional if the changes in an organization will represent a goodness of fit between the larger demand for change and growth and the organization's capacity to meet that demand, translate it, and give it form and substance (**FIGURE 8-6**).

▶ The Capacity to Be Relevant

As the digital environment expands its influence on human and organizational life, the response to it creates a new level of leadership demand, especially with regard to innovation. Because of the breadth of big data and the increasing speed and utility of the information infrastructure, just-in-time responses to the demand for change are now the normative pattern of organizational and team behavior. Unlike traditional changes affecting health service in clinical practice, where changes in policy, procedure, and practices could transition over weeks and months, evidence-based practices now operate within an immediacy where data aggregation, evaluation, and information now affect practice instantaneously, with the expectation that change in practice will occur as soon as we know what that change should be. This milieu creates a new understanding of relevance. The capacity to be relevant depends exclusively on the organization and the individual's ability to predict, adapt, and change. Failure to do so now constrains the organization's opportunity to thrive in a sustainable way and its members' ability to adapt their work to meet the accelerating demands of excellence and the accelerating levels of competitive performance spiraling upward and continually challenging all to improve performance.

▶ A Failure of Leadership

Fundamental to all delineations and management of failure is the role of the leader. At the end of the day, in all human dynamic organizations, the role of the leader has the greatest impact on the culture, characteristics, work, and outcomes of the organization (Erickson, 2013). Leadership failure usually encompasses areas of awareness, insight, competence, process, and execution. Each of these arenas demonstrates the critical viability of the substance of leadership and challenges leaders to be continuously aware of their capacity to lead in complex dynamic human systems, perhaps most intensively evidenced in the healthcare arena (Porter-O'Grady & Malloch, 2016).

DISCUSSION

Have you ever personally experienced what you considered a failure of leadership? What were the circumstances that led you to that conclusion? What do you feel was missing in the leader's role? How would have you addressed the particular issue differently with what you have gained from reading this text?

With regard to innovation, there are several areas where leadership capacity can affect the successful process and trajectory of innovation work. Like every other area of organizational undertaking, leadership of innovation is as critical as is the innovator's own efforts at producing an innovation. Leaders are predominantly responsible for creating a context that facilitates the creativity and work effort leading to successful innovation. Without this context and structural and relational encouragement, the innovation process can often starve. Strong innovation leaders are advised to be aware of the critical indicators of the failure of leadership. Although they are many and varied, there are a few significant arenas of leadership that have the broadest impact on either facilitating or constraining effective innovation in an organization:

- Failure to predict: As previously outlined, the ability of the leader to demonstrate predictive and adaptive capacity is critical to the success of an innovative organization. Organizations live within a broader context. This context exemplifies a constant vortex and continual shifting and change in ways that represent the constant, undifferentiated, chaotic convergence of the larger sociopolitical, technological, and economic forces affecting every human system.

   Leaders, recognizing this constant and complex pattern of shift and change, continuously read the environment, looking deeply at the contextual issues influencing the organization in the broader setting with a lens directed to determining meaning and impact on the organizational system. These leaders devote particular and specific energies to this predictive activity as a way of translating environmental concerns and influences with a language that translates them into content that has meaning and value for health leadership and organizational members. This is especially true within the frame of innovation. Because innovation represents a relevant response to contemporary and future demand for enhancement, advancement, and transformation of process and product, it requires that there be a goodness of fit among the changing characteristics of the environment and its impact on the culture and life of the organization, and the organization's innovative response to those demands.

   In this framework, leaders validate their capacity to manage the vagaries of shift and transformation through the mechanism of good translation. This is demonstrated by their own capacity to be available to the changes generated from the environment, to recognize their meaning and impact on the organization and its people, and to respond specifically and particularly in a way that operates in the best interest of the organization and its ability to thrive. This predictive capacity of the leader is central to ensuring the organization's viability and continuous response to environmental and contextual shifts and as a way of ensuring that the organization remains relevant, engaged, and busy constructing the positive creation of a preferred future.

■ Failure of effective communication: Most people who work in organizations are busy fulfilling the activities to which they are assigned. What consumes their attention, for the most part, is the work that they do, the people that they serve, and the impact of their specific energies and activities. Generally, most of the work they do takes their full attention and occupies all of their energies in a way that reflects a focus on the present, current working capacity and the functional activities that complete the obligations of the day. Because work is so demanding in real time for most workers in organizations, their ability to be aware of the future, critical shifts in the environment, the emergence of the new and different, and the changing environmental and social circumstances affecting their long-term work is severely limited.

Recognizing this reality, leaders are constantly aware of the need to translate to the organization and its people the conditions and circumstances generating from the larger context or environment that will have an impact on their role. To do this, the leader ensures that there is an effective and continuous mechanism for communicating the environmental and contextual demands for currency, change, adaptation, and refinement of contemporary practices into new frames and models that best address the emerging issues moving the organization into its future. These mechanisms of communication are defined and structured in a way that make it easy and accessible for organizational members to access what they need to know, be able to incorporate that information into their practices, and collectively challenge contemporary work functions with emerging realities in ways that encourage them to engage and embrace these potentials for change as a fundamental part of their work.

The system of communication facilitated by the leadership includes opportunities for organizational members to participate in environmental scanning, translation, and application of those dynamics. This means workers have an impact on the work world and affect their own efforts and that of their teams in the exercise of the work of the organization. An effective communication system in a responsive organization is exemplified by broad-based participation, ownership, and engagement by all stakeholders who play a role in translating and adapting environmental demands for change into effective work processes and products in the organization.

Leaders create the communication network and pathways within which this information and organizational response processes can be channeled in a way that demonstrates an effective impact on the organization. This effort continues to make innovation viable and sustainable over the long term. Indeed, organizations that have existed over generations have done so through the mechanisms of engagement and ownership at every level, using open communication models and mechanisms for ensuring that meaningful and important decisions and actions and deliberations about potential innovations have both a voice and a place where ideas are acted upon. Here is where the innovator's voice can be legitimately heard and responded to with appropriate supports throughout the organization. Good communication pathways around the innovative process also help facilitate and support the various structural mechanics in the organization.

Sound communication gives form to the innovation, disciplines the process, and ensures that both the mechanics and means that advance the innovation are in place and positioned to accelerate the opportunity for the innovation to thrive. Demonstrated here is the capacity of the organization to continually enable innovation, confirmed by its open and interactive communication infrastructure in a way that encourages, supports, and advances the innovation through its various phases and stages to completion and impact.

■ Failure to engage risk: So much in health care depends on the capacity of its leaders to manage risk. Historically, emphasis on danger and threats to the safety of patient care have resulted in organizations that are in many ways fundamentally risk averse. This constant focus on ensuring that patients remain safe and that harm is avoided and prevented at all costs creates a mental model in an organizational milieu that sees risk as a threat and endangerment to the viability of patient care and the stability of the healthcare organization. While it is important for patients to remain safe and for the work environment to generate the highest-level potential for patient safety, that environment of patient safety should not be confused with the capacity of the organization to engage essential and necessary risk as it addresses constructing its future.

Risk cannot be eliminated. While risk can be effectively managed, in the course of human events there is always a measure of risk and the potential for that risk to influence decisions, actions, and impacts (Shaw, 2014). Good leaders recognize the value of risk. Embedded deep inside risk is the potential for improvement, enhancement, and creativity. Indeed, the future of the organization depends on its ability to engage risk, manage it well, and use its dynamics as a generator for creativity and innovation in a way that enhances the organization's opportunity to thrive. For the organization's capacity to succeed over the long term, its members' ability to identify, manage, and utilize risk in decision making, planning, and executing innovation processes is critical (Sundheim, 2013). The leader provides mechanisms and methods for the safe engagement of risk at every level of the organization, with an emphasis that 90% of the engagement of risk needs to occur at the point of service where most of the opportunity for creative insight and innovation occurs.

Good leaders use risk management tools, such as scenario planning, as a way of helping to create a safe environment for exploring, experimenting, and challenging the potential deeply embedded in risk in ways that can be translated to the benefit of the organization. Through the use of case and scenario activities at every level of the organization and in ways that reflect the obligation of strategic, operational, tactical, and functional roles in the organization, patient care is ultimately positively affected throughout the organization.

Leaders make sure that through scenario or case-based work, external drivers and influences are clearly outlined and articulated, financial and economic indicators and implications are thoroughly vetted, the veracity and strength of a strategy and/or tactic is tested in safe conditions, new possibilities are considered, and process mechanisms can be generated and safely tested to determine their viability and efficacy. The leader providing this kind of a platform in the innovative process ensures that innovation is incorporated as a regular expectation of the work of everyone in the organization and is structured in the organization in a way that ensures its utility and viability as a fundamental and functioning part of the work of the organization.

■ Failure to admit failure: As this chapter clearly attempts to emphasize, failure is a normative, functioning part of the role of leadership in assessing the viability and effectiveness of the innovation process inside the system. Failure is not a deficit for either the organization or the individual if managed properly and with careful leadership wisdom.

Failure serves as a metric, helping leaders know precisely where they are on a specific trajectory related to any innovation. Incremental failure lets the individual and innovation team know about the veracity and appropriateness of any particular element in the innovation dynamic. Failure helps leaders understand, through the use of specific enumerated evaluation elements, where the innovation is currently and its potential along with the choices and actions that can facilitate that potential. Failure also helps leaders identify what does not work, what is no longer appropriate, when a change in course needs to occur, or when a process or project has reached a terminal point in its current trajectory. All of these are objectives and viable tools that suggest to the leader subsequent choices and adjustments in the innovation process necessary to sustain and support it.

The requisite of failure is that it be used objectively as a tool. Failure must constantly be identified as a part of the metrics that assess the trajectory of an innovation and help determine choices and actions that need to be taken as a result of the information that a failure provides to leaders of the innovation process. As outlined previously in this chapter, if failure is engaged as a productive and positive tool set for defining the success of a particular innovation trajectory, the emotional and personal content often affiliated with it can be minimized and potentially eliminated. In this case, it is the obligation of leaders to create that objective and safe approach to the utility of failure as an objective and meaningful tool along the continuum of innovation work. Leaders who do not create this safe and productive capacity for the use of failure metrics actually contribute to the emotional trauma and debilitation. Negative feelings and responses to failure in the organization should come as no surprise to leaders if their organizational members are failure sensitive and risk averse. If the leadership climate generates and supports those negative sentiments and punishes or creates an adverse response to notions, mechanisms, processes, and outcomes that result from the aversion to risking and failing, then debilitating failure is guaranteed. Failure is good only if it is perceived as good and only if it produces values that result in better decisions, more effective action, and exciting processes and products that demonstrate the positive use of failure analytics as a part of the process of producing a dynamic outcome (**FIGURE 8-7**).

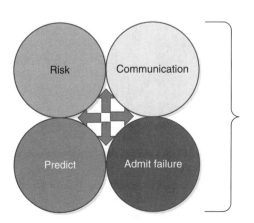

FIGURE 8-7 A failure of leadership.

DISCUSSION

When considering the leadership of innovation, what particular personal skill sets do you bring to the engagement of innovation? As this chapter closes, what specific skills do you need to focus on developing in your capacity to embrace failure as an objective tool for managing innovation? How will you test your new and developing skills in your leadership role?

🔍 CASE EXAMPLE: LEADERSHIP

Leticia Morgan, RN, BSN, had been approached by one of her staff members with a new digital device and software that would help monitor the movement of geriatric patients in their homes and inform the geriatric continuum of care nurse coordinator if the patient was involved in a safety risk activity. The nurse has been working on this idea for the last couple of years, and now she is ready to move her idea into a useful product. The nurse inventor had kept Leticia informed during every stage of her idea creation, but Leticia had paid only cursory attention to the progress. Now this nurse was approaching her to determine if there were any formal steps or processes she needed to go through in the organization to access supports and systems that might help take her invention to production.

Leticia had heard about her health agency's interest in facilitating monitoring the care of homebound patients but was not sure how it worked. When she heard about the innovation development process, Leticia thought it was very complicated and detailed and was directed mostly to helping physicians develop practice innovations within their own specialties to advance their technology and financial partnership with the health organization. Leticia was pretty sure they would not be interested in any nursing idea that did not appear to make much difference in nurses' work. Leticia informed the nurse inventor that it might be wiser for her to find a patent or invention organization outside the health agency that might be interested in an invention like hers because the organization's resources were tight and there would not be much support inside the system. The nurse inventor was discouraged, leaving the conversation with Leticia believing that her potential innovation was not significant enough to pursue and feeling that perhaps she should simply let it go.

Discussion

Leticia and the nurse inventor practiced in an organization that did have an organized and structured innovation process. Leticia assumed that from what she had understood about process, it was directed more to position inventors who had a larger stake in the financial impact for themselves and the organization. Leticia further assumed that the invention was not significant enough for further consideration and directed the nurse inventor elsewhere. This scenario can be replicated in a number of health organizations across the country and creates some real challenges for inventors and a potential limitation on the possibilities and implications for an innovation that should get to see the light of day.

Questions

1. What do you think of Leticia's original relationship with the nurse inventor during the idea stage over the past 2 years?
2. How thorough do you think Leticia's understanding of the agency's innovation process was, and how did that influence her advice to the nurse inventor?

3. If you were the nurse leader in Leticia's place, what series of activities and interactions would you have with the nurse inventor? What stages or phases of the innovation process might you facilitate for the nurse inventor's efforts?
4. How many levels of failure are you able to identify in this scenario? (Keep in mind that there is evidence in this scenario of failure at the systemic, departmental, leadership, and individual levels.)
5. What steps would you take to address the failures you identified in question 4 to keep these kinds of failures from occurring again and instead facilitate an environment of innovation supportive of invention?

▶ Summary

From an objective perspective, the only role that failure plays is in the evaluation and assessment of organizations' and individuals' movement to success and thriving. The incongruent fear of failure generally expressed by leaders and others does not come near representing the significance of the value of failure as a metric along the trajectory of the journey to successful innovation. Instead, engaging and embracing failure as a viable and useful measure of progress is a much more realistic and valuable perspective of the role of failure and one that provides great utility in the innovation process. Leaders must confront individual and organizational apprehensions regarding the role of failure and make issues related to the management of failure a fundamental part of the leadership development process. If the mechanisms and characteristics of failure are utilized as positive tools in evaluating the mechanisms and processes of innovation, a more disciplined, appropriate, and meaningful experience of innovation development can be generated in individuals and in the organization. Failure is a tool, not a condition.

References

Akintoye, A., Goulding, J., & Zawdie, G. (2012). *Construction innovation and process improvement.* Ames, IA: Wiley-Blackwell.

Anderson, N., & Costa, A. C. (2010). *Innovation and knowledge management.* Los Angeles, CA: Sage.

Bennis, W. G., Sample, S. B., & Asghar, R. (2015). *The art and adventure of leadership: Understanding failure, resilience and success.* Hoboken, NJ: Wiley.

Bolman, L. G., & Deal, T. E. (2013). *Reframing organizations: Artistry, choice, and leadership* (5th ed.). San Francisco, CA: Jossey-Bass.

Cleary, J. (2014). *The Cambridge companion to Irish modernism.* New York, NY: Cambridge University Press.

Davila, T., & Epstein, M. (2014). *The innovation paradox: Why good businesses kill breakthroughs and how they can change.* San Francisco, CA: Berrett-Koehler.

Erickson, J. I. (2013). Reflections on leadership talent: A void or an opportunity? *Nursing Administration Quarterly, 37*(1), 44–51. http://dx.doi.org/10.1097/NAQ.0b013e3182751610

Guzzini, E., & Iacobucci, D. (2017). Project failures and innovation performance in university-firm collaborations. *Journal of Technology Transfer, 42*(4), 865–883.

Harford, T. (2012). *Adapt: Why success always starts with failure.* New York, NY: Farrar, Straus & Giroux.

Hoque, F., & Baer, D. (2014). *Everything connects: How to transform and lead in the age of creativity, innovation, and sustainability.* New York, NY: McGraw-Hill Education.

Kale, V. (2015). *Inverting the paradox of excellence: How companies use variations for business excellence and how enterprise variations are enabled by SAP.* Boca Raton, FL: CRC Press.

Kumar, M., & Kumar, N. (2016). Three dimensions of service recovery: Examining relationships and impact. *Supply Chain Management, 21*(2), 273–286.

LaRusso, N., Spurrier, B., & Farrugia, G. (2015). *Think big, start small, move fast: A blueprint for transformation from the Mayo Clinic Center for Innovation.* New York, NY: McGraw-Hill Education.

Ledema, R., Verma, R., Wutzke, S., Lyones, N., & McCaughan, B. (2017). A network of networks: The governance of deliberative approaches to healthcare improvement and reform. *Journal of Health Organization and Management, 31*(2), 223–236.

Ormerod, P. (2010). *Why most things fail and how to avoid it.* New York, NY: Wiley.

Owens, T., & Fernandez, O. (2014). *The lean enterprise: How corporations can innovate like startups.* Hoboken, NJ: Wiley.

Porter-O'Grady, T., & Malloch, K. (2016). *Quantum leadership: Building better partnerships for sustainable health* (4th ed.). Burlington, MA: Jones & Bartlett Learning.

Shaw, R. (2014). *Leadership blindspots: How successful leaders identify and overcome the weaknesses that matter.* San Francisco, CA: Jossey-Bass.

Sills, D. L., Wolf, C. P., & Shelanski, V. B. (1982). *Accident at Three Mile Island: The human dimensions.* Boulder, CO: Westview Press.

Sundheim, D. (2013). *Taking smart risks: How sharp leaders win when stakes are high.* New York, NY: McGraw-Hill.

Talukder, M. (2014). *Managing innovation: Adoption from innovation to implementation.* Surrey, UK: Gower.

Tawfik, A., Rong, H., & Choi, I. (2015). Failing to learn: Towards a unified design approach for failure-based learning. *Educational Technology, Research and Development, 63*(6), 975–994.

U.S. Congress, Senate Committee on Commerce, Science, and Transportation, Subcommittee on Science, Technology, and Space. (1986). *Space shuttle accident: Hearing before the Subcommittee on Science, Technology, and Space of the Committee on Commerce, Science, and Transportation, United States Senate, Ninety-ninth Congress, second session, on space shuttle accident and the Rogers Commission report, February 18, June 10 and 17, 1986.* Washington, DC: US Government Printing Office.

von Held, F. (2012). *Collective creativity: Exploring creativity in social network development as part of organizational learning.* Wiesbaden, Germany: Springer.

Weberg, D. (2017). Innovation leadership behaviors: Starting the complexity journey. In S. Davidson, D. Weberg, T. Porter-O'Grady, & K. Malloch (Eds.), *Evidence-based innovation in nursing and health professions.* Cambridge, MA: Jones & Bartlett Learning.

Wilson, H., Gole, J., Bharat, M., & Jitendra, M. (1916). Value-based Healthcare. *Advances in Management, 6*(1), 1–8.

CHAPTER 9

Leading Innovation and Performance Improvement for High-Performing Systems

Daniel Weberg, Jung G. Kim, and John Myovich

CHAPTER OBJECTIVES

Upon completion of this chapter, the reader will be able to:

1. Describe and differentiate the performance improvement and innovation in high-reliability organizations operating in complex systems
2. Use performance improvement and innovation methods to address organizational strategic and change management issues.
3. Analyze the role of the leader in performance improvement and innovation in a high-reliability organization operating in complex systems

Author Note: The goal of this chapter is to discuss the leadership needed to combine innovation and performance improvement. Although the chapter will describe the process of both, it is not the goal of the chapter to train you in the performance improvement (PI) or innovation process. Therefore, we have provided references and links for further exploration of either process within the chapter.

▶ Introduction

High-reliability organizations are always moving, always evolving, and always iterating to maintain safety, sustainability, relevance, and organizational performance (LaPorte & Consolini, 1991; Roberts, 1990; Vogus & Singer, 2016; Vogus & Sutcliffe, 2007). Organizations become highly reliable when ideas, information, and people are brought in, incorporated into the workflows despite complex conditions that create barriers, and have feedback loops to promote continuous improvement. In health care, organizations adopt learning and information through two main modalities: innovation and performance improvement (PI). These processes help organizations balance strategic effectiveness (PI) and strategic flexibility (innovation). Combining incremental improvements and breakthrough change is associated with significant improvement over focusing on performance improvement alone (Terziovski, 2002). However, failure to adopt innovation and PI are commonly observed because organizations are unable to implement them properly (Mintzberg, 1994; Shortell & Kaluzny, 2006).

The relationship between innovation and PI is symbiotic. Innovation is the process by which organizations adapt to change by generating new ways of work, value, and outcomes. PI is the process by which organizations properly identify, refine, and optimize existing processes to improve and spread reliability, efficiency, and effectiveness (Langley et al., 2009). From a complex adaptive systems point of view, innovation is the organization's movement into chaos and uncertainty, while PI is the counterweight toward stability and optimization. The role of the innovation process is exploration, and the role of PI is exploitation. These arguments imply PI as being detrimental, but in the advent of scarce resources in the healthcare delivery setting, exploitation taps into existing processes and maximizes value and resources. For example, leaders would incorporate PI to exploit a hand-washing process improvement to get 99% compliance, thus getting every ounce of value out of existing workflow processes. On the other hand, Innovation would explore ways to decrease the transmission of infection through alternative patient contact should infection control efforts require a radical solution. In high reliability organizations, both PI and innovation serve as a check and balance as they keep the organization on the edge of chaos by pulling each other from extreme stability (stagnation) or falling into total chaos (see **FIGURE 9-1**).

However, if an organization overemphasizes innovation, it will have a pipeline of new and disruptive ideas that continually flow, but it will lack the ability to optimize them into efficient or effective workflows (imagine drinking from the firehose). If an organization is overly focused on PI, it will refine and optimize existing work but divert resources away from creating new and needed disruptions to adapt to environmental pressures. While both are driven by organizational change to add value into strategic planning, they operate on either end of a spectrum. PI, at its core, is focused on optimization of existing processes and improving their reliability, which essentially means it's focused on eliminating waste and variation. In essence, PIs diagnose work processes to eliminate the statistical insignificant work and outliers to maximize the highest probability of success (see Figure 9-1). On the other side, innovation is heavily focused on identifying the outliers and positive deviants that are producing unexpected successes in systems that may be broken yet challenge the status quo. These conceptual descriptions help make the point that PI and innovation are symbiotic but very different organizational change processes to maintain movement and adaptation.

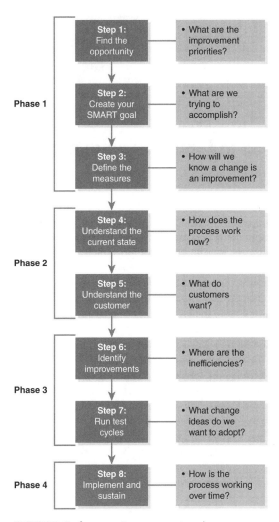

FIGURE 9-1 Performance improvement road map.

We recognize that PI and innovation, in practice, are fluid tactics and often substituted for each other. This is a critical mistake when diagnosing opportunities to incorporate change. High-reliability organizations and their leaders understand the nuances of both strategies and the when, why, and how to use each, and perhaps simultaneously, to achieve the desired outcomes. High-performing leaders also understand that leadership behaviors, team dynamics, and organizational characteristics are attributes that must be considered to successfully implement PI and innovation.

This chapter will describe the foundations of PI and innovation; outline the practice-based tools to implement each; help leaders understand the structures, resources, and processes; and identify outcomes and goals required of leaders to integrate them into a high-performing organization. The chapter will answer the question: How do leaders in organizations within complex systems approach PI and innovation to reduce uncertainty and create high-performing systems?

DISCUSSION

Reflect on healthcare organizations you have worked with. How many have innovation departments? How many have improvement departments? Describe the leadership, team members, and focus of the two groups. How are they similar or different?

▶ The Need to Combine Exploration and Exploitation

History has taught us that siloing innovation and improvement (aka PI) into different departments and accountabilities has not been successful. Boer and Gertson (2006) argue that no matter what organizational change theory you might subscribe to, the combination of innovation and improvement activities in organizations is necessary. The goal of this combination is to have an ambidextrous organization that can adapt organically when new ideas are needed and leverage more resources when the organization needs to optimize those ideas.

For leaders, the combination of these two processes is not as simple as creating a PI team trained in Lean or Six Sigma, and an innovation team that uses human-centered design. Many organizations have those, and healthcare organizations are widely known for having innovation and PI teams. The challenge is to integrate the two teams, processes, and learnings into a dynamic that fuels organizational performance. In essence, it is that ability which creates new strategies and then optimizes those strategies. Even at the point of care, the combination of innovation and improvement is important. The unpredictable environment creates a need for quicker strategic reaction in patient care yet requires optimal decision making to ensure the patient's safety. Frontline caregivers need to know when to standardize process and when to question the status quo. Evidence-based practice (EBP) is an excellent example of this dynamic in action.

EBP embodies the combination of performance improvement and innovation. When clinicians challenge the status quo and ask, "Is there a better way?" they are tapping into the innovation process. They review literature, incorporate patient preferences, include their care team ideas, and develop a best possible evidence intervention for the problem at hand. That is innovation. Then, as they introduce the new intervention, they need to tap the PI process to test, optimize, measure, and refine the work to meet the desired outcome of the evidenced change.

Often in organizations, innovation and improvement get in the way of each other. This may be because they report to different leaders, they are seen as antithetical, or competing organizational priorities displace one process over another. PI often lies with operational leaders such as chief operating officers (COOs) who are motivated by short-term performance targets, whereas innovation is often led by chief executive officers (CEOs) who look to longer term aims and need a safe zone to test pilot and learn from failure. In the end, both PI and innovation are tied together by the strategic goals of an organization, linked by both short- and long-term goals. And leave no doubt, the balancing of these two is not always clear cut. You are combining the organic and mechanistic parts of a complex system while trying to make optimal decisions.

▶ Organizational Evolution toward High Performance

Established organizations with a long history have been shown to evolve over time, first focusing on operations and evolving through improvement and finally becoming innovative and future focused (Boer, Kuhn, & Gertsen, 2006). Thus, the high-performing organization would be able to combine efficiency, quality, flexibility, speed, and innovation. We can observe the need for evolution in reverse, in shorter time periods, when examining the changes that a start-up organization must undergo as it moves from innovation to efficient business models (see **FIGURE 9-2**). Whether the leader is starting an organization or influencing change in an existing one, the skill of improvement and innovation are essential.

This chapter discusses the need for innovation and improvement to support continued organization and team adaptation to the changing pressures of the healthcare industry. Notice that the processes are very similar and use similar terms, tools, and methods to arrive at fundamentally different outcomes because these processes of PI and innovation are both part of the continuum of change. High-performing organizations are excellent at change. Whether the change is the refinement of execution or the disruption of innovation, organizations that are able to challenge themselves, use rigorous change processes, and operationalize those processes across the entity will outcompete, outperform, and outlive the competition. In health care, these organizations will be rewarded with better patient outcomes, higher employee satisfaction, and better performance than those organizations that cling to efficiency alone. This is not a matter of semantics; remember, innovation and improvement are fundamentally different in focus and if mismanaged can lead to system failures. Leaders need to understand when to use PI, innovation, or both, and incorporate the tools to help with decision making.

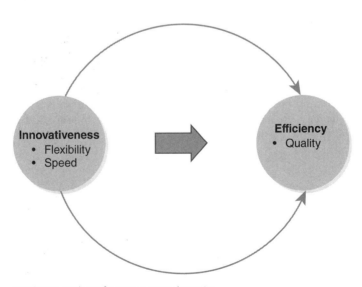

FIGURE 9-2 High-performing system dynamics.

Current Focus or New Focus

The current state is our daily reality and competes for attention. The workflows, products, and processes we use today will always be the starting point for change. The leader and his or her team must determine what the change entails and define the desired outcome of that change. Using an analogy, teams can help determine if they need improvement or innovation by simply asking, "Are we trying to make the light bulb brighter or find a new source of light?" If you are trying to make the light bulb brighter, then you are working on efficiency. This most likely is going to require improvement. If the desired outcome is primarily efficiency gains, then the leader needs to assemble a team to work on improving processes. This will include PI experts using the PI process to refine and remove waste from the system.

If you are looking for new sources of light, you need innovation. Since the desired outcome is finding new sources of light, the team will need to focus on creativity and the innovation process with a team made up of diverse groups who are grounded in the evidence around light generation. If the leader misaligns the teams in this case, the result could be wasted work and an outcome that does not meet the organization's needs, and teams becoming frustrated with the misuse of talent.

The Best Best versus the Worst Best

Similar to the light bulb question, leaders can assess problems from the lens of the change continuum. Has the problem reached its "best best" efficiency? Take hand-washing initiatives in health care as an example. Continually, across all organizations, the percentage of hand-washing compliance remains staggeringly low considering that it's a simple process. In some organizations, despite significant focus by improvement, direct observations, and even punishment, rates go no higher than 70%. That means 70% of the time, clinicians wash their hands when required. Significant resources have been used to solve this issue and it's stuck at its best best using the current state. This is a problem ripe for innovation to resolve.

For leaders, when a problem has been given significant resources, including improvement efforts, and still remains below the desired outcome, it may be time for innovation. Innovation allows you to break from the current state and achieve what innovators call the "worst best." The worst best is the result of a successful innovation process that creates a novel solution to the problem and sets a new baseline for which to improve upon. This new baseline in the case of hand washing might be just 71%, but because it's a radically new process, the room for improvement could be much greater. You are now trying to gain from a new worst best, using PI, to achieve a new best best.

Big Hairy Audacious Problems: A Case for Using PI and Innovation

Leadership must navigate ambiguity and unpredictability. Some problems, like those mentioned previously, lend themselves to PI or innovation with just a little gray area of unknown. Other problems are so complex that they require the use of both PI and innovation working in tandem to solve. These types of problems usually require creating the new and improving the known. For example, if a health system were to undertake reimaging the design, user experience, and inner workings of its primary care clinics, that system may want to utilize both innovation and improvement. That system may want to use innovation to imagine new clinic designs, technologies, and user experiences while using improvement to refine appointment scheduling, check-in procedures, and teamwork workflows. For leaders to combine the efforts, evidence, and processes of PI and innovation, it is important to understand and further explore these two areas separately.

▶ Leading PI

PI hinges on the strategic direction of one's organization in response to changes needed to adapt and survive in the healthcare environment (Scott, Ruef, Mendel, & Caronna, 2000). Since it's based on short-term outcomes using measurable goals that connect to the overall strategic direction of an organization, PI sets a scientific-based standard on how to improve reliability, decrease variability, and (especially important for healthcare settings) prevent harm to patients (Shortell & Kaluzny, 2006). These characteristics of PI help optimize organizational strategies by improving information flows from the front line to the executive and help you, as a leader, identify and facilitate the feedback loops to continuously improve your organization's goals. This makes understanding the organizational goals up front a critical step to implement PI. And first and foremost, it should be based on the patients' (or customers') needs.

In general, PI first asks the following questions: (1) Is our strategy on track? (2) How can we perform better? and (3) Are there more effective and efficient ways of working? These questions will ignite your PI journey on how to find opportunities for improvement and diagnose the existing work processes to maximize your PI goal's success.

Leading your team's PI journey can be illustrated as a road map that includes five key phases with eight steps. Each step includes action steps, outcomes identified, and tools needed to support accomplishing the step:

Phase 1: Target Area for Improvement

This phase helps identify a specific goal that your organization, program, or daily operations want to achieve. It essentially helps you create a bull's-eye target so your PI efforts are specific enough to achieve accuracy, and when you implement, you maintain precision to keep hitting the target.

■ Step 1: Find the Opportunity: What Are the Improvement Priorities?

Identifying PI opportunities depends on your assessment of your organizational strategy and prioritizing them. The Strategy Driver Diagram (**FIGURE 9-3**) will help you identify your goal, the drivers that help achieve that goal, and finally the focus areas that are measurable. The results will then unveil a specific goal. These may unveil multiple goals to which you then must prioritize by assessing your PI's potential effort and impact. The Balanced Scorecard (https://www.balancedscorecard.org/BSC-Basics/About-the-Balanced-Scorecard) will capture focus areas with specific targets by scoring how much effort is needed

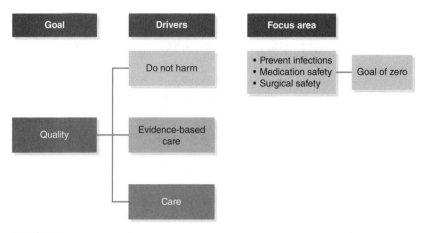

FIGURE 9-3 Strategy driver diagram.

to ensure that your strategy is being executed, and in a meaningful way. The result will help you estimate the return on investment (ROI) that will help you as a leader to see variation or shortfalls with current organizational performance and target opportunities to improve.

- ACTION:
  - ○ Assess your strategies and current performance
  - ○ Evaluate, prioritize, and select an improvement opportunity
  - ○ Estimate the ROI impact/benefits of improvement
- OUTCOMES:
  - ○ Major strategic areas identified and prioritized area for PI selected
  - ○ ROI drafted
- TOOLS:
  - ○ Strategy Driver Diagram
  - ○ Balanced Scorecard
- Step 2: Create Your SMART Goal: What Are You Trying to Accomplish?

Clarifying your PI goal early in your efforts is critical. The overall aim statement is essentially the goal you identified in Step 1. Expanding on this will become your SMART goal, which is a single statement that explains what your team is aiming to achieve: S: Specific on what will be improved without operational definitions or acronyms; M: Measurable for current and desired performance; A: Attainable for the team to accomplish; R: Reflects the voice of the customer; and T: Time bound that sets the dates to which the goal will be achieved over a series of project timeline milestones. Once your aim statement and SMART goal are established, identifying who will support you through sponsors and PI implementation teams follows. Analyzing these stakeholders helps to unpack the resources needed and determine whether your PI goal is achievable. To keep these elements in one place, drafting a Project Charter (http://www.ihi.org/resources/Pages/Tools/QI-Project-Charter.aspx) is a helpful tool to frame and communicate your PI effort.

Step 1. Expanding on this will become your SMART goal, which is a single statement that explains what your team is aiming to achieve: S: Specific on what will be improved without operational definitions or acronyms; *M*: Measurable for current and desired performance; *A*: Attainable for the team to accomplish; *R*: Reflects the voice of the customer; and *T*: Time bound that sets the dates to which the goal will be achieved over a series of project timeline milestones

- ACTION:
    - ◦ Create your PI overall AIM and SMART goal
    - ◦ Identify your PI scope, team, and project timeline milestones
    - ◦ Identify and analyze stakeholders
- OUTCOMES:
    - ◦ Project charter drafted
    - ◦ Stakeholder analysis
- TOOLS:
    - ◦ Project charter

■ Step 3: Define the Measures: How Will You Know a Change Is an Improvement?

This is the last step for this phase in targeting an area for PI by defining your measures of improvement and starting to gather data to "benchmark." Improvement can mean many things to different stakeholders, so defining it by its operational definition is a good way to start as you define your measures. Improvement is the result of some change where the results are positive, relevant, and sustainable, based on what is important to your organization. They can be illustrated by charts, dashboards, formal reports, etc. Ideally, you want to utilize results that are over time and embraced by as many stakeholders as possible. Once you have defined improvement, looking for existing measures that inform your organization's improvement is next. Here, you will examine whether you have the three key measurement categories: outcome (measures whether you are achieving your SMART goal), process (measures that check if your processes lead up to the outcome measure and are strongly correlated with your outcomes), and balancing (measures if there are unintended effects to your PI effort, whether positive or negative). Once your measures have been identified, these can be drafted into your project charter.

An example of these family of measures can be observed with managing patients' cardiovascular health. An outcome measure could be controlling for hypertension, the process measure would be monitoring blood pressure, and the balancing measure would check if more patients who increase their blood pressure monitoring are prescribed more beta-blockers. As you look for measures in your organization, you can start benchmarking previous performance to get a sense of the history. This will help you also refine Step 2 as needed. You may also discover that you don't have a system that currently collects the measures you need. Here is when you will need to develop development assessments.

- ACTION:
    - ◦ Defining what improvement means
    - ◦ Identifying or developing key measures: outcome, process, balancing
    - ◦ Gather baseline (aka "benchmarking")
- OUTCOMES:
    - ◦ Measures identified and drafted into the project charter
    - ◦ Baseline data collected
- TOOLS:
    - ◦ Project charter

Phase 2: Assess/Define Current Processes

This second phase looks at the mechanisms in your workflow processes from both the delivery and receiving end.

■ Step 4: Understand the Current State: How Does the Process Work Now?

First establishing your current state will help you identify areas to further take advantage of high value and to remove those that are low. To start, the following diagnostic tools will help leaders understand and visualize the current processes by deconstructing the process steps and discovering where PI opportunities may lie.

The systems of process mapping (http://www.ihi.org/communities/blogs /5-steps-for-creating-value-through-process-mapping-and-observation) illustrate workflow processes by visualizing each step, clarify the requirements to achieve each step, and show the interdependencies across the workflow process. You start from left to right, mapping out the first workflow step with arrows leading up to the final. Ideally you want to include how much time each step took and the resources expended at each step. And, most important, you want to go to where the work is actually done and do this as a team exercise. The key benefit of a process map is that it helps with the mental model that defines workflow. Do we think we all do our work the same way? The process map will help clarify discrepancies before you get too far into your PI and identify the value of each step as your team reviews the process.

Another useful diagnostic tool that identifies major causes of process flow defects is a visual chart based on the Pareto principle (Institute for Healthcare Improvement, 2017a). This cause and effect principle is more commonly referred to as the "80/20 rule" where 20% of the causes drive 80% of the effect. The Pareto chart is a simple bar chart (Institute for Healthcare Improvement, 2017a) that identifies a small handful (20%) of contributing factors, helps focus your PI efforts, and supports your rationale to implement your targeted PI within your organization. The Institute of Healthcare Improvement provides an array of PI tools that can be adapted to your organization (Institute for Healthcare Improvement, 2018).

- ACTION:
  - ° Create a system of process mapping (or collect data for a Pareto chart)
  - ° Analyze the value of each process in the map (or review the Pareto chart to identify which factor to focus on)
- OUTCOMES:
  - ° Current state identified
- TOOLS:
  - ° Detailed process map
  - ° Pareto chart

■ Step 5: Understand the Customer: What Do Customers Want?

Because change is complex and individuals embrace it differently, understanding your customer's voice helps you clarify the most optimal solution for all stakeholders, not just what you or leadership perceive is right for the customer. Identifying who will be affected by your PI is a critical assessment of the current step. If your stakeholders don't understand the rationale for change, even the most beneficial PI goal will fall to the wayside. Capturing the customer's voice can be achieved in various ways, but the goal should be to engage, and, ideally, collaborate as much as possible. Interviewing only or brainstorming from afar as you assess the current state are weaker methods that can diminish your customer's voice.

Once you've identified your stakeholder's voices, translating them to organizational strategies is key to align resources and leverage effort. The Voice of the Customer Template (http://www.ihi.org/communities/blogs/5-steps-for-creating-value-through-process-mapping-and-observation) will help you identify stakeholder categories, their needs, and how they align with organizational strategies. Revising your Prioritization Matrix will also help target your PI efforts as you incorporate your stakeholders' voices.

- ACTION:
  - º Identify and engage the customer
  - º Translate the customer voice to organizational strategies
  - º Revise your prioritization matrix
- OUTCOMES:
  - º Voice of customer is measured and prioritized
- TOOLS:
  - º Voice of the customer template
  - º Prioritization matrix

Phases 3 and 4: Identify Improvement Opportunities and Evaluate Your Small Tests of Change

These phases finalize your PI planning and ready your team to implement small tests of change.

- Step 6: Identify Improvements: Where Is the Waste/Variation/Inefficiencies?

  Finding waste, variation, and inefficiency is a systematic way to identify the underlying processes and the final step in prioritizing your PI efforts. To identify these hidden forces, understanding how to recognize these low-value elements is challenging but critical. High-reliability organizations have the systems to illuminate these areas immediately. But there are low-fidelity tools that can be used immediately as well. The detailed process map in Step 4 is one. Another is the fishbone diagram (https://www.youtube.com/watch?v=mLvizyDFLQ4) that outlines the causes and effects, commonly known as root cause analysis and a central element found in Lean (D'Andreamatteo, Ianni, Lega, & Sargiacomo, 2015; Institute for Healthcare Improvement, 2017b). As you finalize your PI target areas, consider the lowest hanging fruit to test your improvement efforts on a small scale and prepare your stakeholders for change. These fruits can be identified by visiting areas within your organization or even those external. Then draft a change management plan that incorporates the voices of your stakeholders, along with a communication plan for your pilot sites that you will test in Step 7. This preparation for change will foster awareness of why you are implementing PI and give your stakeholders an opportunity to have their voice heard.
  - ACTION:
    - º Analyze the current work process for waste and variation reduction, and improving workflow
    - º Revisit the detailed process map to identify targeted areas to test at a small scale ("lowest hanging fruit")

    ◦   Draft your change management plan using the voice of the customer template
- OUTCOMES:
  ◦   Prioritized change opportunities have been identified
  ◦   Stakeholders' readiness and communication plan have been implemented
- TOOLS:
  ◦   Fishbone diagrams
  ◦   Prioritization matrix/Pareto chart
  ◦   Detailed process map
  ◦   Voice of the customer template

■ Step 7: Run Tests Cycles: What Change Ideas Do You Want to Adopt?

Although Steps 1–6 may feel like a lot of planning, they help prioritize and reinforce the principles of PI that create a scientific "environment" to implement and enable measurable change. Step 7 runs the test cycles of small change to pilot your PI and identify what you want to adopt, adapt, or abandon. Step 7 is framed by the Plan-Do-Study-Act (PDSA) test framework that is commonly found in today's healthcare setting (Shortell & Kaluzny, 2006). *P*: Plan the questions to be asked and plan the methods to measure your predictions; *D*: Do implement your tests of change while collecting data; *S*: Study your results by comparing them to your initial predictions and asking what you learned; and *A*: Act on what worked or did not by finalizing your decision on what you want to adopt, abandon, or change for another test cycle. The PDSA's key features are that it is based on continuous improvement, identifies the most critical elements that have an impact on your desired outcome, and creates a mini cycle of improvement that is easier to implement (a three-step change vs. eight steps). Your PDSA cycle goes as follows: the first cycle tests a small-scale change; followed by cycle 2, which may test different conditions; followed by cycle 3 that scales up promising findings, etc. Measurement over time through Run or Control Charts (http://www.ihi.org/education/IHIOpenSchool/resources/Pages/AudioandVideo/Whiteboard13.aspx) are key tools to track your progress.

> *P*: Planning the questions to be asked and planning the methods to measures your predictions; D: Do implement your tests of change while collecting data; S: Study your results by comparing them to your initial predictions and asking what you learned; and A: Act on what worked or did not by finalizing your decision on what you want to adopt, abandon, or change for another test cycle.

Similar to a clinical trial that tests an experimental therapy over multiple phases, PDSA aims to implement change that can be sustained. Step 7 may be seem like an overlap of Steps 1–6, but the key feature is that it's a subset of the first six steps that allows you to implement several "mini" PIs at once.

- ACTION:
  ◦   Implement your prioritized change opportunities using PDSA
  ◦   Analyze data from PDSA to evaluate the impact of prioritized change opportunities
  ◦   Determine which prioritized change opportunities will be scaled up for larger efforts

- OUTCOMES:
  - PDSA cycle completed for each prioritized change opportunities
  - Evidence identified for most effective prioritized change opportunities
- TOOLS:
  - PDSA Test Framework
  - Run or control charts

Phase 5: Large-Scale Improvement: Implement and Spread Improved Processes

The final phase is to "spread and sustain" as you understand the magnitude and increase your confidence in making an impact with your PI. Understanding if your PI effort has met its projected benefit whether it is transferable across as many relevant parts of your organization as possible are key elements to spreading and sustaining your PI effort.

- Step 8: Implement and Sustain: How Is the Process Working over Time?

  As you scale up and spread your successful PI efforts from Step 7, consider how you will promote and implement for a larger audience. Is your PI clear and simple to implement? Does it give flexibility through a menu of activities that you found successful in Step 7? And are the new audiences ready to adopt change?

QUESTIONS TO ASK ARE:

1. Does the improvement fill a need?
2. Does it make a difference?
3. Is it evidence based, where we have a clear association and correlation between the improvement and the outcome?
4. Is the bundle or intervention tightly constructed?

An experienced operational leader models the appropriate level of inquiry and problem solving in a performance dialogue with colleagues. For issues with known solutions, a leader will hold individual operational managers accountable to fix it. However, if the performance issue has no known solution or it exists throughout the system, the leader will initiate an improvement charter and follow the PI approach to solving the problem. This requires going back to diagnostic tools including run charts and revisiting the voice of the customer.

However, in complex systems where uncertainty and chaos are everywhere, diagnosing your organization's level of certainty to allocate the necessary requirements and resources is critical. The Stacey diagram (**FIGURE 9-4**) is one tool that is helpful in this situation so that you can find agreement with your stakeholders when implementing change across a system (Stacey, 1996). It highlights five approaches for spread and diffusion. Selecting the right approach is dependent on the degree of agreement and the degree of certainty or the solution. If a solution is well known and the change is simple, then just doing it is the best approach. If the solution is more complex and requires agreement among the stakeholders, then testing, replicating, and defusing is the best approach.

FIGURE 9-4 Stacey chart.

Data from Stacey, R. D. *Strategic management and organisational dynamics: The challenge of complexity.* 3rd ed. Harlow: Prentice Hall, 2002.

Last, planning your PI's sustainability is the key to continuous improvement and long-term organizational success (Wiltsey Stirman et al., 2012). A good sustainability plan will have clear owners identified, measures, cadence for monitoring status, a communication plan, and a documented process. Owners of the process will be especially critical, and effective leaders will have engaged with the appropriate stakeholders, identified and recognized champions, and celebrated successes. As a leader, ensuring that the engagement process is attended to helps to build on prior successes and avoids reinventing the wheel.

- ACTION:
  - Scale up and spread your small tests of change by promoting and implementing your prioritized change opportunities
  - Engage and train team on new processes
  - Identify and remove old processes
  - Create and implement a sustainability and monitoring plan for continuous improvement and maintaining voice of customer (VOC)
  - Celebrate your successes
- OUTCOMES:
  - Implement, spread, and communicate your large-scale improvement
  - Evaluate your large-scale improvement over time and remove old processes
  - Engage with your team and customers
- TOOLS:
  - Run and control charts
  - Voice of the customer template
  - Spread plan and assessment
  - Stacey diagram
  - Sustainability/control plan

As outlined previously, leading PI hinges on team effort by incorporating strategy, measurement, and management to remain effective and increase the propensity for better relationships across the organization. And because its measured success and achievement of goals rely on feedback loops, PI requires innovation to feed it new information from the environment and prevent organizational stagnation. Hence, innovation is a transformative change that creates a new dimension in performance.

DISCUSSION

Reflect on your organization. What problems have been tackled with PI and what was the outcome? What PI is the appropriate method to use? Was it led effectively? What would you have changed?

The process of PI is rigorous and validated to help find solutions, remove barriers, and measure impact. The leadership of PI holds the team accountable to the steps, provides resources and time to complete the process, and paves the way to implement the improvement and spread it across the organization. It is also important not to skip steps or rush the learning process. PI, like innovation, requires time to let the solutions emerge. PI also requires that teams have difficult and honest conversations about what is and is not working in a given system. As you read the next section on leading innovation, compare and contrast the processes.

▶ Leading Innovation

Innovation in organizations involves a change from the status quo that results in a new product or process that adds value. The leadership to create conditions that allow for challenging long-held assumptions, traditions, processes, and work routines is a bit different from that of a high-precision improvement team. As we discussed earlier, the goal of innovation is to explore, grow the organizational network, and build into the unknown. Here we will describe the conditions, processes, and focus that leaders can create to facilitate innovative exploration in organizations.

Innovation, like PI, has a process. One of the most common mistakes leaders make in thinking about innovation is that they believe innovation is simply brainstorming, sticky notes, and inspiration. Real innovation requires the same energy and rigor that is used in the PI processes. The process for innovation aligns well with improvement as they are both types of change that move along a similar trajectory. The phases of innovation are (1) Inspire, (2) Ideate, (3) Impact. Each one of these phases also has iterative processes that accompany them. Inspire includes (a) Understanding the environment and (b) Framing opportunities. The Ideation phase includes (a) Imaging the possibilities, and (b) Prototype solutions. Finally, the Impact stage encompasses piloting solutions and then selecting the solutions that should become operationalized (Salerno, de Vasconcelos Gomes, da Silva, Bagno, & Freitas, 2015; Bazzano, Martin, Hicks, Faughnan, & Murphy, 2017).

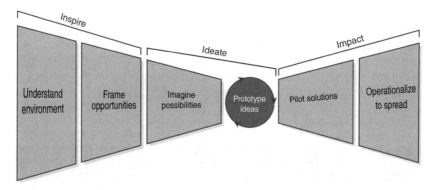

FIGURE 9-5 Innovation process model.

Because innovation is creating something new, the process is less linear and requires the leader to be flexible in jumping forward and backward in the process based on the learnings, failures, successes, and organizational dynamics. Each phase of the innovation process requires a set of tools and leadership focus to be successful (see **FIGURE 9-5**).

Inspire
Understanding the Environment
The goal of this process is to better understand the current state of a given focus area and begin to imagine the areas where innovation might disrupt that process for the betterment of the system, patient, or clinical team. The inspiration phase begins with a sense of curiosity and alignment with what is occurring in the organization's environment. One myth of innovation is that there is an aha moment where a lone innovator dreams up a solution for a complex problem. The reality is that leaders and innovators who are successful have a deep understanding of the world they work in. For healthcare innovators this is represented in the culmination of schooling, practice experience, trial and error, and keen observation skills that combine to form a world-view of the system. Innovators see the connections between seemingly unconnected parts and try to better understand those connections through information gathering, network building, and formal or informal ethnography. When understanding the environment, innovation teams must utilize the best evidence available, including evidence-based materials such as research, articles, experts, and users of the system. It is not enough to simply observe and experience; the evidence should be reviewed.

> When understanding the environment, innovation teams must utilize the best evidence available, including evidence-based materials such as research, articles, experts, and users of the system.

By using these skills and experience, innovation leaders are always seeking to understand their environment and the opportunities for disruption that lie within. The process of understanding the environment is usually much less structured than other parts of the innovation process. Individuals understand their environments differently and create worldviews in the context of their experiences. To catalyze an innovation process, however, the innovation leader must begin to focus the team on topical areas or risk having chaotic idea generation. At this stage, topical areas can be large and undefined. For example, home health, telehealth, clinic visits, and member experience are broad categories that can help begin to focus the team efforts without restricting inspiration. When in the Understanding the Environment process, the innovation leader needs to create a diverse team with many different viewpoints, create a safe place to share experiences, and be an expert in linking experiences to the focus of the innovation effort.

Framing the Opportunities

The next process in the Inspire phase is to begin to further refine the areas where innovation might best make an impact. For example, you may have chosen home health as the environmental category and now you can further refine the focus to parts in the process that need disruption. Both framing opportunities and understanding the environment can benefit from the process of journey mapping (Rosenbaum, Otalora, & Ramirez, 2017). This is the process by which you create a map of the experience from a certain point of view. The difference between a journey map and a process map (from PI) is that a journey map focuses on the emotions experienced during the process and not only on the touchpoints in the process. Figure 9-1 shows how to combine PI and Innovation tools. A journey map also contains the ideation of an ideal journey from the eyes of the user. Once completed, the map shows both the idealized journey that could be and the emotions experienced in the current process with which the team can determine the discrepancies between ideal and current state. These discrepancies then provide the opportunities to focus innovation efforts (see **FIGURE 9-6**).

After determining the areas of opportunities using a journey map, the innovation team should frame the opportunities further by using "How might we?" questions geared at solving the discrepancies between the ideal journey and the current state. For example, when kicking off an innovation process, the team may design several questions that enhance team focus while still giving freedom to think radically (see **TABLE 9-1**). In the case of a home health example, a journey map was created showing frustrations from patients in scheduling home appointments. The

TABLE 9-1 Strategy Driver		
	Process Maps (PI)	**Journey Maps (Innovation)**
Focus	The company	The customer/user
Output	Company's internal processes, functions, activities	The customer experience, emotions, point of view
Terminology	Company specific	Customer's language
Team members involved	Process mapping specialists and specific departments	All groups involved in the customer experience

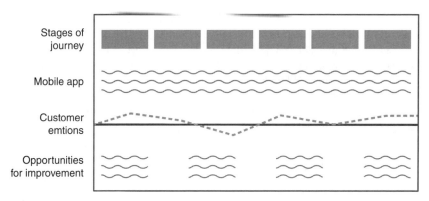

FIGURE 9-6 Customer journey map.

following questions might help frame areas of opportunity: *How might patients use technology to receive care at home? How might members interact with care teams during everyday life without appointments?* Each one of these questions allows for focus and for possibilities.

Ideation

Now that you understand the environment and framed opportunities, it is time to move into the Ideation phase. This phase is most often associated with innovation and often becomes the first step in the process for novice innovation leaders. It is very important to note that you cannot ideate without the Inspiration phase. If ideation becomes the first process in your innovation work, you will have just created the conditions for useless brainstorming, unformed focus areas, and frustrated innovation teams because the relevance of the innovation is not appropriate for the need (Hernández, 2017). In essence, you are betting that your innovation work will have an aha moment instead of informing it to make a rigorous and informed innovation attempt.

Imagine the Possibilities

With a journey map in hand and your guiding "How might we?" questions listed, the next part of the process is to imagine the possibilities. There are several methods to imagine the possibilities including rapid brainstorming. Rapid brainstorming occurs when you facilitate a diverse and informed team to rapidly generate ideas, solutions, and connections related to the "How might we?" questions. The goal of rapid brainstorming is to generate a quantity of ideas and not get stuck in the feasibility of the ideas. The more ideas generated, the better the next step will go. It is also essential in the rapid brainstorming process to ensure that ideas are simply generated and not judged by others. This allows for the divergent connections of the so-called aha moment to be allowed and captured.

Once ideas are captured, the team should begin to categorize ideas in themes and look for connections between ideas. Similar ideas should be clumped together for review. Once those themes are identified, the team should begin to place them on a possibility impact map (see **FIGURE 9-7**).

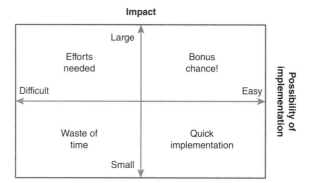

FIGURE 9-7 Payoff matrix.

Once ideas are placed and consensus is reached, the hard work of deciding which solutions fit the organizational will to move forward begins. This can be done through a variety of ways, from voting to executive preference. The most important goal is to pick solutions that match the organization's appetite for risk and can be accomplished with supporting resources. Selecting ideas that may be outside the need, resources, or support may never be successful, no matter how great they are. It is important to push the boundaries but with a mind for maintaining energy and movement of the work.

Prototype Ideas

The next stage of the innovation process is to take the selected ideas and prototype them. Prototyping is creating a low-fidelity version of the idea using minimal resources. If you are prototyping a product, you can use cardboard, glue, and markers to build an idea of what the product might look like, then use simulated interactions where imagination and discovery are used to mimic how people might interact with the product. If you are innovating on a process or workflow, using role-playing in a mock-up space can help with prototyping. If you are innovating the design of a space, you can use moveable materials like cardboard walls and balsa wood to create the initial space and rapidly iterate changes without massive construction bills. Prototyping creates a physical representation of the idea for people to react to.

The role of the innovation leader in this phase is to support the innovation team with resources, time, and space for prototyping. While prototyping can occur almost anywhere, it is essential that the team be given the time to iterate, fail, and create multiple prototypes with which users can react. These prototypes will ultimately support the creation of the pilots. If the leader allows the team to skip prototyping, the result is that more expensive piloting work will become the source of prototypes. This is more costly and less flexible to change, which may result in a poorer solution fit. You can learn more about prototyping at https://www.usability.gov/how-to-and-tools/methods/prototyping.html.

Impact

The final stage of the process for innovation is Impact. Impact is where ideas are brought to life, measured, and then spread across an organization. This part of the Innovation process is very similar to the PI PDSA process. We will discuss the

Piloting solutions phase in this chapter. The step of operationalization to spread is worthy of its own book, and much research has been done on this process in the book *Diffusion of Innovations* by Everett M. Rogers.

Pilot Solutions

After working through the prototyping process, the team members must now take their innovation solution and pilot it in a sample population. Pilots can range in size depending on the solution, budget, and need for feedback. For some complex innovations, small pilots in a single hospital unit, clinic, or a small department may be needed. The purpose of the pilot is to test the solution in a real setting, gather user feedback, and measure the impact of the solution on users and staff. The role of the leader in the pilot phase is to help remove barriers to implementing a pilot within the organization and to ensure rigorous measurement of the solution in practice. Many times the pilot stage is where innovation dies because the organization is unwilling to support a change in their departments. The leader must use their networking skills, influence, and storytelling to communicate the need for the innovation, the possible outcomes of the innovation, and the resources needed to make the pilot successful.

The other issue that arises in the pilot stage is a lack of intentional measurement of the outcomes associated with the pilot. The pilot measurement must be linked directly to the "How might we?" question and the problem the team is trying to solve. The measurement should include cost, business, and process metrics. For example, a pilot to decrease the number of interruptions a nurse has in passing a medication should include some of the following metrics: time of medication pass compared to old process, cost of solution, number of medication errors before and after, staff satisfaction, barriers to use, number of interruptions before and after.

Without intentional and rigorous measurement, the pilot may not be viewed as a success and further adoption could be questioned. Leaders must resist the tendency to just measure process. For example, only measuring if nurses liked the new process or that patients felt safer would not yield the metrics to inform further implementation. Business and cost metrics should always be included in the innovation pilot. The work of determining measurement is tough but will support the decision of whether the innovation is worth continuing or not.

The innovation process is iterative and fluid work to inspire questions, ideate solutions, and implement changes, all with an eye to evidence and measurement. The leader's work is to facilitate, participate, and coordinate the efforts across the system. While the leader can be part of the process as a participant, it is important that the leader does not impose his or her will on the project. Rather, the leader should remain open to the emergence of the innovation through the rigor of the innovation process. The most essential role of the leader of innovation is to ensure that the innovation process is rigorous and founded in evidence and not a session of sticky notes and uninformed brainstorming.

DISCUSSION

Describe a time you participated in an innovation session. Did it follow the Inspire, Ideate, Impact model? Compare and contrast your experience in the innovation session to this model. What could have been improved?

Conditions for Innovation

There are several conditions that support the process of innovation and ensure that it is rigorous. Innovation leaders are those that create the conditions for creativity, conflict, ideation, and evidence to combine in dynamic ways to yield new value to organizations and/or populations. This is more than holding unstructured brainstorming sessions in which participants imagine the possibilities and place sticky notes on walls. Innovation is a science, and a process that requires the commitment of people, resources, and time to do right. In our experience, organizations in health care routinely fail at innovation because they lack an understanding of innovation and have failed to create conditions in which innovation can thrive. Based on this experience and the evidence of innovation success, we are proposing that leaders consider creating conditions in their organization to ensure that innovation is successful in the context of the PI/Innovation relationship.

Strategic Alignment of Dedicated Innovation Teams

While performance improvement is tied to the strategic plan of an organization and its microsystem, innovation has a tendency to go rogue. Healthcare organizations specifically have aligned PI with quality, operational success, and error reduction efforts intentionally while leaving innovation to flounder without alignment to any real strategy. Innovation teams are usually placed in the office of the CEO, Information Technology, or some other department that is far from the frontline work that needs to be innovated. By placing these innovation teams in organizational pockets, the teams struggle to understand how their disruptive work actually fits with organizational directions.

While it might seem well intentioned to place innovation teams far from the meddling of eager executives and operational leaders, this only serves to isolate the innovation teams, resulting in reduced networking, poor diffusion of innovation, and misaligned innovation efforts. Many times, innovation leaders try to protect their creative teams by shielding them in the manners mentioned previously. This is understandable, and some care is needed to keep innovators in their creative space. Instead of isolating the team, we recommend caring for the innovator using this reference (Unterschuetz, Hughes, Nienhauser, Weberg, & Jackson, 2008). Isolating innovators and innovation teams can be the worst possible scenario for innovation teams to face. Also, innovation does not always flow from a single innovation team but rather from individuals and other groups throughout the organizational network. The challenge for the innovation leader is to create structure to enhance specific innovation team alignment and to harness the collective power of innovators throughout the organizations. This builds the innovation network within the organization and distributes innovation work throughout. The leader's role is to harness innovation across the system, not to compartmentalize it into a corner.

Innovation teams are good at big disruption work. They are wholly focused on challenging assumptions and building new insights to push the organization forward. These teams need to be embedded in the core strategic decision-making processes of the organization. For example, Lockheed Martin created an innovation team to deliver on highly strategic and difficult contract requests from the military. These teams were given more freedom to fail, disrupt the bureaucracy, and push faster without intense scrutiny, all while still being held accountable to budget, timelines, and deliverables. The innovation team reported high into the organization but was strategically leveraged to tackle the most complex and ambiguous challenges from the customer. Simply improving the propeller plane did not get them jet engines. They needed space to build the new while learning from the known.

Leaders can learn from stories like Lockheed Martin and others when developing innovation alignment (Rich & Janos, 2013).

1. Place the innovation team in the organization so that it has influence to key strategic decision makers (formally or informally).

2. Allow innovation teams to tackle really complex and ambiguous problems while maintaining accountability for budget, timelines, and deliverables. (Constraints catalyze innovation.)

3. Allow for the bureaucracy to flex to support innovation. Allow some disruption in budget cycles, hiring processes, and pay incentives to support innovation.

4. Support a learning culture by rigorously documenting innovation work and reflecting on failures along the way.

5. Care for your innovators as they keep your organization moving, and doing so requires significant personal and professional energy.

The innovators and innovation teams in your organization require the leader to support and care for them. Innovators frequently challenge the norm, push against organizational structure, and routinely encounter resistance and barriers in their efforts. These can be taxing to individuals, and leaders should understand that innovators need frequent feedback and support to continue their work. The five steps mentioned previously provide some examples for how leaders can support innovators in their work, but the most important tool a leader has to keep innovation flowing in his or her organization is using open and transparent communication practices. Keeping innovators informed of organizational struggles, successes, politics, and needs will help align the resulting innovations for success.

▶ Leader's Role in Creating High-Performing Systems

The leader's role is that of the coordinator and facilitator. In complex problem solving, the leader needs to utilize excellent communication in building the teams, communicating the goals, and facilitating how the PI and innovation teams will interact. The leader can almost guarantee failure by giving vague directions, such as simply telling the PI team to improve stuff and the innovation team to be innovative. The leader's work is to examine the overlap and facilitate clear and frequent communication between the teams on how the work informs one another. This can be done through frequent joint meetings in which the teams discuss their work to date and share the artifacts of their processes. For example, the PI team may share a process map of an issue, and the innovation team may share a similar journey map. Those two artifacts of the work can show the breakdowns in the process while also demonstrating the emotions the users feel while going through the process. Together, the process map and the journey map provide an even clearer picture of the problem than what either process might gain in isolation. All too often these teams are isolated and speak different change languages. This creates artificial conflict and misunderstandings that might inhibit the organization's adaptation. Leaders must be willing to translate, co-ordinate, and communicate across these arbitrary boundaries to improve the system.

Organizational leaders of change can use three tools to assess what processes should be deployed in problem solving. Sometimes the choices are simply defined and other times they require using PI and innovation to gather information for problem definition and ultimately deployment. The leader should not be afraid to combine innovation and improvement teams in problem solving as long as the leader creates clear expectations, provides clear problem definition, and facilitates meaningful interactions between the two teams.

DISCUSSION

Make a list of problems in your organization. Categorize them by which process might be best used to solve them: PI, innovation, or both. Provide a few sentences describing your decision rationale.

The complexity, uncertainty, and evolving nature of the healthcare delivery landscape require leaders to understand where and how their own organization's variation, performance gaps, and stagnation occur. This creates a demand for leaders to foster conditions for high performance, reliability, and ultimately more certainty in complex systems. Leading under these conditions requires being aware of what's going on outside your organization's walls and having the ability to explore and exploit innovations and other evidence-based approaches to improve as needed. This chapter outlined how to be aware of your organization's strategy, understanding the differences between innovation and PI, and how to lead in each by incorporating the five phases and eight steps of PI:

1. Target Area for Improvement
2. Assess/Define Current Processes
3. Identify Improvement Opportunities
4. Evaluating Your Small Tests of Change
5. Large-Scale Improvement: Implement and Spread Improved Processes and the three phases of innovation:
   1. Inspire
   2. Ideate
   3. Impact

Leaders now have a toolkit to equip their teams to identify when innovation or improvement is needed.

References

Associates in Process Improvement (API). Model for Improvement. Retrieved from www.apiweb.org.

Balanced Scorecard Institute. (n.d.). Balanced scorecard basics. Retrieved from https://www .balancedscorecard.org/BSC-Basics/About-the-Balanced-Scorecard

Bazzano, A. N., Martin, J., Hicks, E., Faughnan, M., & Murphy, L. (2017). Human-centered design in global health: A scoping review of applications and contexts. *PLOS One, 12*(11), e0186744.

Boer, H., Kuhn, J., & Gertsen, F. (2006). Continuous innovation: Managing dualities through co-ordination. *Continuous Innovation Network. WPS, 1.*

D'Andreamatteo, A., Ianni, L., Lega, F., & Sargiacomo, M. (2015). Lean in healthcare: A comprehensive review. *Health Policy, 119*(9), 1197–1209. https://doi.org/10.1016/j.healthpol.2015.02.002

HarvardX. (2017, April 19). How to create cause-and-effect diagrams [Video file]. Retrieved from https://www.youtube.com/watch?v=mLvizyDFLQ4

Hernández, E. (2017). Brainstorming. In *Leading Creative Teams* (pp. 57–74). Berkeley, CA: Apress.

IHI Multimedia Team. (2015). 5 Steps for Creating Value Through Process Mapping and Observation. Retrieved from http://www.ihi.org/communities/blogs/5-steps-for-creating-value-through-process-mapping-and-observation

Institute for Healthcare Improvement. (2017a). QI essentials toolkit: Pareto chart. Retrieved from http://www.ihi.org:80/resources/Pages/Tools/ParetoDiagram.aspx

Institute for Healthcare Improvement. (2017b). QI tools: Cause and effect diagram. Retrieved from http://www.ihi.org:80/resources/Pages/Tools/CauseandEffectDiagram.aspx

Institute for Healthcare Improvement. (2018). Tools. Retrieved from http://www.ihi.org:80/resources/Pages/Tools/default.aspx

Institute for Healthcare Improvement. (2019). Control charts. Retrieved from http://www.ihi.org/education/IHIOpenSchool/resources/Pages/AudioandVideo/Whiteboard13.aspx

Institute for Healthcare Improvement. (n.d.). QI project charter. Retrieved from http://www.ihi.org/resources/Pages/Tools/QI-Project-Charter.aspx

Langley, G., Moen, R., Nolan, K., Nolan, T., Norman, C., & Provost, L. (2009). The improvement guide: A practical approach to enhancing organizational performance (2nd ed.). San Francisco, CA: Jossey-Bass.

LaPorte, T. R., & Consolini, P. M. (1991). Working in practice but not in theory: Theoretical challenges of "high-reliability organizations." *Journal of Public Administration Research and Theory: J-PART, 1*(1), 19–48.

Mintzberg, H. (1994, January–February). The fall and rise of strategic planning. *Harvard Business Review.* Retrieved from https://hbr.org/1994/01/the-fall-and-rise-of-strategic-planning

Rich, B. R., & Janos, L. (2013). Skunk works: A personal memoir of my years of Lockheed. Boston, MA: Little, Brown, and Company.

Roberts, K. H. (1990). Some characteristics of one type of high reliability organization. *Organization Science, 1*(2), 160–176. https://doi.org/10.1287/orsc.1.2.160

Rogers, Everett M. (2009). Diffusion of innovations (5th ed). New York, NY: Simon & Schuster.

Rosenbaum, M. S., Otalora, M. L., & Ramírez, G. C. (2017). How to create a realistic customer journey map. *Business Horizons, 60*(1), 143–150.

Salerno, M. S., de Vasconcelos Gomes, L. A., da Silva, D. O., Bagno, R. B., & Freitas, S. L. T. U. (2015). Innovation processes: Which process for which project? *Technovation, 35*, 59–70.

Scott, W. R., Ruef, M., Mendel, P. J., & Caronna, C. A. (2000). *Institutional change and healthcare organizations: From professional dominance to managed care.* Chicago, IL: University of Chicago Press. Retrieved from https://books.google.com/books?id=vomaHpFVcOAC

Shortell, S. M., & Kaluzny, A. D. (2006). *Health care management: Organization, design, and behavior.* Clifton Park, NY: Thomson Delmar Learning.

Stacey, R. (1996). *Complexity and creativity in organizations.* San Francisco, CA: Berrett-Koehler.

Terziovski, M. (2002). Achieving performance excellence through an integrated strategy of radical innovation and continuous improvement. *Measuring Business Excellence, 6*(2), 5–14.

Unterschuetz, C., Hughes, P., Nienhauser, D., Weberg, D., & Jackson, L. (2008). Caring for innovation and caring for the innovator. *Nursing administration quarterly, 32*(2), 133–141.

Vogus, T. J., & Singer, S. J. (2016). Creating highly reliable accountable care organizations. *Medical Care Research and Review: MCRR, 73*(6), 660–672. https://doi.org/10.1177/1077558716640413

Vogus, T. J., & Sutcliffe, K. M. (2007). The safety organizing scale: Development and validation of a behavioral measure of safety culture in hospital nursing units. *Medical Care, 45*(1), 46–54. https://doi.org/10.1097/01.mlr.0000244635.61178.7a

Wiltsey Stirman, S., Kimberly, J., Cook, N., Calloway, A., Castro, F., & Charns, M. (2012). The sustainability of new programs and innovations: A review of the empirical literature and recommendations for future research. *Implementation Science: IS, 7*, 17.

SECTION 3

Trends and Issues

CHAPTER 10

The Best Way to Predict the Future Is to [Co]Create It: A Technology Primer for Healthcare Leaders

Richard Booth, Gillian Strudwick, Josephine McMurray, Adam Morse, Ryan Chan, and Timothy Zhang

CHAPTER OBJECTIVES

Upon completion of this chapter, the reader will:

1. Gain awareness and explore future technological trends as related to nursing leadership in health and health care.
2. Obtain deeper insight related to the emergent competencies, skills, and knowledge required by nurse leaders to leverage and amplify the use of future digital health technology.
3. Identify new opportunities for leaders to build innovative models of care in increasingly digitized and automated environments.

▶ Introduction

Over the last decade, there has been substantive growth in the use of various types of information and communication technology (ICT) across all areas of society and health care. Currently, in many clinical and health-related settings in North America, various types of technologies are increasingly commonplace, including electronic health records (EHRs), patient portal technology, point-of-care devices, electronic whiteboards, and other forms of digital health technology. While the exploration of technological innovations in the nursing profession has existed for decades within nursing informatics literature, the recent rapid spread of the latest types of various digital health technologies has begun to generate entirely new areas of opportunity for the profession. For instance, the growing interest in artificial intelligence (AI), robotics, and other personalized/precision healthcare approaches are all examples of nascent healthcare innovations that are viewed as disruptors to the status quo and yet are not widely understood or embraced in the profession. Although it is difficult to make accurate predictions related to these kinds of technologies and their incorporation into elements of nursing and healthcare practice, their influence has already been felt in other related industries where humans and technological innovations come together to generate a product or deliver a service. According to studies, automation technology has been forecasted to have an impact on anywhere from one-third to one-half of North American jobs in the coming decade (Manyika et al., 2017; RBC, 2018), although, the nursing profession appears to be somewhat protected from the rise of automation (Frey & Osborne, 2013; Muro, 2017) witnessed in other industries such as manufacturing, retail, and food services. Other emergent technologies like AI have been recognized as having significant potential to have a direct impact on elements of the nursing role, including clinical decision making, clinical documentation, and aspects of the nurse-client relationship (Booth, 2016; Sensmeier, 2017; Strudwick & Xie, 2018).

While it is important to explore the proposed impacts of emergent digital health technologies on the larger nursing profession, the cohorts of nurses who must be at the forefront of this evolution are *nurses in leadership positions*. Increased environmental complexity, professionalization, and shared accountability have shifted our understanding of leadership to more distributed models (Bolden, 2011; Fitzsimons, Turnbull James, & Denyer, 2011). By definition, these models imply a shift away from hierarchical archetypes with command-and-control leadership toward relational, shared, and team-based leadership models, which recognize each nurse's independence and autonomy within his or her own practice (Remus, 2016a). Subsequently, nursing leadership will be conceptualized and defined in this chapter as a relational entity exercised by nurses. This concept is found, demonstrated, and represented through a complex array of human, environmental, and contextual interactions both within and between organizations. Even so, other and somewhat more concrete definitions of nurse leaders exist. For example, nurse leaders are often defined as being those with the ability to influence their peers; further, formal leadership positions sometimes afford nurses with human and financial resource management responsibilities.

Given the increasing diffusion of digital health technology that has the potential to shape and reshape various elements of the nursing role and its related practice (Glasgow, Colbert, Viator, & Cavanagh, 2018), the remainder of this chapter will explore the domain in the following three ways: (1) the chapter will deconstruct the nursing leadership implications of when humans and emergent digital health technology interact, (2) it will analyze various types of emergent digital health technology that are suggested to be of material importance to health care and the nursing profession of the future, and (3) it will provide implications for nursing leaders to prepare the profession and health care for the opportunities and challenges brought on by these types of emergent digital health innovations.

> Definition of Leadership
> While leadership denotes the characteristics of an individual, relational leading refers to the ability of persons in relationship to move with engagement and efficacy into the future. . . To be sure, individuals may be designated as leaders, but the process of leading is ultimately relational. (Gergen, 2009, p. 333)

▶ Digital Health Technology and Nursing Leadership

To date, research completed in the nursing informatics domain has explored the role of nursing leadership in the development, implementation, usage optimization, and sustainment of health technology (Amendola, 2008; Collins, Phllips, Yen, & Kennedy, 2017; Hart, 2010; Kassam, Nagle, & Strudwick, 2017; Kennedy & Moen, 2017; Kleib & Nagle, 2018; Remus, 2016a; Remus & Kennedy, 2012; Strudwick, Booth, Bjarnadottir, Collins, & Srivastava, 2017; Yang et al., 2014). A primary focus of this work has been on the type and level of nursing informatics competencies that nurse leaders must hold to be effective in their roles within organizations. Much of this work has also focused on EHR systems, and nursing leadership's ability to advocate for systems and processes that support the work of nurses, rather than detract from it. The evolution of this work has paved the way for the emergence of chief nursing informatics officers (HIMSS, 2016), a relatively new role with a strong leadership focus in nursing informatics.

While this area of inquiry has generated valuable insights related to the use of health information systems in practical settings, the predominant foci of this body of literature has been very much centered on the various competencies required by nursing leadership to help enable interaction with the system life cycle of ICT used within institutional healthcare settings (Collins et al., 2017; Kassam et al., 2017; Kennedy & Moen, 2017; Simpson, 1994; Staggers, Gassert, & Curran, 2001; Westra, Delaney, & Delaney, 2008). Further, the current cross-section of informatics-related competencies for nursing leadership has been grounded in contemporary interpretations of what healthcare environments look like, including where various technologies exist to serve, and be used by, nurses and other clinicians to conduct clinical activities (Collins et al., 2017). As outlined by Kassam et al. (2017), "without informatics competent nursing leadership, organizations run the risk of not being able to obtain expected returns on investments or garner the potential safety and quality benefits of ICT for clinical care delivery" (p. 4). The authors reinforce this statement by declaring that if nursing leadership does not inform the system life cycles of ICT, then "patient care and nursing practice may be inadvertently compromised" (p. 4). Unfortunately, although various informatics competencies have existed in the nursing literature for decades, the uptake and adoption of these competencies into nursing leadership have been remarkably slow. Therefore, nurse leaders today may not hold the necessary informatics knowledge, notwithstanding the more advanced competencies required to be able to effectively provide strategic and tactical leadership related to the adoption and use of ICTs.

Given the current low levels of informatics and ICT competency diffusion among nursing leadership ranks (Kassam et al., 2017; Westra et al., 2008), the true value that health ICT can bring to clinical practice and the nursing role has yet to be fully realized in contemporary healthcare practice. Regardless, while there appears to be a lack of wide-scale diffusion of nurse leader informatics competencies related to mainstream clinical ICT like EHRs and data standards, new and emergent digital health technologies that have the potential to fundamentally refabricate models of care have begun to appear en masse. As outlined by Remus and Kennedy (2012), nursing leaders now require entirely *new* types and kinds of competencies as a result of the shifting paradigms of healthcare practice toward a more holistic and patient-centric model of care, driven by clinical intelligence afforded by emergent digital health technologies (Remus & Kennedy, 2012).

"Value . . . clinician's involvement at all appropriate phases" (Westra et al., 2008, p. 806)

"Recognize the relevance of nursing data for improving practice" (Simpson, 2013, p. 285)

"Change management for health information technology" (Yen, Kennedy, Phillips, & Collins, 2017, p. 275)

One artifact that underlies most of the previously established nursing informatics competencies for leadership is the alignment of these competencies with past and present-day interpretations of the healthcare system and its related structures. Consequently, the majority of informatics competencies have been viewed using interpretations centered around hospital or acute care settings and described from the perspective of how leadership can be involved as a change agent for other clinicians, support aspects of the technology life cycle, provide direction related to health system utilization and interoperability, and conduct necessary education and research to ensure the sustainment of the innovation. While all these aspects will be important within the healthcare system moving into the future, the authors of this chapter suggest that updated competencies for nursing leaders that are sensitive to emergent digital health technologies need to be generated to future-proof elements of the nursing profession for the decades to come (Archibald & Barnard, 2018; Booth, 2016). Given the potential of many emergent digital health technologies to augment or recast existing models of care in all areas of the healthcare system, a more relational approach to viewing the role of leadership in this domain must be considered. While there are numerous relational approaches that have been explored in nursing literature on leadership in complex and adaptive healthcare environments (Booth, McBride, & Tietze, 2015), for the purposes of this chapter the conceptual lens of *sociomateriality* (Orlikowski & Scott, 2008) will be used to accentuate two key perspectives: (1) to explicate how the presence of various commonly unseen digital health technologies currently exert force within the larger healthcare ecosystem, and subsequently the nursing role, and (2) to provide nursing leaders with a conceptual lens to both identify and explore various social, technical, and environmental factors within the processes of healthcare, in an effort to generate future opportunities for the nursing profession.

Sociomateriality

Sociomateriality is a conceptual lens that seeks to explore the relationships between *social* and *material* (i.e., sociomaterial) in everyday life (Leonardi, 2012; Orlikowski & Scott, 2008). As a neologism combining both words *social* and *material*, the conceptual lens of sociomateriality seeks to highlight how many social elements of humans are shaped, modified, and influenced by various *material* (i.e., technology, objects) entities in the environment. For example, the use of an EHR is commonplace in many contemporary healthcare environments. An EHR system is comprised of various pieces of hardware, software, and other devices that nurses and other clinicians use to document and plan various aspects of patient care. While the EHR system is arguably a collection of *material* entities (i.e., hardware, software, peripherals) that cannot perform human-like tasks or behaviors (e.g., provide reassurance to a patient, change a wound dressing, etc.), the EHR represents or facilitates many human activities within the context of health care. For instance, an EHR shapes many *social* aspects and behaviors of nursing care—including clinical documentation processes, the workflow of clinicians during their shift to interact with the system, and requiring specific user training to learn how to use the system effectively. Subsequently, while the EHR is uniquely a *material* thing, its presence, role, and function within the clinical context highly influences many *social* aspects of humans, including the nursing role and delivery of care.

While the importance of material objects having an influence on social systems is notable, one of the central aspects of sociomateriality is that social aspects also have importance and the ability to shape material entities. That is, humans have the potential to shape technology, as much as technology has the ability to shape humans (Booth, Andrusyszyn, Iwasiw, Donelle, & Compeau, 2016). The reciprocal nature of sociomateriality means that proponents of this conceptual lens are always sensitive to the fact that to truly examine any phenomena, examination of both the *social* and *material* factors of a given situation, with equal relational emphasis, is required.

Although being able to explicitly identify and define various social and material entities of importance can be cumbersome at times, it is suggested that the real value of this conceptual lens is realized when a deeper understanding related to the complex relationship between social and material entities are recognized. Since nursing care is composed of a complex array of decision making, skills, and interactions with both people and various types of equipment, a sociomaterial lens can help to better describe and explain how sometimes complex processes within the profession go unnoticed or unexplained. For instance, the impacts of an EHR implementation on a clinical environment that previously operated without electronic records is a superb example of how the merger of various social and material elements come *together* to generate a new reality. From a social perspective, the implementation of an EHR into a clinical environment can fundamentally alter and evolve various social processes, including clinician workflows, clinical decision making, and interactions with patients. From a material perspective, the EHR implementation may lack interoperability with other medical equipment in the context or require retrofitting physical areas of the clinical environment and its related infrastructure. For instance, a sociomaterial observation in this EHR implementation would be that nurses generate practical work-arounds or deviations in their use of the system, either as a response to poor usability of the EHR or to realign with a clinical workflow that existed pre-EHR implementation. While the practical work-arounds or deviations inspired by the EHR implementation contain both social (e.g., nurses' decisions to generate work-arounds to the EHR system) and technical aspects (e.g., poor usability of the EHR system), the end result of nurses attempting to revert to previously established work patterns is an emergent sociomaterial outcome. Essentially, it becomes difficult to tease apart whether the *social* or the *material* elements of the EHR implementation caused the work-arounds to be generated by the nurses, given the active blurring of both social and material factors in the situation.

While the use of a sociomaterial conceptual lens is important for nursing leaders who wish to generate deeper insights into human and technical relationships within contemporary healthcare contexts, the authors of this chapter suggest that due to the proposed influence and significance of certain emergent digital health technologies that are forecasted to scale in the coming decades, a sociomaterial lens will be required to *fully* appreciate the impacts of these innovations. Given the increasing embeddedness of many emergent digital technologies, more and more humans are becoming increasingly interlinked with technology in a seamless, ubiquitous, and sometimes unseen fashion. Although nursing has historically provided insights into the development, maintenance, and upkeep of various health information systems in organizational settings, the growing repertoire of digital technology outside the immediate span of control of nursing leaders is as empowering as it is potentially troublesome. To date, nursing leadership involvement (and general nursing involvement, for that matter) in many technology-enabled emerging models of health care are few and far between. With the growing use of AI, robotics/automation, personalized medicine, and wearables/biometrics, the blurring between what is *social* and what is *material* will become even more nuanced moving into the future. Therefore, to *see* this new and quickly approaching reality, it is advocated that nursing leaders leverage a conceptual lens such as sociomateriality to: (1) recognize how the increasing merger and blurring of social and material entities within healthcare practice is becoming amplified through emergent digital health technology and (2) use this lens to generate new roles for the nursing profession, which operate in the uncontested space of a future healthcare system that has not yet been defined or, in many cases, conceptualized. Hopefully, through an exploration of emergent digital health technology in the forthcoming sections, the value of using sociomateriality as a conceptual lens to elucidate new opportunities for the profession, led by nursing leaders, will become evident.

REFLECTION SCENARIO 1

Reflect on an environment in a clinical context that could benefit from the generation of insights for future planning and resource allocation. How could this be accomplished by deconstructing the environment using the ontological lens of sociomateriality?

For instance, the role of the *visiting clinician* has become an established piece in various home-care models of health care. In this model of care, clinicians (e.g., nurses) travel to a patient's home and deliver a range of clinical assessments and treatments in the home environment. While this model of care has evolved over the last few decades with the advancement of health technology in many areas (e.g., mobile access to EHRs, cellular technology to assist with mileage reimbursement calculations incurred by the clinician, etc.), clinician workflows and other related processes have remained largely unchanged. When considering this environment with a sociomaterial perspective, the role of the home-care clinician is a worthy example to be deconstructed due to its robustness and inherent complexities. From a *social* perspective, the roles of humans (e.g., clinicians, patients, family members, etc.) and the related interactions between these human agents is primarily predicated on face-to-face, in-person interactions. While various *material* technological innovations such as telemedicine and other virtual health approaches currently exist, their usage within home-care settings (as of 2019) is limited. Many of these *material* technological innovations could fundamentally evolve the deeply related processes and dynamics between clinicians and patients, but the current models of home-care delivery have been resistant to change the *social* nature of the clinician-patient relationship dynamic. Although some blurring between various *social* and *material* entities in home care has begun to occur in certain places (Piraino, Byrne, Heckman, & Stolee, 2017; Royackers, Regan, & Donelle, 2016), the overall resilience of the traditional face-to-face clinician-patient experience is impressive. This speaks to a range of hidden factors and forces that have likely assisted the continuance of this approach, despite various technical *material* innovations (i.e., videoconferencing, telepresence robotics, Internet-enabled collaborative coordination platforms, etc.) which could all be leveraged to virtualize elements of the visiting clinician role.

▶ Emergent Digital Health Technology

... [W]e probably will see little change to clinical practice from AI [artificial intelligence] in the next 5 years. We should certainly see changes in 10 years, and there is a real prospect of massive change in 20 years. For students starting medicine today, by the time they are mid-career, substantial technology-induced disruption will have occurred. Predicting where disruption is most likely to occur is hard, but if it feels routine today, then it is likely to be a target for the machine tomorrow. (Coiera, 2018, p. 10)

Given the nascence of many emergent digital health technologies and our limited understanding of their influence on healthcare work and delivery, we will provide an operational definition of each, appreciating the fact that as they mature, their use in, and impact on, health care will be co-constructed with nurses. For the purposes of this chapter, *digital health technology* will be used to describe a wide range of emergent, disruptive innovation that is used for health(care) purposes. Digital health technologies include not only software, but also integrated systems of software within hardware, such as wearables, or platforms that enable the interaction between numerous types of hardware and software. While digital health technologies include a vast and diverse range of innovations, one foundational characteristic is that they possess *significant disruptive potential* to traditional or contemporary healthcare processes, workflows, and structures. Although the magnitude of impact generated from these digital health technologies is unclear, it suffices to say that many of these emergent innovations have the potential to transform the nursing profession in both direct and indirect fashions. Due to this potential, this section of the chapter will describe a range of digital health technologies that have been forecasted to become mainstream elements of a future, consumer-driven healthcare ecosystem. To do this, two approaches will be taken: (1) a description and analysis of

the emergent digital health technology will be provided, and (2) the forecasted impacts of these nascent digital health technologies along with the related healthcare
value chains they may propagate will be examined in terms of healthcare processes
and system service evolution.

Conventionally, healthcare technology has been controlled, governed, and
managed by traditional healthcare structures and systems. For instance, EHRs,
point-of-care devices, and other medical devices commonly used in healthcare processes have been historically implemented, managed, and utilized by healthcare providers in the delivery of various health services. While this kind of health technology
will continue to exist (and its importance is not to be underrated), a newer generation of emergent digital health technology has begun to apply pressure to both the
traditional conceptualizations and processes of the healthcare system. Responding
to a range of societal, technological, and healthcare forces, this newer generation
of emergent digital health technology commonly embraces a consumer-centric,
personalized, and on-demand nature. While many emergent digital health technologies interact with traditional healthcare structures and their related technology systems, not all do. With the shifting demographics of health consumers (i.e.,
Millennials/Generation Z), a growing societal familiarity with the use of sophisticated mobile ICT, and an increasing desire to use services that provide personalized
and on-demand functionality, many of the emergent digital health technologies discussed in the following section do not currently align with contemporary healthcare
practices or processes. Further, many of these emergent digital health technologies
will (or already have) generated entirely new models of health(care) funding, practice, and delivery. While it is unclear which emergent digital healthcare technologies
will have the most significant impact on the nursing profession, at the time of this
writing, the following selection provides some of the greatest existential threats to
the status quo.

Artificial Intelligence and Machine Learning

One of the most discussed and advanced emergent digital health technologies
of the coming decade is AI. While definitions of AI are diverse and commonly
discipline-specific, the Encyclopedia Britannica defines the term as "the ability of a
digital computer or computer-controlled robot to perform tasks commonly associated with intelligent beings" (Encyclopedia Brittannica, 2018). A more contemporary and industry-employed definition of AI arises from Amazon, which outlined AI
as a "field of computer science dedicated to solving cognitive problems commonly
associated with human intelligence, such as learning, problem solving, and pattern
recognition" (Amazon, 2018). A key tenet of many AI definitions is that this type
of technology attempts to mimic the cognitive functions of a human, including various human traits like learning, problem solving, and curiosity. While AI is a vast
discipline, the term *AI* will be used in this chapter to outline a range of digital health
technologies that have the ability to, by themselves or through cooperation with
other humans and non-human systems (e.g., other health technologies), to autonomously generate decisions or outcomes. AI-enabled technology possesses specialized software algorithms that are continuously improving based on both previously
and newly learned data and prompts to increasingly operate and function independently and autonomously. This technology is commonly associated with *machine*

learning where the computer is able to identify patterns and change its behavior based on learned information. This *self-learning* allows it to modify and improve its own understanding of phenomena and to make predictions based on that understanding (Amazon, 2018).

To date, many technologies are supported by elements of AI and machine learning (e.g., advertisement personalization on the Internet, facial recognition technology embedded into mobile phones, etc.). While there is a significant continuum in the power and abilities of AI-enabled technologies, the growing abilities and predictive capabilities of these forms of technology have begun to trickle into healthcare innovations in a significant fashion. One of the most well-known AI systems currently operating in health care is likely IBM Watson. Commercially launched in 2013, IBM Watson is an AI computing system that has been modified to operate with healthcare data. IBM Watson is able to quickly analyze large data sets, generate insights from this data, and then present actionable insights back to human users who can use this information to improve decision making. A key element of IBM Watson is that the system can analyze and manage vast data repositories and generate insights on both structured and unstructured data in a way that human decision-making capabilities could never manage (IBM, 2018). Essentially, IBM Watson is able to identify trends and patterns and offer evidence-informed solutions to humans through complex analytical approaches with massive amounts of data, well beyond the cognitive capabilities of a human.

Although the diffusion of IBM Watson and other AI-enabled decision-making tools for health care has only just begun, the influence of AI and other machine-learning approaches can be viewed in other aspects of society in a much more material fashion. Personalization algorithms used by most social media platforms (Just & Latzer, 2017; Narayanan et al., 2018), targeted marketing applications on the Internet (Aluri, Price, & McIntyre, 2018), and other facial recognition technologies commonly embedded in mobile phones (Kaplan & Haenlein, 2018) are all examples of AI used in daily life. One aspect of AI that sometimes remains unclear to healthcare professional audiences is the fact that systems that use this kind of technology are commonly unseen or subtle in their operation. With improvements in technology, AI-enabled devices are starting to emerge in health(care) practice, informing traditional healthcare structures (e.g., clinical decision support), but they are also stimulating entirely new domains and models of care (e.g., personalized health trackers, personalized wellness applications). For the purposes of nursing leadership, understanding the value and impact of these kinds of technologies on both traditional and nontraditional healthcare environments is important, as the likelihood that most future health technology will be embedded with some element of AI and machine learning is high.

Robotics/Automation/Service Drones

While robotic and automation technology has existed in health care for decades (i.e., robotic surgery, patient lift technology) to amplify many ranges of specific tasks required by humans, most of these forms of innovation have required direct human input to operate or use (Davenport & Kirby, 2015). Since robotic and automation technology can be developed to fulfill virtually any task within many conceivable environments, a detailed description of all types of robotic and automation technology in health care is well beyond the scope of this chapter; instead, a more detailed examination of the next generation of robotics and automation technology that possess AI and other aspects of autonomous functionality will be described.

To date, the growth and evolution of robotic and automation technology in society has been impressive. It has been forecast that nearly 30–50% of all Canadian and American employment in the coming decade will be affected by aspects of automation in the workplace (Manyika et al., 2017; RBC, 2018). Although deeper predictions and analyses of how robotics and automation will influence the profession of nursing have been conducted, it would seem that the profession is reasonably future-proofed against direct and immediate augmentation by these forms of innovations (Frey & Osborne, 2013; Muro, 2017). Nonetheless, with the growing potential and technical functionalities of many robotic and automation technologies currently in existence or planned for development, the nursing profession must deeply reflect on its own role and the skills and value it brings to health care.

Currently, the use of robotic and automation technology in healthcare settings has been largely observed within traditional healthcare structures, such as acute-care and institutional settings. Notwithstanding the current generation of robotic technology used in many clinical procedures (i.e., surgery) or automated processes (i.e., lab specimen processing), future innovation in this space is predicted to augment the current roles of humans in new and innovative ways. For instance, some hospitals have recently introduced social robots: AI-enabled robots whose purpose is to interact and sometimes befriend humans. Trial runs of a humanoid robot, Pepper, acting as a greeter is currently underway at hospitals around the world (see **FIGURE 10-1**; Crowe, 2016; Humber River Hospital Foundation, 2018); MEDi—a small humanoid robot—is currently being tested as a pain management intervention for pediatric patients (McIntyre, 2018); service drone robots (see **FIGURE 10-2**) are currently used by a number of hospitals globally to automate the delivery of supplies and other materials throughout the organization (UNC Health Care, 2018); and robots are seeing use as social companions in long-term care and nursing home environments (Riek, 2017).

FIGURE 10-1 Example of Pepper, a social robot that has been used as a hospital greeter.
© Antonello Marangi/Shutterstock

FIGURE 10-2 A service drone robot delivering medications on a hospital unit.
© Andy Dean Photography/Alamy Stock Photo

While the current generation of autonomous robotics and other service drones are still limited in terms of functionality, their potential to augment, evolve, and disrupt various health(care) processes within both traditional and nontraditional healthcare structures is significant. To date, the rapid diffusion of intelligent robotic technology can be seen in consumer-level smart-speaker products like Amazon Echo and Google Home, and also service drones that complete basic cleaning chores (i.e., iRobot's Roomba) and home automation (i.e., domestic Internet-of-thing-connected devices like thermostats, lights, and security cameras). Although these forms of emergent digital health technology will likely not change the traditional nursing role in established healthcare structures in the immediate future, robotics and automation innovation have the distinct potential to augment and subtly change aspects of nursing work and culture in the coming decades. Subsequently, it would befit nursing leaders to explore the emergent domain of robotics and automation within both healthcare and societal settings to identify new areas of opportunity that can be leveraged to use these forms of technology to not only amplify elements of the contemporary nursing role (Maalouf, Sidaoui, Elhajj, & Asmar, 2018) but also to generate new nurse-robotic/automation care models that synergistically leverage the best parts of both humans and technology as a means to future-proof the nursing profession in the coming decades.

Big Data

One by-product of digital health technology use is that many of these systems generate large quantities of data through their operations. Unlike a healthcare system underpinned by paper-based records, the use of digital records has allowed healthcare practitioners to generate and aggregate enormous amounts of data regarding patients, staff, healthcare processes, and other measurable aspects related to healthcare delivery. Virtually every other modern industry (i.e., manufacturing, marketing, agriculture) has also experienced similar exponential growth in terms of the collection and aggregation of context-relevant data that can be processed and analyzed to generate insights to inform business operations. In healthcare, the term *big data* has become popularized over the last decade as a term used to define data that both contains large amounts of unstructured data and has outgrown conventional database and warehouse solutions (McBride et al., 2018). Due to the sheer size and complexity of data generated in most modern healthcare interactions, traditional approaches to analysis and data management are not sufficient. Although big data can come in many different forms and originate from a variety of contexts, the 3-V mnemonic has been commonly used to identify the concept (McBride et al., 2018):

Big data consists of . . .

Volume: data presenting in significant size and scale that would overwhelm traditional management or analysis approaches

Variety: the data can present in any combination of structured or unstructured forms

Velocity: commonly, big data is accumulated or generated quickly

Specifically, from a nursing outlook, big data offers the profession a massive opportunity to learn more about its role, efficacy, and processes within the healthcare system like never before (Brennan & Bakken, 2015; Westra et al., 2015). Due to emergent health technology such as AI and machine learning, big data can now be processed and inspected to generate insights and hypotheses related to all sorts of health(care) issues—including health human resources allocation, efficacy of nursing care, and many other medically focused morbidity/morality factors related to patient care. Although it is beyond the scope of this chapter to describe the various analytical approaches currently used to inspect and mine big data generated in healthcare contexts, the emerging role of data scientists should be considered as an indicator of the growing importance of the skill sets required by nurses to use existing big data to generate recommendations and insights that guide future nursing practice (Remus, 2016b; Topaz & Pruinelli, 2017). Along with big data generated within traditional healthcare sectors, the established use of big data to guide and direct marketing, sales, and product development can be observed in the robust machine learning and AI developments of most social media and personalized Internet applications currently in existence (i.e., Facebook, Amazon). With the increasing use of personalized healthcare solutions by clients and consumers outside traditional healthcare structures, nursing leadership must pay attention to the importance of generating skills and expertise in analyzing and generating insights from big data. Currently, the nursing profession does not have a critical mass of data scientists within its ranks—this is a significant issue moving into the coming decade, given the aforementioned importance of using data to plan, advise, and respond to emergent societal and healthcare needs (Remus, 2016b; Topaz & Pruinelli, 2017).

Personalized and Precision Medicine

Personalized and precision medicine consists of tools and applications that can be used by both consumers and providers to generate more specific healthcare approaches and treatment plans for individuals. In essence, this concept seeks to use advanced technology to support care models and approaches that are unique to the individual, commonly made more sensitive to the person by utilizing the context of a patient's genetic makeup (Savard, 2013). Although there are differences between personalized and precision medicine, for the purposes of this chapter, both topics will be discussed contemporaneously, as they share common features.

Simply put, personalized and precision medicine approaches use an individual's genetic makeup to help individualize treatments and therapies. While this type of healthcare approach has existed for some time in traditional healthcare structures, only recently has the cost and availability of diagnostic and genetic testing become affordable to allow for the upscaling of this model of care. Currently, personalized and precision medicine approaches have been most commonly used for oncology, respiratory, and other conditions that present consumers with increased morbidity. Outside the traditional healthcare system, a number of third-party industries have emerged over the last five years that offer consumers *do-it-yourself* approaches to personalized and precision medicine. Companies such as 23andMe, uBiome, and Navigenics are all businesses that offer various direct-to-consumer genetic testing solutions. To use one of these services, a consumer simply sends a DNA specimen (commonly saliva) to the organization. After a fee payment, the company generates a personalized medicine breakdown of the individual's genetic makeup, commonly including risk factors identified in their genetics related to various health conditions and illnesses. To date, the company 23andMe has sequenced over 5 million consumers and recently partnered with a large pharmaceutical company to use the aggregated data generated from these 5 million customers to aid the development and design of new drugs (Fox, 2018).

As an emergent digital healthcare technology that is being used by both traditional and nontraditional healthcare structures, the scaling of personalized and precision medicine approaches is of importance to nursing leaders who wish to ensure that clients receive the most ethical and targeted healthcare approaches. To date, there remains many unanswered legal, ethical, and privacy considerations related to the use of genetic information to personalize healthcare approaches—it would befit nursing leaders to reflect on the growing use of these kinds of healthcare approaches and generate new opportunities for nursing to ensure relevancy in these emergent care models.

Hybrid and Virtual Healthcare Models/Telepresence

With the growing use of ICT in all aspects of society and health care, it is no surprise that virtual healthcare models of care have become mainstream in certain healthcare delivery models. Clinical specialty areas such as home care, primary healthcare, and psychiatry have witnessed impressive growth over the last decade in relation to many forms of telemedicine and virtual healthcare (Francisco & Archer, 2015; Owens, 2018). Through these sorts of virtual healthcare approaches, clinicians commonly use various types of videoconferencing technology to remotely assess and treat consumers. While telemedicine has existed in traditional healthcare structures for decades, virtual healthcare models have expanded over the last decade, roughly corresponding with the increase and popularity of social media technology. Currently, there are many virtual healthcare solutions that exist, supported by hospitals, community healthcare centers, and public health agencies. For instance, the Ontario Telemedicine Network (OTN) provides provincial-level telemedicine/videoconferencing abilities for all hospitals and most rural and remote clinics spread across the province (OTN, 2015). Through OTN's network, consumers can be remotely connected to various providers and healthcare specialists, which can amount to significant savings in travel and logistics for consumers who can remain in their homes and still receive equitable access to health services. More recently, other innovative solutions have emerged to fill gaps in the healthcare system between traditional structures afforded by hospitals, community health centers, and public health. For instance, the development of a virtual primary healthcare application operated by Maple affords users the ability to quickly connect on demand to a physician via a mobile phone application (Owens, 2018). Through this interaction, the physician can assess the consumer and, in some cases, diagnose and write prescriptions for a variety of conditions or illnesses.

While some virtual care models utilize fully distributed approaches to engagement with a client, other more hybrid approaches seek to leverage ICT to amplify elements of nursing. One such model is eShift, a home-care model where nurses remotely monitor up to six clients through a web-based platform from the point of care in the home (Royackers, Regan, & Donelle, 2016). In this model of care, personal support technicians who operate within the home environment of the client are able to execute a wide range of care actions and tasks, as delegated by the remote supervising nurse. This model of care has resulted in increased patient comfort, increased efficiency in staffing resources, increased capacity, and decreased hospital readmission rates (SWLHIN, 2017). Although these models demonstrate a significant evolution of the nursing role from contemporary home-care practices, the ability of the nurse to manage and coordinate the care for numerous patients, through the amplification of their abilities using the eShift technology and partnerships with unregulated healthcare technicians, is a dynamic worthy of deeper examination by the profession.

Finally, one extension to a purely virtual healthcare approach is the use of *telepresence* technology. The definition of *telepresence* is "a set of technologies, such as high definition audio, video, and other interactive elements that enable people to feel or appear as if they were present in a location which they are not physically in" (Beal, 2018). Within health care, the use of mobile telepresence technology that affords a user the ability to move and interact with a remote environment has become used in some care settings (see **FIGURE 10-3**). Although various telepresence approaches have been used for decades within health care, more recent cost-effective telepresence robots and devices have entered the marketplace, providing opportunities for clinicians to use these kinds of devices to physically navigate around remote buildings and facilities to interact with people and context, at a distance (Becevic et al., 2015; Koceski & Koceska, 2016). With the increasing power and availability of telepresence robotics, nursing should explore the role of this kind of logical extension to videoconferencing technology for use in nursing roles where possessing the ability to navigate a remote environment or location can both facilitate the nurse-client relationship and the ability to assess the client.

Smart Cities and the Internet of Things (IoT)

Juniper Research (2016) has predicted that the number of connected *things* (e.g., devices, sensors, smart speakers, etc.) will reach over 46 billion in 2021, a 200% increase since 2016. This linking of digital and physical realms is enabled by increasingly inexpensive sensors collecting and transferring data from physical systems to information and communication systems that process, control, and manage processes through feedback loops. These networks become *smart* when *things* are able

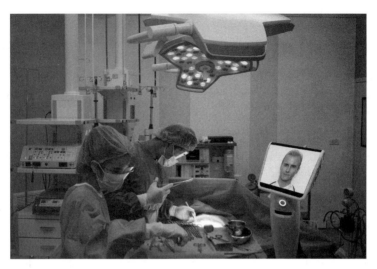

FIGURE 10-3 Telepresence robotics provide users with the ability to communicate and navigate autonomously in remote locations.
© Monopoly919/Shutterstock

to "sense, compute, communicate, and integrate seamlessly with the surrounding environment" (Borgia, 2014). The IoT vision, particularly related to health care, has yet to successfully emerge, but the rate of innovation in hardware, data processing, data storage, and 5G networks enabling data movement is rapid. The issues of security and privacy surrounding IoT devices and networks, a major matter of concern for both private citizens and independent organizations, are particularly troubling in the healthcare sector. This includes issues related to the invasiveness of the connected networks that can sometimes hear, see, sense, and transmit data to third parties; questions surrounding who owns the data that is transmitted; and what the data is used for are just some of the modern-day concerns related to many IoT technologies. As the era of connected, *intelligent* implantable devices becomes a reality (Teshome, Kibret, & Lai, 2018), issues involving the ownership and governance of data collected from individuals while they are in the healthcare system will have to be addressed.

IoT-powered or *smart* cities that seamlessly and ubiquitously improve the lives of their citizens through the promotion of more sustainable eco-friendly practices and health services that are delivered in response to individuals' actual needs (determined by data from wearables or interactions with city structures) still face many challenges (Kamel Boulos & Al-Shorbaji, 2014). However, as the technology that helps to collect and synthesize this data continues to mature and becomes cheaper, hyperconnected smart cities will become a reality. Building out the infrastructure to capture data at a population level has the potential to contribute social capital that subsequently redistributes the benefits of digital health technologies also up to a population level. Smart cities have been promoted as a potential antidote to the rising number of older adults, increasing geographic dispersion of families, and economic challenges (Solanas et al., 2014). Providing monitoring and health services in connected or smart homes is seen as a way to anticipate and avoid more expensive forms of care for the elderly and chronically ill.

To date, the nursing function might be characterized as reactive rather than proactive in this area of emergent digital health technology development. While the full power of many *smart* and IoT-connected technologies has yet to have a functional impact on healthcare processes, nurses need to pay attention to this quickly diffusing technology. For instance, with projections that much of health care will occur in the home over the coming decades (Canadian Healthcare Association, 2009; Gleckman, 2016), the use of smart or intelligent IoT devices needs to be considered as not only a potentially significant mechanism to support care but also as a situation in need of deeper exploration in terms of consumer privacy and related home healthcare processes. Nursing needs to play a dedicated and verbal role in ensuring IoT-connected devices, especially those used for healthcare purposes, provide functional, beneficent, safe, and ethical approaches for users and their families.

Blockchain

The healthcare industry has been called the ultimate "data economy" (Tang, Plasek, & Bates, 2018), yet it grapples with increasing costs, smaller labor pools, and an increasingly technologically savvy consumer base that demands transparency and a desire for meaningful engagement in care decisions. Due to this, it is forecast that healthcare systems of the future will need to rely on wearable and embedded technologies to allow machines to manage a mass of day-to-day patient monitoring and related care coordination. Further, these systems will produce large volumes of data, which must be managed to ensure that privacy is protected; the system is secure; and transaction friction is reduced for researchers, healthcare providers, funders, and consumers alike who want to enter, access, exchange, and use this data.

One emergent technology that will likely facilitate many of these future information and data transactions is *blockchain*. Blockchain is the digital version of ledgers or lists of information that have been used to record and manage transactions for centuries. Unlike ledgers and lists of the past, these digital ledgers are permanent, digital blocks of transactions that are encrypted and then linked to other blocks. Blockchain lists and their history are instantly accessible to the network of contributors, validated by timestamps and unique digital signatures that facilitate encryption and anonymity and prevent editing, and have the ability to include constraints or execute actions automatically (i.e., they are smart; Brogan, Baskaran, & Ramachandran, 2018). These ledgers are unable to be changed and can be viewed as a true account of what has happened, similar to a "reference library for finding where something is or when an activity happened" (Disney, 2018). Distributed databases are a foundational element of the emerging cryptocurrency industry, but they are increasingly being considered as a solution to some of the more intractable health conundrums such as the ownership of healthcare records (Disney, 2018), health information systems portability and interoperability (Gordon & Catalini, 2018), tracking of clinical trials' data and medical devices (Andrianov & Kaganov, 2017), pharmaceuticals (Mettler, 2016; Tseng, Liao, Chong, & Liao, 2018), and public health records (Mettler, 2016).

While there are currently numerous barriers to its effective use in health care (Gordon, Wright, & Landman, 2017), nursing leaders need to understand the basic mechanics of blockchain, as forces largely outside health care are driving their adoption and diffusion into various health-related contexts. Consequently, its use in managing healthcare data puts the nurse leader in a central role to ensure privacy, security, and appropriate use safeguards are well-developed before implementation.

REFLECTION SCENARIO 2

Reflecting on the various emergent digital health technologies described in the previous section, as a nurse leader it may be worthwhile to conceptualize how, and if, these innovations may serve as levers or drivers within a future healthcare ecosystem.

Along with theorizing how various emergent digital health technologies will influence the healthcare landscape, identifying partnerships and other relational opportunities with fields such as policy and education to support the use of these innovations is important to consider. For instance, when considering the use of *robotic and automation technology* within various aspects of the future clinician's role, it is worthwhile to consider the following:

1. What will be the direct and indirect effects of the automation of various lower skill, high-intensity tasks within the clinical purview in terms of funding, safety, and health human resources allocation?
2. How will clinical staff be oriented and taught to adapt to the use of these forms of innovation, which may displace roles and tasks once held by other humans?
3. How will nurse leaders collaborate with other developer stakeholders to generate robotic and automation technology that will benefit patient care in mechanisms beyond mere efficiency metrics?
4. How will the development, scaling, and stabilization of robotic and automation technology positively and negatively influence future roles and tasks held by clinicians?

▶ Process, Structures, and Nursing Leadership: Implications for the Profession

In the previous sections, we discussed and analyzed numerous emergent digital health technologies and their potential to disrupt current state healthcare processes and structures. While many of these technologies have yet to be fully realized in terms of development or diffusion within health care, their latency should not be underestimated when planning for the future. To better understand *how* these digital health technologies will affect the nursing role, the profession must better understand how these forms of innovation will influence health(care) structures and processes. In the following section, three main considerations will be explored: (1) how emergent digital health technology will transform the processes and structures of the healthcare system; (2) how embracing a sociomaterial lens will be important to *observe* this new, emergent reality, which will blur social and material processes in all aspects of health care; and (3) how nursing leadership will be required to steward the profession over the coming decades, to leverage these emergent digital health technologies to advance nursing practice.

Health(care) Process and Structure Evolution

While an exact understanding of how emergent, disruptive digital health technology will influence health care is not fully known, insights can be drawn from a variety of works that have explored the future reach and potential of these innovations. According to recent reports (KPMG, 2018; Thimbleby, 2013), there are salient healthcare domains that are expected to experience substantive growth in the coming decades: (1) personalized health care on demand and (2) treatment innovation and hybrid workforces. Each of these domains touches on traditional healthcare approaches of contemporary time periods (i.e., hospitals, community health care, public health), and many of the new and emergent models of care that these domains will utilize have been previously discussed in this chapter. Further, while this chapter has largely discussed various emergent digital health technologies in isolation of each other, the future healthcare processes will likely blur all aforementioned innovations together, in an effort to generate a robust and consumer-centric healthcare ecosystem.

1. *Personalized health care on demand*

    Leveraging various emergent digital health technologies such as IoT, precision medicine, and direct-to-consumer applications, the future healthcare ecosystem will seek to generate a comprehensive value chain for the consumer that is both personalized and on demand. Currently, various smart home technologies, do-it-yourself genetic testing, and virtual primary healthcare applications are markers for the future evolution and synergy among people, technology, and processes in the coming years. The potential of new models of care to emerge to compete against or complement traditional healthcare processes and structures is extremely high—this is especially true in healthcare environments where regulation related to fee structures and service provision is relaxed. How much these emergent models of care will compete or complement traditional services is yet unknown, although, given the quick adoption of virtual primary healthcare solutions, it is likely that these services will act as a disruptive force to the incumbent processes and structures.

    One area that traditional healthcare structures have yet to fully capitalize on is *wellness*, as opposed to almost exclusively focusing on *illness* (KPMG, 2018). Future care models focused on providing personalized and on-demand health care will purposefully seek to provide a value structure to the consumer that spans both wellness and illness. From the redevelopment of home and domestic environments to provide wrap-around support through various sensors and IoT devices to wearable and other biometric applications that assist the consumer in generating personalized wellness recommendations, the future model of care will include a denser focus on the sustainment of wellness, as much as a focus on illness.

2. *Treatment innovation and hybrid workforce*

    Much like the drive toward personalized services that are available on demand, future healthcare models will also seek to use AI, machine learning, and robotics to amplify the abilities of healthcare providers. Even at the time of this writing, the rise of AI and machine learning in health care has become a mainstay in certain aspects of practice (Coiera, 2018). Undoubtedly, future models of care will leverage various elements of AI and machine learning to learn from past evidence, processes, and systems to generate future recommendations. Contemporary examples such as personalized/precision medicine indicate that wider use of these kinds of emergent digital health technologies is inevitable within many areas of healthcare practice, especially when the amount and complexity of data and information (i.e., big data) surpasses human cognitive abilities.

While AI and machine learning for large-scale predictive data mining and analysis is important, the use of this kind of innovation within robotic and automation technology is a reality that must be appreciated in the physical sense. Although it may seem radical to suggest (at the time of this writing) that nurses and other clinicians will *physically* interact with non-human, artifically intelligent robotic agents in the provision of health care to a variety of consumers across the healthcare system, this future-state reality is likely no more than a decade or two away. Contemporary examples of healthcare-specific service drones and robotic assistants currently exist in the media and published literature (Ahn, Lee, & MacDonald, 2015; Humber River Hospital Foundation, 2018; UNC Health Care, 2018). While the clunkiness of many robotic assistants currently in existence may not inspire confidence for the future, it is important to consider that these forms of non-human agents will be developed and inserted into clinical processes and workflows to accomplish specific tasks through and between contemporary healthcare structures that are currently occupied by humans. As an existential threat to various current-day clinician healthcare delivery roles and activities, deeper appreciation for the use of AI-enabled robotics and other automation technology *needs to be explored immediately by the profession.* While the nursing profession is somewhat sheltered from the immediate effects of robotic and automation technology as related to the main core nursing skills and knowledge possessed by its membership (Frey & Osborne, 2013; Muro, 2017), other aspects of the nursing role are not. For instance, a range of skills, tasks, and cognitive functions conducted by nurses can likely be augmented or disintermediated by specialized robotic and AI software (Booth, 2016; Coiera, 2018). This could include basic knowledge tasks such as the transcription of information, certain routine clinical tasks, and other high-repetition tasks that offer low-value yield within the care experience. While a contentious proposition to suggest that some elements of the nursing role could be "up for grabs" by non-human robotics and AI agents, this reality is not so farfetched when juxtaposed against other knowledge-intense industries that have successfully scaled the use of these kinds of innovations in their daily operations (i.e., publishing, news/media, manufacturing, financial industry; CGP Grey, 2014). Regardless of the interpretation of whether this potential disintermediation of elements of the nursing role by AI and robotics is a *good* or *bad* trajectory, the profession at large needs to understand the impending force that these forms of innovation will apply in both direct and indirect ways. Subscribing to the status quo as a mechanism to ensure future relevancy and permanence of the nursing role is likely a poor course of action given the disruptive potential exhibited by these innovations.

Sociomaterial Lens for the Future

Throughout this chapter, sociomateriality has been highlighted (and advocated) as a lens that practitioners and nurse leaders can use to *see* the future healthcare environment and its related structures. Essentially, the blurring and hybridization of human and technological roles in the future healthcare system will become more nuanced and powerful than ever. With disruptive innovations amplifying and expediting this phenomenon of blurring between humans, technology, and processes, nursing leaders will need a conceptual lens that allows the theorization of new realities where the *social* and *material* are considered concurrently. For instance, a modern-day example of a sociomaterial phenomenon is an individual's online presence, as represented through e-mail, social media platform interaction, and all other digital footprints available on the Internet. While someone's digital footprint online is very much a *material* entity, it also contains a fair amount of *social* identity. Attempting to suggest that someone's online identity is separate from her or his physical identity, especially at the time of this writing in 2019, is especially cumbersome given the blurred nature of how people interact with the Internet and their reliance on its functionality to represent themselves in the absence of their physical selves (i.e., LinkedIn profile). It is proposed that an individual's online presence as an example of a nuanced sociomaterial representation is *just the beginning* of the blurring and complex entanglement of social and material entities in daily life.

In essence, a sociomaterial lens allows a nursing leader to both conceptualize and appreciate human-level agency in the generation of action and also the agency a technology or material entity can convey within a given context or phenomenon. While it is difficult to suggest that material entities can possess humanlike *agency* to perform an action, the upcoming generation of emergent digital health technology will possess the technological agency and capacity that may resemble that of humans in many respects. The illusion of cognition, problem solving, and learning through experience are all elements of various robotic technology expected to diffuse into elements of health(care) in the coming decades (Broadbent, 2017; Taipale, de Luca, Sarrica, & Fortunati, 2015). Therefore, while it may seem presumptuous to suggest that non-human agents like robots and AI-enabled technology will possess *agency* in the truest humanlike sense, they will possess their own capacity to exert force, presence, and certain levels of autonomy upon or within their given operational environments.

REFLECTION SCENARIO 3

To see the significance and role of future healthcare models that use AI and robotic technology, it will be important for a nursing leader to have the ability to view the phenomena from a sociomaterial lens.

For instance, picture a futuristic scenario where an AI-enabled robotic drone, featuring autonomous functions and the ability to follow basic verbal instructions conveyed by humans, has been implemented in a clinical environment to assist nurses and other clinicians in restocking shelves and supplies. At first glance this robotic supply drone may seem innocuous, but the operational, maintenance, workflow, and other safety considerations it engenders should be considered by a nurse leader. Although some of these considerations are common concerns with any newly implemented technology, using a sociomaterial lens to inspect the situation yields even deeper considerations worthy of discussion. For instance:

1. How does the AI operate—does the robot self-learn or is its AI limited to a set array of decisions and outcomes?
2. What reach does the robot have into other digital or electronic record systems—can the robot potentially modify or update records automatically without human intervention or cross-reference?
3. How do humans *actually* perceive their relationship with the drone—is the robot viewed as a cumbersome technology or a useful tool, or is it anthropomorphized through the provision of a name, personality, and other human-level characteristics defined by its users?
4. How do work processes change when the robot is unexpectedly absent or may be negatively affecting previously existing workflows—do humans successfully readapt or develop work-arounds?
5. How do humans *react* when the robot fails or makes a mistake—what level of confidence and *trust* do human users impart and expect from the robot, and *who* is accountable for errors or adverse events?

Nursing Leadership

The coming generation of emergent digital health technology, including but not limited to some of the examples discussed previously in this chapter, poses significant implications for the nursing profession—specifically to the nursing role and nursing leadership. As the influx and diffusion of technology become more prominent, it will inevitably influence the traditional nursing role in any number of fashions, including the probable dissolution of certain nursing activities and tasks while simultaneously generating new roles and opportunities for nurses. Traditionally, the nursing profession has been somewhat reluctant to generate modifications to the nursing role when new technology has been introduced into clinical settings. However, with the rise of emergent digital health technology and its impending impact on the nursing profession, nursing leaders must be mindful that hesitation to proactively plan for the future will limit the potential opportunities these forms of innovation may bring to the nursing role. Therefore, in addition to those in formal leadership positions, nurses in various roles and capacities must also be actively invited and involved in the discussions related to emergent digital health technology. The lack of a comprehensive and meaningful discussion related to these technologies and their influence on the nursing role will prevent the profession from moving past the status quo and do a disservice to the nursing profession, nursing practice, and healthcare delivery in future decades.

From a nursing leadership perspective, leaders can no longer view these forms of technology and innovation as neutral or static entities. While a neutral or static conceptualization of technology in the profession might have sufficed in the past, the disruptive potential of many emergent digital health technologies described in this chapter will yield significant direct and indirect impacts on the profession and healthcare structures that have never been experienced before. Consequently, viewing these forms of technology as static entities or merely as neutral, passive tools that the profession can use to generate action fails to appreciate the dynamic, sociomaterial nature these innovations facilitate. To embrace a future of this magnitude and complexion, nursing leaders will need to have both the awareness and insight to recognize, shape, and guide the development of these sorts of visible and hidden emergent digital health technologies to understand and appreciate the benefits and challenges they will bring to all aspects of healthcare work. Along with exploring the impact of emergent digital health technology upon the profession, a simultaneous examination of the consumers and their presence within this emerging dynamic is also required. For instance, what role(s) will consumers take within these new models of care, what influence will these interactions have on consumer health and wellness, and what influence (if any) will the consumer possess in directly shaping how the data generated from these models of care are used, monetized, and aggregated with other data sources? From a nursing perspective, nursing leaders need to immediately advocate for nurse involvement in all aspects of conversation around these kinds of emergent digital health technologies. Without this type of active engagement, the nursing profession will not develop the necessary grounding, skills, or embeddedness within the domain to functionally move beyond the current status quo in terms of the profession's involvement in health(care).

To begin this transformational process, the authors of this chapter recommend nursing leaders complement their current knowledge of traditional informatics competencies with a deeper, sociomaterial understanding of how these emergent digital health technologies will evolve many aspects that are sensitive to the nursing role. Essentially, the profession needs to develop deeper competencies for leadership that reflect on the potential impact, interaction, and agency possessed by emergent digital health technologies, and how their forces will be represented upon processes, structures, and interactions in health(care). Further, as emergent digital health technology with AI and other autonomous capabilities begin to scale within health(care) processes, nursing leadership will need to view these non-human agents as possessing power, presence, and the ability to shape and reshape processes. Failure to appreciate the nuanced dynamic between humans and technology as a competency will prevent nursing leaders from fully leveraging these emergent innovations in a proactive and productive fashion for the betterment of the profession and consumers. Without this sort of proactivity, nursing will miss a sizable opportunity to generate new roles within the future health(care) ecosystem, which will undoubtedly operate in the interstitial spaces between what is social and what is material.

▶ Conclusions

The emergent and unpredictable nature of new technologies must engender competencies in nursing leaders that address second-generation capabilities such as the ability to gather, analyze, and manipulate disparate data for decision making, as well as working alongside *intelligent* non-human entities and technologies that possess AI. Furthermore, the very resilience of healthcare organizations and structures is predicated on the abilities of future leaders to understand challenges emerging from the digital economy such as cybersecurity and technology-enabled ethics and compliance as related to the profession of nursing and the healthcare system.

Overall, this chapter has elevated the discussion of emergent digital health technology beyond its impact on the nursing profession in general and advocated for the development of a nursing epistemology related to those who choose to lead the profession's response to technological change. The sociomaterial lens used throughout the chapter seeks to explain to future leaders of the profession the interdependent nature of sometimes invisible digital health technology assisting, amplifying, and at times underpinning various healthcare structures and processes. In effect, nursing practices and future innovations will have an impact on each other, and nursing leaders must be prepared to actively engage in the discourse of whether and how technologies should be further adopted and embedded into the nursing role. While there must be a convergence around competencies for 21st-century nursing leaders and beyond, it is also contingent on current nursing leaders to clearly communicate the importance of the nursing perspective in the development of, and response to, technological evolution. Without this type of leadership, the profession may miss a vital opportunity to become agents of change in this quickly evolving domain—a domain where remaining static is incompatible with a prosperous or productive future.

References

Ahn, H. S., Lee, M. H., & MacDonald, B. A. (2015). Healthcare robot systems for a hospital environment: CareBot and ReceptionBot. In *2015 24th IEEE International Symposium on Robot and Human Interactive Communication (RO-MAN)* (pp. 571–576). https://doi.org/10.1109/ROMAN.2015.7333621

Aluri, A., Price, B. S., & McIntyre, N. H. (2018). Using machine learning to cocreate value through dynamic customer engagement in a brand loyalty program. *Journal of Hospitality and Tourism Research, 43*(1), 1–23. https://doi.org/10.1177/1096348017753521

Amazon. (2018). What is artificial intelligence? Retrieved from https://aws.amazon.com/machine-learning/what-is-ai/

Amendola, M. L. (2008, July). An examination of the leadership competency requirements of nurse leaders in healthcare information technology. *ProQuest Dissertations and Theses,* 156.

Andrianov, A., & Kaganov, B. (2017). Blockchain in clinical trials—the ultimate data notary: Assessing the benefits of using blockchain technology as a notary service in the network sharing of clinical data. *Applied Clinical Trials, 27*(8), 16.

Archibald, M. M., & Barnard, A. (2018). Futurism in nursing: Technology, robotics and the fundamentals of care. *Journal of Clinical Nursing, 27*(11–12), 2473–2480. https://doi.org/10.1111/jocn.14081

Beal, V. (2018). Telepresence. Retreived from https://www.webopedia.com/TERM/T/telepresence.html

Becevic, M., Clarke, M. A., Alnijoumi, M. M., Sohal, H. S., Boren, S. A., Kim, M. S., & Mutrux, R. (2015). Robotic telepresence in a medical intensive care unit: Clinicians' perceptions. *Perspectives in Health Information Management, 12,* 1c.

Bolden, R. (2011). Distributed leadership in organizations: A review of theory and research. *International Journal of Management Reviews, 13*(3), 251–269. https://doi.org/10.1111/j.1468-2370.2011.00306.x

Booth, R. G. (2016). Informatics and nursing in a post-nursing informatics world: Future directions for nurses in an automated, artificially-intelligent, social-networked healthcare environment. *Canadian Journal of Nursing Leadership, 28*(4), 61–69. https://doi.org/10.12927/cjnl.2016.24563

Booth, R. G., Andrusyszyn, M., Iwasiw, C., Donelle, L., & Compeau, D. (2016). Actor-network theory as a sociotechnical lens to explore the relationship of nurses and technology in practice: Methodological considerations for nursing research. *Nursing Inquiry, 23*(2), 109–120. https://doi.org/10.1111/nin.12118

Booth, R. G., McBride, S. G., & Tietze, M. (2015). Scientific and theoretical foundations for driving improvement. In S. G. McBride and M. Tietze (Eds.), *Nursing informatics for the advanced practice nurse: Patient safety, quality, outcomes, and interprofessionalism* (pp. 47–80). New York, NY: Springer.

Borgia, E. (2014). The internet of things vision: Key features, applications and open issues. *Computer Communications, 54*, 1–31. https://doi.org/10.1016/j.comcom.2014.09.008

Brennan, P. F., & Bakken, S. (2015). Nursing needs big data and big data needs nursing. *Journal of Nursing Scholarship, 47*(5), 477–484. https://doi.org/10.1111/jnu.12159

Broadbent, E. (2017). Interactions with robots: The truths we reveal about ourselves. *Annual Review of Psychology, 68*, 627–652. https://doi.org/10.1146/annurev-psych-010416-043958

Brogan, J., Baskaran, I., & Ramachandran, N. (2018). Authenticating health activity data using distributed ledger technologies. *Computational and Structural Biotechnology Journal, 16*, 257–266. https://doi.org/10.1016/j.csbj.2018.06.004

Canadian Healthcare Association. (2009). *Home care in Canada: From the margins to the mainstream.* Ottawa: Author.

CGP Grey. (2014). Humans need not apply. Retrieved from https://www.youtube.com/watch?v=7Pq-S557XQU

Coiera, E. (2018). The fate of medicine in the time of AI. *The Lancet, 6736*(18), 10–11. https://doi.org/10.1016/S0140-6736(18)31925-1

Collins, S., Phllips, A., Yen, P.-Y., & Kennedy, M. K. (2017). Nursing informatics competency assessment for the nurse leader: The Delphi study. *JONA: The Journal of Nursing Administration, 47*(4), 212–218. https://doi.org/10.1097/NNA.0000000000000467

Crowe, S. (2016). Pepper robots working at Belgian hospitals. Retrieved from https://www.roboticsbusinessreview.com/rbr/pepper_robots_working_at_belgian_hospitals/

Davenport, T. H., & Kirby, J. (2015, June). Spotlight on man and machine. *Harvard Business Review,* 59–65.

Disney, H. (2018). It's time to get smart about blockchain in healthcare. Retrieved from https://pharmaphorum.com/digital/its-time-to-get-smart-about-blockchain-in-healthcare/

Encyclopedia Brittannica. (2018). Artificial intelligence. https://www.britannica.com/technology/artificial-intelligence

Fitzsimons, D., Turnbull James, K., & Denyer, D. (2011). Alternative approaches for studying shared and distributed leadership. *International Journal of Management Reviews, 13*, 313–328.

Fox, M. (2018, July 25). Drug giant Glaxo teams up with DNA testing company 23andMe. *NBC News.* Retrieved from https://www.nbcnews.com/health/health-news/drug-giant-glaxo-teams-dna-testing-company-23andme-n894531

Francisco, K., & Archer, N. P. (2015). *The impact of telemedicine on primary mental health care in Canada.* Hamilton, Canada. Retrieved from http://hdl.handle.net/11375/17714

Frey, C. B., & Osborne, M. A. (2013). *The future of employment: How susceptible are jobs to automation?* Oxford, UK: Oxford Martin School, University of Oxford.

Gergen, K. (2009). *Relational being: Beyond self and community.* New York: Oxford.

Glasgow, M. E. S., Colbert, A., Viator, J., & Cavanagh, S. (2018). The nurse-engineer: A new role to improve nurse technology interface and patient care device innovations. *Journal of Nursing Scholarship.* https://doi.org/10.1111/jnu.12431

Gleckman, H. (2016, October 21). Long-term care is increasingly becoming managed care at home. *Forbes.* Retrieved from https://www.forbes.com/sites/howardgleckman/2016/10/21/long-term-care-is-increasingly-becoming-managed-care-at-home/#341d183e106d

Gordon, W. J., & Catalini, C. (2018). Blockchain technology for healthcare: Facilitating the transition to patient-driven interoperability. *Computational and Structural Biotechnology Journal, 16*, 224–230. https://doi.org/10.1016/j.csbj.2018.06.003

Gordon, W., Wright, A., & Landman, A. (2017, February 9). Blockchain in health care: Decoding the hype. *New England Journal of Medicine Catalyst.* Retrieved from https://catalyst.nejm.org/decoding-blockchain-technology-health/

Hart, M. D. (2010). A Delphi study to determine baseline informatics competencies for nurse managers. *CIN—Computers Informatics Nursing, 28*(6), 364–367. https://doi.org/10.1097/NCN.0b013e3181f69d89

HIMSS. (2016). CNIO job description. Retrieved from https://www.himss.org/sites/himssorg/files/himss-cnio-job-description.pdf

Humber River Hospital Foundation. (2018). Meet Pepper, Humber River Hospital's humanoid robot. Retrieved from https://www.hrhfoundation.ca/blog/pepper/

IBM. (2018). IBM Watson. Retrieved from https://www.ibm.com/watson/about/index.html

Juniper Research. (2016). IoT connections to grow 140% to hit 50 billion by 2022, as edge computing accelerates ROI. Retrieved from https://www.juniperresearch.com/press/press-releases/iot-connections-to-grow-140-to-hit-50-billion

Just, N., & Latzer, M. (2017). Governance by algorithms: Reality construction by algorithmic selection on the Internet. *Media, Culture and Society, 39*(2), 238–258. https://doi.org/10.1177/0163443716643157

Kamel Boulos, M. N., & Al-Shorbaji, N. M. (2014). On the Internet of things, smart cities and the WHO Healthy Cities. *International Journal of Health Geographics, 13*(1), 1–6. https://doi.org/10.1186/1476-072X-13-10

Kaplan, A., & Haenlein, M. (2018). Siri, Siri, in my hand: Who's the fairest in the land? On the interpretations, illustrations, and implications of artificial intelligence. *Business Horizons.* https://doi.org/10.1016/j.bushor.2018.08.004

Kassam, I., Nagle, L., & Strudwick, G. (2017). Informatics competencies for nurse leaders: Protocol for a scoping review. *BMJ Open, 7*(12), 1–4. https://doi.org/10.1136/bmjopen-2017-018855

Kennedy, M., & Moen, A. (2017). *Nurse leadership and informatics competencies: Shaping transformation of professional practice in forecasting informatics competencies for nurses in the future of connected health.* Amsterdam, Netherlands: IMIA and IOS Press. https://doi.org/10.3233/978-1-61499-738-2-197

Kleib, M., & Nagle, L. (2018). Psychometric properties of the Canadian Nurse Informatics Competency Assessment Scale. *CIN—Computers Informatics Nursing, 36*(7), 359–365. https://doi.org/10.1097/CIN.0000000000000437

Koceski, S., & Koceska, N. (2016). Evaluation of an Assistive Telepresence Robot for Elderly Healthcare. *Journal of Medical Systems, 40*(5). https://doi.org/10.1007/s10916-016-0481-x

KPMG. (2018). *Healthcare reimagined: Innovation trends, predictions and actions for healthcare leaders.* Retrieved from https://home.kpmg.com/au/en/home/insights/2018/01/healthcare-reimagined-report.html

Leonardi, P. M. (2012). Materiality, sociomateriality, and socio-technical systems: What do these terms mean? How are they related? Do we need them? *SSRN Electronic Journal.* https://doi.org/10.2139/ssrn.2129878

Maalouf, N., Sidaoui, A., Elhajj, I. H., & Asmar, D. (2018). Robotics in nursing: A scoping review. *Journal of Nursing Scholarship, 1985.* https://doi.org/10.1111/jnu.12424

Manyika, J., Lund, S., Chui, M., Bughin, J., Woetzel, J., Batra, P. . . . Sanghvi, S. (2017, December). Jobs lost, jobs gained: Workforce transitions in a time of automation. *McKinsey Global Institute,* 1–160. https://doi.org/10.1002/lary.20616

McBride, S., Powers, C., Gilder, R., Rhodes, W., Sobel, A., & Philips, B. (2018). "Big data" and advanced analytics. In S. McBride and M. Tietze (Eds.), *Nursing informatics for the advanced practice nurse: Patient safety, quality, outcomes, and interprofessionalism* (2nd ed., pp. 653–682). New York, NY: Springer.

McIntyre, C. (2018, February). The University of Toronto's nursing program: VR, robots and more— University of Toronto students research robots and games to mitigate pain. *Macleans.* Retrieved from https://www.macleans.ca/education/medi-robocare-toronto/

Mettler, M. (2016). Blockchain technology in healthcare: The revolution starts here. *2016 IEEE 18th International Conference on E-Health Networking, Applications and Services, Healthcom 2016,* 16–18. https://doi.org/10.1109/HealthCom.2016.7749510

Muro, M. (2017). *Digitalization and the American workforce.* Washington DC: Brookings Institution.

Narayanan, V., Barash, V., Kelly, J., Kollanyi, B., Neudert, L.-M., & Howard, P. N. (2018). Polarization, partisanship and junk news consumption over social media in the US. *ArXiv.* https://doi.org/10.1029/2004JD005113

Orlikowski, W. J., & Scott, S. V. (2008). Sociomateriality: Challenging the separation of technology, work and organization. *The Academy of Management Annals, 2*(1), 433–474. https://doi.org/10.1080/19416520802211644

OTN. (2015). OTN, about us. Retrieved from https://support.otn.ca/en/about-us

Owens, B. (2018). Telemedicine on the rise but lagging in Canada. *Canadian Medical Association Journal, 190*(38), E1149–E1150. https://doi.org/10.1503/cmaj.109-5634

Piraino, E., Byrne, K., Heckman, G. A., & Stolee, P. (2017). Caring in the information age: Personal online networks to improve caregiver support. *Canadian Geriatrics Journal: CGJ, 20*(2), 85–93. https://doi.org/10.5770/cgj.20.271

RBC. (2018). *Humans wanted: How Canadian youth can thrive in the age of disruption.* Toronto, Canada: Royal Bank of Canada.

Remus, S. (2016a). Advancing the digital health discourse for nurse leaders. *Studies in Health Technology and Informatics, 225*(January 2016), 412–416. https://doi.org/10.3233/978-1-61499 -658-3-412

Remus, S. (2016b). The big data revolution: Opportunities for chief nurse executives. *Canadian Journal of Nursing Leadership, 28*(4), 18–28.

Remus, S., & Kennedy, M. A. (2012). Innovation in transformative nursing leadership: nursing informatics competencies and roles. *Nursing Leadership (Toronto, Ont.), 25*(4), 14–26. https:// doi.org/10.1177/0894318413500313

Riek, L. D. (2017). Healthcare robotics. *Communications of the ACM, 60*(11), 68–78. https://doi .org/10.1145/3127874

Royackers, A., Regan, S., & Donelle, L. (2016). The eShift model of care: Informal caregivers' experience of a new model of home-based palliative care. *Progress in Palliative Care, 24*(2), 84–92. https://doi.org/10.1179/1743291X15Y.0000000006

Savard, J. (2013). Personalised medicine: A critique on the future of health care. *Journal of Bioethical Inquiry, 10*, 197–203. https://doi.org/10.1007/s11673-013-9429-8

Sensmeier, J. (2017). Harnessing the power of artificial intelligence. *Nursing Management, 48*(11), 14–19. https://doi.org/10.1097/01.NUMA.0000526062.69220.41

Simpson, R. L. (1994). Nursing informatics core competencies. *Nursing Management, 25*(2), 18–20.

Simpson, R. L. (2013). Chief nurse executives need contemporary informatics competencies. *Nursing Economic$, 31*(6), 277–87; quiz 288. https://doi.org/10.1017/CBO9781107415324.004

Solanas, A., Patsakis, C., Conti, M., Vlachos, I., Ramos, V., Falcone, F. . . . Martinez-Balleste, A. (2014). Smart health: A context-aware health paradigm within smart cities. *IEEE Communications Magazine, 52*(8), 74–81. https://doi.org/10.1109/MCOM.2014.6871673

Staggers, N., Gassert, C. A., & Curran, C. (2001). Informatics competencies for nurses at four levels of practice. *The Journal of Nursing Education, 40*(7), 303–316. Retrieved from http://www.ncbi .nlm.nih.gov/pubmed/11596683

Strudwick, G., Booth, R. G., Bjarnadottir, R. I., Collins, S., & Srivastava, R. (2017). Exploring the role of the nurse manager in supporting point-of-care nurses' adoption of electronic health records: Protocol for a qualitative research study. *BMJ Open, 7*(10), e018129. https://doi.org/10.1136 /bmjopen-2017-018129

Strudwick, G., & Xie, L. (2018). Incorporating technology meaningfully into the clinical encounter: A nursing perspective. *Nursing Informatics Bulletin, 11*(11), 9.

SWLHIN. (2017). eShift. Retrieved from http://healthcareathome.ca/southwest/en/Getting-Care /Getting-Care-at-Home/eshift

Taipale, S., de Luca, F., Sarrica, M., & Fortunati, L. (2015). Robot shift from industrial production to social reproduction. In J. Vincent, S. Taipale, B. Sapio, G. Lugano, & L. Fortunati (Eds.), *Social robots from a human perspective* (pp. 11–24). New York, NY: Springer. https://doi.org /10.1007/978-3-319-15672-9

Tang, C., Plasek, J. M., & Bates, D. W. (2018). Rethinking data sharing at the dawn of a health data economy: A viewpoint. *Journal of Medical Internet Research, 20*(11), e11519. https://doi .org/10.2196/11519

Teshome, A. K., Kibret, B., & Lai, D. (2018). A review of implant communication technology in WBAN: Progresses and challenges. *IEEE Reviews in Biomedical Engineering.* https://doi.org /10.1109/RBME.2018.2848228

Thimbleby, H. (2013). Technology and the future of healthcare. *Journal of Public Health Research, 2*(3), e28. https://doi.org/10.4081/jphr.2013.e28

Topaz, M., & Pruinelli, L. (2017). Big data and nursing: Implications for the future. *Proceedings of the Nursing Informatics Post Conference 2016, 232*, 165–171. https://doi.org/10.3233/978-1 -61499-738-2-165

Tseng, J. H., Liao, Y. C., Chong, B., & Liao, S. W. (2018). Governance on the drug supply chain via gcoin blockchain. *International Journal of Environmental Research and Public Health, 15*(6). https://doi.org/10.3390/ijerph15061055

UNC Health Care. (2018). The TUG robots are coming. Retrieved from http://news.unchealthcare .org/empnews/2018/jan-25/the-tug-robots-are-coming

Westra, B. L., Clancy, T. R., Sensmeier, J., Warren, J. J., Weaver, C., & Delaney, C. W. (2015). Nursing knowledge: Big data science—implications for nurse leaders. *Nursing Administration Quarterly, 39*(4), 304–310. https://doi.org/10.1097/NAQ.0000000000000130

Westra, B. L., Delaney, C. W., & Delaney, C. (2008). Informatics competencies for nursing and healthcare leaders. *AMIA . . . Annual Symposium Proceedings/AMIA Symposium. AMIA Symposium*, 804–808. https://doi.org/10.1016/j.outlook.2007.05.005

Yang, L., Cui, D., Zhu, X., Zhao, Q., Xiao, N., & Shen, X. (2014). Perspectives from nurse managers on informatics competencies. *The Scientific World Journal, 2014*, 3–7. https://doi .org/10.1155/2014/391714

Yen, P.-Y., Kennedy, M. K., Phillips, A., & Collins, S. (2017). Nursing informatics competency assessment for the nurse leader. *Journal Nursing Administration, 47*(5), 271–277. https://doi .org/10.1097/NNA.0000000000000478

CHAPTER 11

Incorporating New Evidence from Big Data, Emerging Technology, and Disruptive Practices into Your Innovation Ecosystem

Rayne Soriano and Daniel Weberg

CHAPTER OBJECTIVES

Upon completion of this chapter, the reader will be able to:

1. Describe emerging sources of data to inform evidence-based practice (EBP).
2. Discuss leadership competencies to support new sources of evidence.
3. Compare and contrast new sources of evidence and their value to EBP leadership.

▶ Introduction

Against the backdrop of healthcare challenges and linking hospital reimbursements to the quality of care, the need to efficiently access information to maintain and improve quality measures is heightened by benchmarking across organizations and public reporting by hospitals to consumers, insurers, and regulatory bodies (Centers for Medicaid and Medicare Services, 2014; Chassin, Loeb, Schmaltz, & Wachter, 2010; National Quality Forum, 2014; The Joint Commission, 2014). Drivers to improve the quality, safety, and value in the U.S. healthcare system have focused on transformational efforts through channels such as accessing and utilizing data as a staple for health learning (Institute of Medicine, 2010), improving systems for safety (Institute of Medicine, 2000), achieving high-reliability organizations (Chassin & Loeb, 2011), and adopting health information technology (HIT; Institute of Medicine, 2000, 2012) through groundbreaking and widespread efforts like the implementation of electronic medical records (EMRs), thus producing exponentially more data for using complex mathematical algorithms to find answers in big data sets and using those sources of evidence to employ disruptive practices to improve outcomes.

▶ Information at the Caregivers' Fingertips

Traditional sources of evidence for EBP methodologies have focused on comprehensive systematic reviews, randomized control trials (RCTs), peer-reviewed journals, and other formal research. As technology becomes more and more integrated in health care, new sources of data are available in near real time at caregivers' fingertips, just like new sources of data are available to consumers through the Internet in mobile devices, to help augment more traditional sources of data. These new sources of data serve as a platform allowing frontline clinicians to innovate at the point of care in near real time, thus completely disrupting the current EBP timelines of 17 years from research to practice. In the backdrop of complex and busy environments in health care, whether in acute care hospital settings or crowded primary care clinics, the onus is on HIT vendors in partnership with clinical informatics, and innovation teams to develop seamless and contextual solutions to access information and avoid adding to the information fatigue resulting from growing technology in health care.

Cross-industry, department, and system collaboration requires different leadership behaviors than the pure operational work that many nursing and healthcare leaders focus on. The development and implementation of solutions that bring new sources of data to the bedside in real time, and the cultural and staff support that is required to adopt and sustain such efforts, call for the ability to view and translate complex systems, understand and enable nonlinear workflows, and understand that all data is not created equal.

▶ New Sources of Data in Health Care

As more health information technologies are implemented in healthcare settings across the continuum of care, emerging sources of data have also grown, surrounded by the promise of interoperable systems, portable health information, and improvements in information access leading to better quality care. There are three broad categories of data that are providing new sources of evidence for disruptive practices in health care and shifting the paradigm of EBP to instantly available, accurately curated information that enables frontline caregivers and organizational leaders to more quickly make decisions, intervene for better outcomes, and potentially control costs and quality in more dynamic and innovative ways.

The first source of new evidence is the ubiquitous use of EMRs to gather, sort, and display data about patients. The second source of new evidence is the emerging categories of wearable devices that collect social and physiological data on individuals and send that data wirelessly to healthcare providers. The third source of new evidence comes from the output of complex mathematical algorithms that can churn and process massive data sets and find patterns, linkages, and visualizations that lend new insights to previously buried information. This chapter will discuss these new sources of evidence, their impact on innovation, and the leadership competencies needed to use new sources of data to implement disruptive strategies.

EMRs as a Source of Evidence and Innovation

The U.S. healthcare environment is complex, with challenges in quality, safety, efficiency, and value. Furthermore, healthcare spending in the United States is greater than in any other industrialized country (Squires, 2012). Despite the mounting financial investment in health care, the system is plagued with issues that continue to deteriorate the quality of care, such as medical errors (Van Den Bos et al., 2011), overtreatment, failures of care coordination, failures in execution of care processes, administrative complexity, pricing failures, fraud, and abuse (Berwick & Hackbarth, 2012). In the backdrop of ongoing incidences of patient falls, hospital-acquired pressure ulcers, and medication errors in the acute care environment, a critical focus of hospital quality is on nurse-sensitive measures that are indicators of ensuring that nursing care is carried out in a safe and evidence-based manner.

New Data Contribution

As a tool to support real-time access to information needed for quality monitoring in general, and for nurse-sensitive quality measures in particular, the EMR has been implemented in many hospitals as part of a mandate under the Health Information Technology for Economic and Clinical Health (HITECH) Act. The U.S. Department of Health and Human Services (2013) defined EMRs as real-time, patient-centered records that make information available instantly, bringing together everything about a patient's health in one place. Beyond the implementation of EMR systems, the meaningful use initiative was developed as an incentive program to ensure that EMRs are used according to standards that achieve quality, safety, and efficiency measures (Centers for Medicare and Medicaid Services, 2013).

One of the most significant structural developments for reinforcing information access has been the implementation of EMRs in hospitals. Evaluating caregiver experiences in using EMRs is important for highlighting opportunities and challenges in utilizing the tool for accessing information to enable quality monitoring. The features and applications within EMRs can also facilitate their use. Studies examining the applications and features of technology in health care have evolved from focusing on specific work functions to focusing on measures of EMR functionality for driving meaningful use in increasing quality, safety, and efficiency. Studies that have examined the features and applications of technology in the healthcare setting have looked at specific functions and various roles, such as continuous patient monitoring by nurses (Jeskey et al., 2011); data gathering and quality monitoring for operational leaders (Bradley et al., 2003); electronic information systems for planning, organizing, and staffing for managers (Lammintakanen, Saranto, & Kivinen, 2010);

and EMRs. Under EMRs, specific functions that were studied include the use of electronic patient support materials and ordering tests, procedures, and drugs (DesRoches, Donelan, Buerhaus, & Zhonghe, 2008), and electronic documentation of medications, vital signs, ongoing assessment data, and progress notes (Kossman & Scheidenhelm, 2008; Moody, Slocumb, Berg, & Jackson, 2004). Findings from these studies have shown that using the EMR must be facilitated through the availability of useful applications and features, such as the ability to document clinical care efficiently and retrieve data for monitoring patient care. With the quality, safety, and efficiency drivers of using EMRs, meaningful use has set the bar for EMR features to higher standards for achieving these outcomes. This raises questions as to how clinicians develop the skill sets to access information using these features in light of the challenges with preparation and training, as well as the structural challenges, and barriers to EMR adoption.

Challenges to Utilization

Despite significant evidence-based interventions and innovations to address major healthcare quality issues such as falls and pressure ulcers, the translation and implementation of that evidence to the frontline caregivers remains a significant problem. Even with the installation and use of EMR systems, clinical decision support remains fragmented from the complex workflows that govern patient care. This fragmentation of information and workflow began with the first EMR systems because these early systems were merely databases and billing support systems that contained clinical notes. As the systems evolved, teams of information technology professionals in healthcare organizations have attempted to optimize the user interface, data structures, and data linking in relevant ways to support care and the care team members. As these optimizations have continued, it has become possible to link evidence-based information that has been vetted through the EBP process directly to care interventions that nurses, physicians, and other care providers are implementing at the point of care. For example, partnerships among third-party content vendors that serve as clinical practice guidelines for nursing plans of care can be integrated into the EMR and activated via decision support engines to highlight the required assessments and interventions based on the most current evidence.

The literature suggests that EMRs as a source of information may be underutilized, with reports of structural and system challenges and process work-arounds that have led to increased complexity and challenges for providers in accessing information due to the persistence of paper documentation and nonintegrated systems (Ash & Bates, 2005; Keenan, Yakel, Dunn Lopez, Tschannen, & Ford, 2013).

In light of the benefits and features of EMRs for improving access to information for quality measures, there is an emerging body of literature from hospital settings with varying sample sizes that reveals EMR use as problematic for caregivers based on national surveys, large federal and academic health systems, and users from individual hospitals. Structural challenges with accessing information in the EMR include problems filtering information, lack of context-sensitive decision support and issues with the usefulness of the data, lack of usable functionality, lack of interoperability, lack of technical support, slow system response, need for multiple screens, overuse of check boxes and copy-and-paste documentation, and various system interface challenges (**TABLE 11-1**).

TABLE 11-1 EMR Data Issues and Consequences

Structural Challenges to Information	Consequences
Trouble filtering information	Information overload, clinician confusion, irrelevant information displays, wasted time
Useless data	Information overload, inefficient chart review, poor analysis
Lack of context	Faulty information interpretation
Slow system response	Wasted time, frustration, poor user adoption
Complex displays	Inefficiency, poor data input, poor analysis
Poor technical support	User frustration, work-arounds
Overuse of check boxes	Inaccurate charting, mindless data entry
Challenges with interfaces	Inefficiency, poor data input, frustration, confusion

Despite the availability of functions that enable automation of work tasks and meaningful use, studies have emerged showing that technology can also be a source of increasing complexity in health care and may not be easy to use, leading to potentially negative implications for all, including healthcare leaders. To highlight the effects of technology in healthcare environments, Alexander and Kroposki (2001) performed a longitudinal study comparing technology over a 10-year period and found a significant change in the complexity of technology on three dimensions: instability, uncertainty, and variability. As a result of this complexity, a study of electronic information system use by nurse leaders revealed participants described their concerns with information technology addiction and that system outages would lead to stoppages of clinical processes due to the overreliance on technology (Lammintakanen et al., 2010). Two studies also found perceptions that technology increases the workload for staff (Kossman & Scheidenhelm, 2008; Lammintakanen, Kivinen, Saranto, & Kinnunen, 2009), leading nurse leaders to defer from using the systems themselves and delegating any computerized work to those with training in computers and information processing (Lin, Wu, Huang, Tseng, & Lawler, 2007).

There needs to be a focus on system usability and work processes to support the use of information systems, integrated systems are needed for information flow to assist users with efficiently accessing information and guiding them with decision support, and information access and processing skills need to be developed beyond basic computer skills. Without intentional training and better design in EMRs, the leaders of our healthcare systems will be unable to stay informed and adaptable as the complexity of the healthcare environment increases.

Summary of EMRs as a Data Source

The EMR has been an impressive innovation that has facilitated transformations in care through digital documentation. New data that has been generated by EMRs has allowed nurses and other team members to collaborate, share information, and alert one another about care variations, patient needs, and assessment information. Challenges still remain in the implementation of EMRs and the structuring of data contained within them. Billions of dollars are being spent in the "optimization" of these archaic systems and despite new design features and upgrades, EMRs still largely resemble glorified spreadsheets. Leaders need to facilitate processes that match the workflow to documentation systems and support new informatics competencies to fully utilize this rich source of new evidence. It is no longer acceptable for leaders to defer informatic and technology competencies to others.

▶ The Disruption of Evidence Model

Technology is disrupting the ways evidence is being sourced, consumed, and interpreted in health care. In general, the foundation of evidence (data) is being decentralized from large organizational labs, data centers, and healthcare practitioner offices to the homes of the patients. Industry and innovators are sponsoring this dramatic shift with billions of dollars given to healthcare entrepreneurs for novel solutions and industry-funded competitions to build future technologies. One example is a competition to create a working Star Trek tricorder, a single handheld device that can gather vital signs and other data, that a patient can use without the need for clinical expertise or training. Companies are rapidly creating wearable devices that gather all vital signs, including blood pressure, and that are the size of a wedding ring.

The gathering of clinically accurate data from patients in their everyday life is very different from how medicine captured data in the past. From these new tools will come massive amounts of data into the system, and leaders will need to create new ways of interpreting and linking this data into real-time evidence for clinicians to use. For practitioners and healthcare organizations to stay relevant, they must be aware of the democratization of data and develop ways to leverage it for better care and new organizational structures (**TABLE 11-2**).

TABLE 11-2 Sources and Challenges of New Evidence		
Tool	**New Evidence**	**Challenges**
EMRs	■ Digital records ■ Analytics ■ Linked decision support ■ Instant information access ■ Relevant data alerts	■ Underutilized tool ■ Inefficient systems ■ Not designed for clinical workflow ■ Lack of technical support ■ Interpretation of unstructured data

Tool	New Evidence	Challenges
Wearable technology and sensors	■ Continuous monitoring of patient data (vital signs, activity, etc.) ■ Longitudinal data sets ■ Data while patient is away from care team	■ Too much data ■ Reliability concerns ■ Relevancy of data to diagnosis and treatments ■ Security and accuracy of data ■ Accuracy of tools to collect data
Big data	■ New links among variables ■ Predictive analytics ■ Population health insights ■ Pragmatic intervention recommendations	■ Privacy ■ Emerging field ■ Technical support and relevancy

Wearables and Patient-Entered Data

With consumerism of health care growing, there is an emerging trend wherein healthcare organizations are taking advantage of the ubiquity of mobile devices, the Internet, and social media to effect healthy behaviors through virtual means via partnerships with the retail industry. The wearable and patient-entered data revolution has democratized data and freed it from the constraints of paper charts, inefficiently designed mainframe EMRs, and the back-office medical practices, and placed it into the überaccessible Internet cloud. Here, the data can be accessed by the whole care team and across systems, crunched by complex algorithms, and used to link personal data to clinical diagnoses, treatment outcomes, and preventive care. But even with the ability to quantify health through these technologies, self-efficacy and motivation remain ongoing challenges.

DISCUSSION

What can be done to integrate and sustain wearable technologies in consumers' lives? Where is the balance between privacy and linking health behaviors to avenues like social media?

Beginning with fitness and diet applications that consumers use to track their health goals, healthcare organizations and application vendors are expanding these tools to quantify overall health, and even utilize gamification and fashion to motivate people to sustain the use of these wearable technologies (Chan, Estève, Fourniols, Escriba, & Campo, 2012; Dobkin, 2013). Patient-entered data is collected and aggregated in many different ways. Wearables are a category of devices that people can wear and that both actively and passively collect data. Examples of wearables include activity trackers like Fitbit, wirelessly connected insulin pumps, and U.S. Food and Drug Administration (FDA)–cleared vital sign monitors like Withings products, among others.

New Data Additions

Wearables are capable of capturing and continuously transmitting millions of data points to create a quantified picture of an individual's activity, habits, vital signs, and body metrics. These discrete and massive data sets have never before been possible in medicine, and they disrupt the very foundations on which diagnosis, treatment, and interventions are founded. They also bring incredible capabilities out of critical care units and into the home. Steinhubl, Muse, and Topol (2015) described some wearables that can optically assess cell microvasculature to continually and accurately measure blood pressure. It is now possible to see every step, every heartbeat, and every brain wave a patient may have in the course of a day and link that data, through complex algorithms, to measures of stress, anxiety, cardiac health, and more. Even large technology companies like Apple are partnering with academic institutions to use wearables as a research data-gathering tool. Apple and Stanford University enlisted millions of iWatch users to take part in a longitudinal study evaluating users' electrocardiograms. These types of massive data sets will provide insights into the normal and abnormal variation of vital signs over time. The longitudinal data may disrupt our current understanding of patient conditions because our current understanding is largely based on episodic encounters. Wearables will help usher us into an age where care can be evaluated and delivered anywhere.

Banaee, Ahmed, and Loutffi (2013) suggested that wearable data will provide the fuel to support big data analytics to mine physiological data and determine new patterns, relationships, and anomalies. Uncovering these new anomalies provides new insights to care, frees evidence from RCT studies, and opens data up to real-time assessment by frontline caregivers. From this freedom of data, practitioners can potentially change care interventions instantly while simultaneously viewing instant impacts to the patient's physiology. Wearable data may provide a new modality for real-time EBP implementation.

Another way wearables are changing how evidence is consumed in care is by freeing once-siloed data from the hands of clinicians and into the view of patients. No longer is vital sign data held in a paper folder in the file room—now, real-time trending of activity, diet, and physiology are available at any time to the patient. This freedom of data is affecting how patients self-manage chronic conditions. Fox and Duggan (2013) found that 62% of patients with two or more chronic conditions track their health either by paper or in their heads. Aitken and Gauntlett (2013) suggested that patients who track their health metrics via a mobile app would have an increased compliance percentage. Chiauzzi, Rodarte, and DasMahapatra (2015) suggested that using monitoring devices can make a direct and real-time impact on self-management of patients with chronic conditions. Patients who received data from their monitoring efforts were more likely to change behaviors related to lifestyle. Wearable data is providing a real-time feedback loop to practitioners and patients to support change and adaptation. Now patients, along with the care team, can monitor for abnormalities and patterns in the data and work together to alert one another to issues or successes with treatments.

With the expansion of wearable and mobile technologies, healthcare organizations and third-party vendors are exploring ways to filter and leverage the data from these devices to integrate them into their preventive health plans and provide caregivers with insights about their patients' adherence to care plans and prescriptions. Examples include applying wearable devices in the surgical environment to improve efficiencies and safety (Shantz & Veillette, 2014) to utilizing wearable technologies for assessing daily activity, and fall risk for older adults (Najafi, Armstrong, & Mohler, 2013). As wearable technologies continue to develop in the clinical arena, healthcare providers and organizations will need to form strategies to embrace the new data from these sources so it can be meaningfully used in their patients' care.

Challenges of Wearables

Along with the potential of wearable technologies to have an impact on clinical outcomes and patient engagement, challenges are emerging. The struggles of extracting and utilizing meaningful insights from information systems today is compounded by the introduction of new sources of data. This makes the caregiver's role even more stressful and hard to carry out as more and more data is sent to already overloaded practitioners.

Another area of concern includes increasing regulatory oversight and compliance (Chan et al., 2012). Many devices on the market today are focused on consumers, not specifically on health care. Consumer-grade devices may not be as accurate in data collection, and they cannot be used for clinical diagnosis unless they are FDA approved. Devices used for general wellness, such as weight tracking, fitness, and relaxation, are not currently regulated by the FDA. On the other hand, devices that make specific claims about treating a recognized disease or medical condition will require FDA approval. This approval process also creates a barrier for many companies that have limited funding. This barrier may be short-lived as large tech giants enter the marketplace and drive more efficient regulation.

There are social factors that can also affect the validity of the data. Patients who obsess over their own body metrics and instant interventions for any abnormal value, regardless of clinical validity, can hamper adoption of the technology by care teams and insurers (Swan, 2013). There are also questions about the validity and motivation to track personal data to meet treatment goals. Some patients may inaccurately report data or place the wearable on a family member or friend to get data that might be acceptable to the clinician and avoid confrontation about the lack of adherence to treatment plans.

These social, regulatory, and logistic issues related to patient-entered data require leaders to continue to innovate and iterate on solutions for the best use of the data. There is no doubt that the wearable revolution is a new source of data for EBP and innovation in health care. Samples of very early but innovative programs have begun to crop up in the industry, and they are supported by large consumer companies that allow the technology and mechanisms for adoption to remain inexpensive and easy to use.

🔍 *CASE EXAMPLE*

One example of a program that is using wearables as a source of data and evidence for treatments centers on diabetes management. Data from wireless glucometers is transmitted directly to the complex care case manager, who can review trends over days and months and intervene faster than with the traditional chart review method or patient-reported levels. Data is making the care more efficient and is streamlining workflows.

(continues)

🔍 **CASE EXAMPLE** *(continued)*

This diabetes program demonstrates the synthesis of traditional EBP interventions enhanced by unproven and innovative sources of data to improve outcomes in patients. It is just a matter of time before data points from activity and other wearable data will be linked to clinical outcomes and decision support tools to rapidly improve the care that teams can deliver.

Summary of Wearable Evidence

Wearable data sources are dynamically shifting the sources of evidence that patients and providers have to intervene in their own health journey. Advantages including longitudinal data, continuous monitoring, and information feedback loops. There are challenges with validity, the quantity of data, and processing large amounts of data. Healthcare leaders must continue to innovate and explore new ways of using this evidence to change practice and treatment, and also be open to gaining insights from the patients themselves as they recognize patterns drawn from monitoring their everyday life.

Big Data Analytics

With new sources of data from EMR and wearable technologies, organizations are driven to invest in analytical tools and infrastructure to process and utilize vast amounts of data to deliver efficient, effective, and affordable care. Big data analytics has become the engine driving organizations toward becoming learning institutions through means such as the following: improving decision support at the bedside that is underpinned by data, developing clinical and operational dashboards, supporting predictive analytics for early warning of preventable conditions, and serving as a foundation for research and new partnerships to perform studies that were never possible before the emergence of big data.

Big data is defined by Mayer-Schonberger and Cukier (2013) as the application of math to data sets so large that they cannot be managed by traditional data management tools. By applying complex mathematics, the big data systems process variables across massive data sets to infer probabilities of linkages to one another. Big data is not the creation of artificial intelligence or machine learning, although big data is part of the process that supports those endeavors. Everyday examples of big data can be seen in how driverless cars avoid collisions by processing millions of data points from sensors and translate them into speed and breaking pressures to adjust the car with respect to its surroundings. Google and Amazon use big data to determine search patterns, infer desires, and present the most relevant search findings to the user. How might we use big data in health care and leadership?

Big data is a "buzzword, or catch-phrase, used to describe a massive volume of both structured and unstructured data that is so large it is difficult to process using traditional database and software techniques" (Beal, 2014, para. 1). Big data generally comes from multiple sources and has value when the data sets are integrated and analyzed.

IBM (2015) informs us that we create 2.5 quintillion bytes of data every day. We have generated so much data that 90% of the data in the world today has been created in the past 2 years. Those data come from everywhere: sensors used to gather climate information, posts to social media sites, digital pictures and videos, purchase transaction records, cell phone GPS signals, and more.

Big data tells us *what* is happening but generally fails to tell us *why* it is happening. However, uncovering "what" can be the first step to uncovering "why." Henly (2014) informs us that the dimensionality of big data is huge, that data types are diverse, and that there are innumerable interconnections among the data. Henly stated that instead of using data for explanation, the three goals of big data use are to describe, integrate, and predict. Healthcare organizations can use data science to analyze these large amounts of data to inform decision making.

The complexities of big data are often characterized as three *V*s: volume, velocity, and variety (Thorpe & Gray, 2015):

- Volume represents enormous repositories of data, for example, millions of data pieces collected from millions of patient electronic health records and other data sources. The low cost of data storage and the increasing use of electronic health records are factors that are encouraging massive data collections.
- Velocity refers to the increasing rate at which data flows into an organization which is often a near real-time stream of data. The data must be analyzed quickly so that appropriate feedback can occur. In some cases, so much data may arrive that useless data must be filtered out and discarded to provide sufficient space for data that are useful.
- Variety refers to the many forms of structured and unstructured data that are collected from numerous sources. Thorpe and Gray (2015) tell us that structured data includes quantitative information that is always entered in the same format across systems, such as a patient's name, address, medical record number, and vital signs. Unstructured data represents qualitative information that is often generated as narrative notations; some identify this as storytelling.

Nursing and other health professions frequently use this type of documentation to describe situations and environmental factors that affect outcomes because flow sheets are generally not designed to accommodate narrative data. Therefore, these types of data are difficult to capture and analyze in a meaningful way. However, artificial intelligence is being used to explore ways to code these textual entries to produce structured data.

Marcus (2014), in a document from the National Institute of Standards and Technology Big Data Working Group, suggests that three other *V*s should be considered in relationship to healthcare data: veracity, variability, and value:

- Veracity refers to the accuracy of the data. Unfortunately, data may be inaccurate when it is generated, or it may lose meaning when it is translated. Therefore, veracity is extremely important when making clinical decisions.
- Variability must be considered when the same information can have different meanings; for example, listing Oxford as a patient's location may refer to Oxford in 23 states or 4 countries. Therefore, it is important to resolve these ambiguities to enhance the accuracy of data analysis.
- Value is enhanced when the aggregation of information into a data set, such as big data, enables analysis to reveal correlations, trends, and patterns across populations that may not be possible when analyzing smaller data sets.

Marcus (2014) informs us that big data analysis is not only useful in answering research questions, but it has been used to develop and test models for predicting outcomes for interventions, costs, and readmissions. The availability of big data and its analysis is an important tool that can be used to identify evidence-based best practices.

The use and analysis of big data in the healthcare industry lags behind industries such as finance, insurance, and pharma. Dan LeSueur from Health Catalyst suggests five reasons that healthcare data are unique and difficult to measure (LeSueur, 2014):

1. Much of the data are in multiple places, and the sources are not interconnected. In healthcare organizations, data may come from electronic medical records; pharmacy, laboratory, and radiology systems; membership databases; and others. It also comes in different formats, such as text, numeric, paper, digital, pictures, and so forth. More sources of data from patient-generated tracking devices, like fitness monitors and blood pressure sensors, will soon be integrated.

2. The data are structured and unstructured. LeSueur (2014) notes that, although electronic medical records provide a platform for consistent data capture, clinicians are used to documenting in ways that are most efficient for them without regard for how the data could eventually be aggregated and analyzed. For example, there are times when documenting in fields of a flow sheet cannot adequately describe a situation. It is easier to write a narrative, even though it is likely that the data will not be captured or useful during data analysis.

3. Definitions are inconsistent and variable. EBP guidelines and new research are coming out every day. The amount of available healthcare data continuously changes, and interpretation is often variable. Reaching consensus on definitions or conditions may be difficult, if not impossible. Therefore, identifying ways to structure the data are challenging.

4. The data are complex and are often derived from multiple sources that are not connected. LeSueur (2014) notes that developing standard processes to improve quality outcomes is one healthcare goal; however, the number of variables makes it challenging. The human body is much more complex, and the variety of data collected from multiple information systems is much more difficult to analyze than in other industries, such as manufacturing.

5. Regulatory requirements are increasing and evolving. LeSueur (2014) posits that traditional approaches to data management do not work in health care because of the complexities previously listed. He writes that health care is unlike industries in which business rules and definitions remain unchanged for long periods of time. LeSueur suggests that "the volatility of healthcare data means a rule set today may not be a best practice tomorrow" (2014, p. 5).

LEARNING ACTIVITY

1. Contact your organization's nurse researcher or the information technology and marketing departments and ask them how big data collection and interpretation have contributed to the organization's plan of action.
2. Knowing that big data tells you the what but not the why (cause), how do you determine cause?

New Data Additions

As caregivers enter more data into EMR systems, electronic histories and preferences are being built for patients as their digital footprints grow in health care. With this wealth of information in electronic systems, clinicians are beginning to leverage the data through real-time decision support systems that pull from variables such as allergies, medication histories, and patient goals and preferences. Through these tools, not only are clinical outcomes improved by giving providers better insights and situational contexts before engaging patients for the first time, but overall service and patient satisfaction are also improved through the personalization of health care (Bates, Saria, Ohno-Machado, Shah, & Escobar, 2014).

The contribution of big data to health care can be seen in several categories. Research is benefiting from big data through the use of predictive modeling to assess clinical trial attrition rates and improve research and development times. Public health is benefiting by analyzing disease patterns and transmissions across large data sets. They are using that data to more accurately target vaccines and provide services during outbreaks. Additionally, big data is supporting EBP by combining and analyzing data from multiple systems, such as EMRs, insurance databases, genomic data, and unstructured narratives, to infer insights into disease risk and care efficiencies (Raghupathi & Raghupathi, 2014).

To better describe how big data is affecting care environments and operations, we will present two case examples. One case study addresses how big data provides decision support and guidance to nurses for nurse-sensitive quality measures. The other case study describes how data and predictive models are helping to support hospital patient throughput operations.

🔍 CASE EXAMPLE: NURSE-SENSITIVE QUALITY MEASURES AND BIG DATA

Nurse-sensitive quality measures are well established through the National Database of Nursing Quality Indicators (NDNQI), a proprietary database of the American Nurses Association (2014), which collects and evaluates unit-specific nurse-sensitive data from acute care hospitals; the National Quality Forum (2004), a not-for-profit, nonpartisan, membership-based organization that works to catalyze improvements in health care; and the Collaborative Alliance for Nursing Outcomes (CALNOC; 2014), which was a state pilot site that ultimately contributed to the development of the American Nurses Association NDNQI.

Hospital falls are a prime example of the importance of nurse-sensitive quality measures. Each fall costs an average of $13,316 per incident (Wong et al., 2011), and between 700,000 and 1 million people in the United States fall in the hospital each year (Ganz et al., 2013). As of 2008, the Centers for Medicaid and Medicare Services no longer reimburses hospitals when certain types of injuries occur while the patient is hospitalized, and many of these injuries occur after a fall. Nurses are primarily responsible for the assessment, intervention, and documentation for fall prevention as part of their care planning process, and organizations are responsible for implementing

(continues)

🔍 *CASE EXAMPLE: NURSE-SENSITIVE QUALITY MEASURES AND BIG DATA*　　*(continued)*

a fall prevention program that includes monitoring, communication, and collaboration (Ganz et al., 2013).

From the data entered into EMRs based on risk assessments and medication administration, alerts and banners warn clinicians of patients who are at high risk for falls, delirium, and other conditions that may lead to their deterioration. Big data technology is able to scan massive amounts of records, run them through complex statistical algorithms, and produce suggested relationships among seemingly disparate data points.

Electronic data care plans and interventions are more collaborative among care team members beyond physicians and nurses because the transparency of information and system alerts and referrals are built to include team members from pharmacy, laboratory, radiology, and behavioral health services to ensure that everyone is at the table to support patients.

🔍 *CASE EXAMPLE: BIG DATA TO OVERSEE CARE AND OPERATIONS*

Above and beyond the use of data at the point of care, organizations are starting to build dashboards and electronic reports to help provide insights into population trends and allow organizations to use information to prioritize care and shift resources in areas with the most need. Within the infrastructure consisting of manual processes and multiple applications that sometimes produce redundant information, it is vital that organizations provide resources and support to operational leaders for them to integrate competencies in information knowledge and skills to oversee the quality of care.

One example of how big data is supporting operations is in the use of command centers and predictive census solutions. Historically, hospital census has been estimated by looking at several past years' numbers and averaging the model to estimate the daily average census on any given day. Very few other data points, aside from historical data, are usually taken into account. With the creation of powerful data analysis tools, such as Tableau and others, data analysts are able to take significantly more data points, such as weather, sporting event schedules, regional data points, and other indicators, to create accurate predictions of emergency department visits, surgery cancellations, and admissions that contribute to a real census. From this data, leaders can more efficiently engage staff departments, allocate resources, and plan for overflow events. This is a significant step up from staffing to a "midnight census."

Challenges of Big Data

Much of the discussion of big data is centered on the possibilities and potential rather than specific measured results. Raghupathi and Raghupathi (2014) stated that big data is an evolving science with great potential, yet there are many challenges to overcome.

Among those challenges they listed are data management practices, ease of use, scalability of platforms, and privacy and security concerns. Recently, several large healthcare organizations have been hacked, resulting in massive data breaches. As big data continues to grow in capability and adoption, security must be of upmost priority.

Summary of Big Data

There are many insights and capabilities that big data and analytics can provide healthcare leaders and care team members. Predictive modeling can help with hospital operations and public health problems. Compiling data from multiple fragmented systems also provides promise of new patterns and connections that can be made. Although there is significant promise in big data capabilities, leaders should be aware of data management and security risks as they deploy these systems. Additionally, leaders should seek to augment decision making with big data technology and not try to replace clinical judgment or critical thinking.

Summary of New Sources of Data in Health Care

As new evidence sources emerge and are continually refined to become more accurate, leaders must be open to unlearning past practices, like staffing from historical data, and develop innovative plans to better use resources that may contrast with past practices. EMRs are providing digitized records that lay the foundation of data for multiple systems to pull from. Wearable technology is providing new sources of patient information that, through big data analytics, will provide care teams with linkages and treatment recommendations never seen before. Big data is an emerging science that shows promise to help leaders, patients, and practitioners connect disparate dots and uncover new meanings among mountains of variables. The new insights generated by new sources of evidence will require a reconfiguration of traditional care and organizational management techniques. Data-driven decision making will become easier to access and implement. Leaders will need new competencies to work in the age of super information. In part, the healthcare leader must exhibit new competencies in informatics and innovation to be successful at optimizing care and leading in highly complex organizations.

▶ Emerging Technology and Other Sources of New Evidence

In addition to EMRs, wearable data sources, and big data analytic capabilities, several emerging technologies are disrupting how data and evidence are collected by patients and providers. According to Wang (2015), investments in health technology–related start-up companies topped $4.1 billion in 2014. Wang observed that

> the top six categories that accounted for 44% of all digital health funding in 2014 were analytics and big data, healthcare consumer engagement, digital medical devices, telemedicine, personalized medicine, and population health management. Personalized medicine, defined as software used to support the practice of medicine customized to an individual's genetics, slid into the top six for the very first time this year. (Wang, 2015)

Among these start-ups are innovative solutions that are changing the landscape of health care and health data. Two case examples provide evidence of disruptive technology that is changing how data and evidence are collected and consumed.

Hype versus Value

With any emerging, unproven technology, one must determine if the risk of piloting a new innovation will add value to the system. Many times this determination is impossible to predict without some level of testing, pilot program, proof-of-concept work, or evidence from other organizations' efforts. However, leaders can use a few tools to assess technologies and determine if they are worth placing bets on.

The first tool is the Gartner Hype Cycle. Gartner is a technology research and consulting firm that has developed a report to assess the usefulness and hype factor of emerging technologies in several industries, including health care (Gartner Hype Cycle, 2015). Technologies are assessed and placed along a hype continuum that can provide a starting point for assessing value. Emerging technologies that are just entering the market are said to be at the Innovation Trigger point. Technologies in that area are virtually untested but show theoretical or early stage success in disrupting the market.

As Innovation Trigger technologies move along the continuum over time, they reach the Peak of Inflated Expectations. At the peak, technologies have accumulated significant discussion about the possibilities and disruptive potential they might offer. For example, when Google Glass, a computer that projects data onto a lens that you wear like glasses, was introduced, early adopters were clamoring to get their hands on one. Healthcare thought leaders hypothesized that Google Glass would be a solution for hands-free documentation, operating room emergency checklists, and even real-time telemedicine consults. After several tests, start-up company solutions, and pilots, Google Glass has only started to catch on. Issues with ergonomics, data reliability, and privacy have slowed its adoption. Technologies at the peak should be considered very carefully with significant due diligence in how they might actually deliver value. Small tests of change are recommended to help with assessments at this stage.

After technologies move through the peak of hype, they slide into the Trough of Disillusionment. This happens as adopters use hyped technology and discover that it may not deliver on all the capabilities that were promised. At this stage, adopters are quickly brought back to reality and must further analyze the value to determine if the technology will deliver on expected outcomes. The trough is a good point to assess if pilots should continue or stop for reassessment. An example of a technology that slid into the trough is EMRs. After the hype and promises that EMRs would streamline workflows, liberate data, and make health care easier and more affordable, the technology slowly declined into the trough as end users realized that workflow, documentation, and data were significantly disrupted and made more complex in the early years after adoption. As realization dawned that they are well worth the investment of dollars, optimization, and time, EMRs have moved to the next stage on the hype curve, the Slope of Enlightenment.

Technologies that have begun to climb the Slope of Enlightenment are moving out of the trough and are showing value to the adopters. Although the value is in the early stage, these technologies might have clinical data or other research to support their value claims. More risk-averse organizations should look to technologies in

TABLE 11-3 Hype Cycle and Innovation Leadership Linkages

Hype Cycle Phase	Description	Innovation Leadership Actions
Technology Trigger	First introduction to the market	Assess technology for potential value; high risk for failure; extra due diligence required
Peak of Inflated Expectations	Media hype begins, activity beyond early adopters starts	Be aware of overhyped technology; relate tech solution to problem you are trying to solve; try small pilots to assess value or wait for others to publish results
Trough of Disillusionment	Negative press begins; capabilities do not match hype; adoption slows	Assess technology's unhyped capabilities and future road map; determine value and ability to meet needs; good time to assess and pilot technologies
Slope of Enlightenment	Value and hype are more aligned; adoption increases and realistic expectations are set	Good time for more risk-averse organizations to assess technology; look for expanding capabilities in technology
Plateau of Productivity	High adoption rate; hype and expectations are close	Look for rapid adoption and fast-track pilots; evidence and value should support technology near this phase; do not spend significant time proving technology, instead focus on workflow integration and value to specific problem

this phase to begin value assessments and pilots. Wearable technology for use in health care is a good example of this phase. Although it has not been fully validated, wearable technology is showing early promise in its impact on health outcomes in research studies.

Finally, technologies will reach the Plateau of Productivity. Here, technologies have user and research validation, and have proven and demonstrated value to the industry. Expectations and values are closely aligned, and adoption has spread significantly. Innovation leaders should look to this phase of technology as a valid solution for implementation. Technologies that have reached the plateau are telemedicine and speech recognition.

Using the Gartner Hype Cycle as a framework for innovation assessment will allow the innovation leader to determine a baseline for adoption (**TABLE 11-3**). It helps the user determine how much time and investment might be needed to prove the value of a technology or determine if the technology is worth pursuing at all. It is important to reflect on what problem you are trying to solve and if technology will enable the solution.

BOX 11-1 Track Emerging Technology

Assessing technology is everyone's responsibility. One way to continually stay on top of emerging technology is to set up informal meetings to discuss the latest trends and determine their hype. Engage staff members, early adopters, and others in the discussion to get a well-rounded view of technology and its potential.

Evidence-Based Assessment of New Data Sources

Assessing technology and new sources of evidence on the Gartner Hype Cycle is only one way to determine innovation value. Leaders who are looking to try new innovations to improve evidence-based care should also critically examine the proposed technology against an EBP framework as well. The Institute for Healthcare Improvement (IHI) has developed a framework for assessing technology and the resulting evidence it produces (Ostrovsky, Deen, Simon, & Mate, 2013).

The authors provide a framework that combines Triple Aim focus areas, level of supporting evidence, investment level, technology type, and end-user criteria. The Triple Aim focus allows leaders to categorize technologies related to what system-level problem they are trying to solve (i.e., patient experience, population health, per capita cost of care). The level-of-evidence criterion allows the team to compare the support for new technologies in the literature. Technologies can be evidence based, evidence informed, or emerging. Technology type and investment level help the team further determine the cost to implement the technology and further define the technology solution. Finally, the end-user criterion helps the team identify who should be included in assessments and pilots of the technology.

By combining the IHI and Gartner tools, organizations will have a consumer- and evidence-based framework to assess technologies and the evidence supporting those technologies. Emerging technology requires leaders to combine tools and frameworks to create assessments because many emerging technologies have little to no formal research supporting them (**BOX 11-1**). Leaders must adapt new ways of assessment and interpretation to foster evidence-based innovation. After technologies are selected and implemented, leaders will need to interpret, manage, and communicate information flowing from the devices and systems. Leaders will need specific informatics competencies, which are described in the next section.

▶ Informatics Competencies for Leaders

To address the emerging advances in health care through HIT, it is important to identify competencies of clinicians in utilizing HIT. The American Nurses Association (2009) published informatics competencies for various levels of nursing leaders, including chief nurses and administrators, as well as operational leaders, to provide guidance to organizations so they can prepare key leaders for the growing use of information and analytics in operations, administration, and financial aspects of their roles. Similarly, the Quality and Safety Education for Nurses (QSEN) organization has developed informatics curricula to bring these competencies to life.

Although many experts in informatics and nursing leadership have contributed their opinions to identify the informatics knowledge, skills, and abilities needed for nurses and nurse or clinical leaders, further studies are needed to tailor the competencies to the actual practices of caregivers. The nurse or clinical leader role spans a wide array of clinical and administrative responsibilities, and leaders need to attain the needed competencies to successfully fulfill their duties, including those that address the use of electronic systems for accessing information. There is a paucity of empirical knowledge about the approaches and strategies that clinical leaders employ, within their already complex and stressful roles, to integrate these competencies to work in today's growing digital healthcare environment. Collins et al. (2017) have continued the initial work to validate informatics competencies that are meaningful to nurse leaders for integrating these areas into their training and onboarding.

This section will describe informatics competencies needed by leaders at the frontline and at the system level. Without skills in interpreting, communicating, and accessing information from multiple systems, leaders will not be prepared for innovative adaptations or EBP.

Frontline Manager Informatics Competencies

The nurse manager role is multifaceted, and the duties and information needs span a range of operational areas that include financial, staffing, human resources, and staff and patient safety. The American Nurses Association provides a comprehensive, but not exhaustive, list of role characteristics that shows their complex nature. Nurse manager priorities are greatly sensitive to external regulatory bodies and benchmarks, which include state and federal nurse-sensitive quality drivers (American Nurses Association, 2014; CALNOC, 2014; National Quality Forum, 2014). Given the impact of the nurse manager on retention, satisfaction, productivity, and outcomes, studies are needed to explore how they access information to support staff retention and satisfaction, productivity measures, and quality outcomes. Yang et al. (2014) focused on the nurse manager role in validating informatics competencies and found factors in developing these knowledge areas for their critical operational role.

Data from electronic sources allows managers to facilitate and grow an evidence-based care environment by enabling three core functions: monitor documentation, monitor practice, and investigate errors through root cause analysis. Competency in these functions allows the manager to enable care teams to gather information in useful ways, translate evidence into practice, determine where errors in the system might be, and facilitate resolution. Managers must rely on several sources to gather information and context for decision making. Electronic methods such as EMRs and other electronic systems can help. Additionally, leaders must rely on their ability to develop relationships with team members to gather information verbally and through observation. Combining these information sources allows managers to understand the context of care, the content of care, and the culture of the team environment (**TABLE 11-4**).

TABLE 11-4 Quality Monitoring Information Sources and Actions					
Sources of Information	Electronic (EMR)	Electronic (Non-EMR)	Verbal	Observation	Paper
Monitoring documentation	Procedures Assessments Tasks Regulatory	Electronic reports	Discussion with staff	Documentation rounds	Paper notes
Monitoring practice	Dashboard Chart auditing tools	Electronic reports	Verbal feedback	Evidence-based bundle interventions Infection prevention Procedures Rounds	Paper audit checklists
Investigating or performing a root cause analysis	Assessments Labs Medications Radiology Notes	Electronic reports	Discussion with staff	Practice variations	Patient complaints

Monitoring Documentation

Monitoring documentation reflects the nurse manager's role in validating that documentation, and also reflects care that is actually provided and that is timely, accurate, and in compliance with regulatory requirements.

Types and Sources of Information Needed to Monitor Documentation

The EMR is the primary source of information used to monitor documentation. The types of EMR documentation monitored include nursing procedures (e.g., restraints, blood administration), assessments (e.g., vital signs, fall risk), nursing tasks (e.g., ambulation), and regulatory mandates (e.g., advance directives). In one study, participants described accessing EMR information from reports they generate and then going into the EMR to monitor documentation by clicking into the various areas of EMR information (Soriano, 2015). Some managers performed these activities, and others delegated some or all of these activities to assistant managers or charge nurses who would report the results back to the manager via e-mail or a paper audit checklist. Participants also reported performing documentation rounds by walking around their units and engaging nurses to review their documentation in the EMR.

It is important to note that the intent, for innovative leaders, is not to demand compliance by monitoring documentation but to facilitate accurate information flow into the system. The difference lies in how managers act on the information they receive from audits, observations, and electronic reports. Leaders with a competency to understand electronic data and personal cues from the team will be able to facilitate learning, feedback loops, and sustained practice changes by building relationships with staff and supporting change with data from electronic means. Using the information from monitoring documentation in more transactional ways (i.e., punishing only noncompliance) will result in staff burnout and turnover (Weberg, 2013).

Monitoring Practice

Monitoring practice reflects the nurse manager's role in validating that care actually happened, in general, beyond the information documented by nurses.

Types and Sources of Information Needed to Monitor Practice

Managers can gather information about the care practices of the team through several sources, including e-mails, electronic reports, direct observation and rounding, and communication with staff and patients. E-mails and electronic reports can be received both automatically and in response to the managers' requests for information from various departments in the hospital, including the quality department, risk management, infection control, pharmacy, and lab. E-mails and electronic reports include information about care practice trends and areas needing improvement, such as (1) scan reports from the pharmacy indicating the use of bar codes to avoid medication identification errors and (2) catheter-associated infection reports from infection control departments indicating when catheters have been in place longer than recommended. Additionally, leaders can gather information by performing rounds to monitor these areas, including observation of evidence-based interventions for quality bundles that include groups of evidence-based interventions for quality measures, such as fall prevention, hospital-acquired pressure ulcer (HAPU) prevention, ventilator-associated pneumonia, catheter-associated urinary tract infections (CAUITs), and central-line-associated blood stream infections (CLABSIs). Leaders can build team relationships by rounding or walking through their units to access information directly by communicating with staff and patients. For example, nurse managers can talk with staff directly about turning patients at risk for pressure ulcers or making sure that medications were scanned prior to administration.

Monitoring practice is an important role for leaders. Data from electronic sources provide the context for intervention by the leader. For example, if reports show increases in falls, pressure ulcers, or other quality issues, leaders can use that information to interact with staff to improve care. Monitoring practice should not be a parental endeavor; instead, the leader should use it to gather information to identify areas where EBP might improve care or in situations and problems that might require innovative solutions. From this information the leader can facilitate change with the team.

Investigating Incidents

Performing investigations reflects the nurse manager's role in investigating incidents, such as patient falls, HAPUs, CAUTIs, and medication errors or discrepancies.

Types and Sources of Information Needed to Investigate Incidents

The information needed to perform investigations was accessed from the EMR, electronic reports of fallouts (areas that need improvement) produced by various departments, reports from incident reporting systems, verbal reports from nursing staff or assistant managers regarding incidents that occurred during the shift, and verbal or written patient complaints. Using the EMR to perform these investigations in combination with getting verbal or written input from staff is essential to understand the context and system inputs. Information accessed in the EMR includes nursing documentation, physician notes, lab results, radiologic results, and medications. This information accessed from the EMR can be used to connect the dots regarding the incident and facilitate a systems view rather than looking for a singular cause.

Incidents involving patient care can be complex and stressful. Leaders and team members should partner to create a culture of growth and learning when errors occur. Leaders can use electronic data to look for patterns in the interactions and systems of care to help find breakdowns that influence error occurrence. Additionally, gathering informal data from team members can also lend insight. Leaders must be competent in both electronic data interpretation and staff relationships to facilitate solutions and more robust, error-free environments of care.

Summary of Frontline Manager Informatics Competencies

As part of their roles in quality monitoring and improvement, nurse managers are required to access comprehensive information from various sources as a basis for assessment, planning, and interventions in their various areas of responsibility (American Nurses Association, 2009). Studies in hospital and individual unit settings have emerged highlighting that the nurse managers' information needs include financial data, supply management data, regulatory standards for quality and safety, patient information for rounds, satisfaction scores, scheduling and staffing data, human resources information, and information about the healthcare climate and population needs for developing and managing projects. The sources of information can be overwhelming for leaders in health care, but becoming competent in researching, validating, and interpreting this information is a core competency of future leaders. There is ongoing work to consolidate informatics competencies for nurse leaders to streamline the adoption into practice (Kassam, Nagle, & Strudwick, 2017). Frontline managers can use data to interpret the context of care and to facilitate innovation and EBP activities to improve quality (**TABLE 11-5**).

TABLE 11-5 Examples of EMR Data to Monitor Practice

Role Component	Monitoring Documentation (EMR)	Monitoring Practice	Investigating or Performing a Root Cause Analysis
■ Examples of information types needed	Procedures: ■ Lines, drains, airways ■ Blood administration ■ Restraints Assessments: ■ Delirium assessments ■ Fall risk ■ Vital signs ■ Weight ■ Nursing assessments ■ Central line assessments Tasks: ■ Ambulation ■ Bundle compliance for infection interventions ■ CAUTI interventions ■ Medication administration Regulatory: ■ Tobacco use ■ Critical lab values ■ Advance directives Observation: ■ Documentation rounds	Electronic reports for quality bundles: ■ CLABSI interventions ■ CAUTI rounds ■ Ambulation rounds ■ Venous thromboembolism rounds Verbal feedback: ■ Staff ■ Debriefings ■ Staff feedback ■ Unit rounds ■ Patient rounds Infection prevention: ■ Hand-washing rounds Procedures: ■ Sedation rounds ■ Bar code scanning reports EMR: ■ Quality dashboard	Electronic reports: ■ Infection report ■ Incident reports ■ Fall report ■ Pneumonia report ■ Urinary tract infection report ■ Pressure ulcer report ■ Pharmacy report EMR: ■ Nursing assessments ■ Vital signs ■ Physician notes ■ Medication information ■ Radiologic information ■ Lab information Verbal information: ■ Talking to staff Paper forms: ■ Patient complaints

▶ Summary and Issues

To move the focus of competencies a layer beyond the frontline healthcare leader, healthcare systems must evolve to be learning organizations, develop robust and consistent information seeking and processing behaviors to leverage growing sources of electronic data and information, and operationalize national quality initiatives such as the Triple Aim.

The Triple Aim is focused on the following dimensions:

- Improving the patient experience of care (including quality and satisfaction)
- Improving the health of populations
- Reducing the per capita cost of health care (Berwick, Nolan, & Whittington, 2008)

As a foundation for improving and sustaining high-quality care, there is an increasing movement by hospitals toward becoming high-reliability organizations through investments in leadership, development of a safety culture, and utilization of robust process improvement tools. As an essential factor for achieving high reliability, organizations must invest in information technology to monitor and sustain quality improvement, consistently measure the safety culture, and utilize improvement tools throughout the organization to synthesize and act on information for quality improvement (Chassin & Loeb, 2011).

Leaders must invest time and effort into understanding data and the sources of data to innovate quality care. Frontline care providers can gather evidence from new technologies, such as wearables, devices, and EMRs, to improve care. Frontline managers and leaders can gather data from reports, systems, and people to facilitate and monitor improvement and quality efforts. Finally, system-level leaders can look for patterns in the data to identify areas, to focus resources for innovation and EBP implementation. To properly train future nurse leaders on these concepts and emerging technologies in the backdrop of their busy schedules, Strudwick, Hubert, and Gehrs (2018) developed an internship and learning plan as a model for organizations to implement informatics competencies into practice.

Finally, new technologies are providing data at a rapid rate. The work to integrate big data into quality improvement by nurse leaders focuses on developing an infrastructure for creating predictive models through the collection of vital signs, continuous alerts, and massive data sets and is changing the way healthcare workers manage patient health and care (Westra et al., 2015). It is imperative that healthcare leaders of the future continue to assess the relevancy of data using the foundations of EBP. This means that leaders should be open to new sources of data that can inform evidence and also keep a critical eye toward validity, reliability, and application of these new data sources. It will require an innovation mind-set to sift through the plethora of technology and data to create new ways of caring for patients, changing the healthcare system, and building EBP.

References

Aitken, M., & Gauntlett, C. (2013). *Patient apps for improved healthcare: From novelty to mainstream.* Parsippany, NJ: IMS Institute for Healthcare Informatics.

Alexander, J. W., & Kroposki, M. (2001). Using a management perspective to define and measure changes in nursing technology. *Journal of Advanced Nursing, 35*(5), 776–783.

American Nurses Association. (2009). *Nursing administration: Scope and standards of practice.* Silver Spring, MD: Nursesbooks.

American Nurses Association. (2014). NDNQI. Retrieved from http://www.nursingquality.org/

Armstrong, K. J., & Laschinger, H. (2006). Structural empowerment, Magnet hospital characteristics, and patient safety culture: Making the link. *Journal of Nursing Care Quality, 21*(2), 124–132.

Ash, J. S., & Bates, D. W. (2005). Factors and forces affecting EHR system adoption: Report of a 2004 ACMI discussion. *Journal of the American Medical Informatics Association, 12*(1), 8–12. https://doi.org/10.1197/jamia.M1684

Banaee, H., Ahmed, M. U., & Loutfi, A. (2013). Data mining for wearable sensors in health monitoring systems: A review of recent trends and challenges. *Sensors, 13*(12), 17472–17500.

Bates, D. W., Saria, S., Ohno-Machado, L., Shah, A., & Escobar, G. (2014). Big data in health care: Using analytics to identify and manage high-risk and high-cost patients. *Health Affairs, 33*(7), 1123–1131.

Beal, V. (2014). Big data. Retrieved from: http://www.webopedia.com/TERM/B/big_data.html

Berwick, D. M., & Hackbarth, A. D. (2012). Eliminating waste in U.S. health care. *JAMA, 307*(14), 1513–1516. https://doi.org/10.1001/jama.2012.362

Berwick, D. M., Nolan, T. W., & Whittington, J. (2008). The Triple Aim: Care, health, and cost. *Health Affairs, 27*(3), 759–769.

Bradley, E. H., Holmboe, E. S., Mattera, J. A., Roumanis, S. A., Radford, M. J., & Krumholz, H. M. (2003). The roles of senior management in quality improvement efforts: What are the key components? *Journal of Healthcare Management, 48*(1), 15–28.

Centers for Medicare and Medicaid Services. (2013). Meaningful use. Retrieved from http://www.cms.gov/Regulations-and-Guidance/Legislation/EHRIncentivePrograms.html

Centers for Medicare and Medicaid Services. (2014). CMS.gov. Retrieved from http://www.cms.gov/

Chan, M., Estève, D., Fourniols, J. Y., Escriba, C., & Campo, E. (2012). Smart wearable systems: Current status and future challenges. *Artificial intelligence in medicine, 56*(3), 137–156.

Chassin, M. R., & Loeb, J. M. (2011). The ongoing quality improvement journey: Next stop, high reliability. *Health Affairs (Millwood), 30*(4), 559–568. https://doi.org/10.1377/hlthaff.2011.0076

Chassin, M. R., Loeb, J. M., Schmaltz, S. P., & Wachter, R. M. (2010). Accountability measures—using measurement to promote quality improvement. *New England Journal of Medicine, 363*(7), 683–688. https://doi.org/10.1056/NEJMsb1002320

Chiauzzi, E., Rodarte, C., & DasMahapatra, P. (2015). Patient-centered activity monitoring in the self-management of chronic health conditions. *BMC Medicine, 13*(1), 77.

Collaborative Alliance for Nursing Outcomes. (2014). CALNOC. Retrieved from http://www.calnoc.org/

Collins, S., Yen, P. Y., Phillips, A., & Kennedy, M. K. (2017). Nursing Informatics Competency Assessment for the Nurse Leader: The Delphi study. *Journal of Nursing Administration, 47*(4), 212–218.

DesRoches, C., Donelan, K., Buerhaus, P., & Zhonghe, L. (2008). Registered nurses' use of electronic health records: Findings from a national survey. *Medscape Journal of Medicine, 10*(7), 164.

Dobkin, B. H., & Carmichael, S. T. (2015). The specific requirements of neural repair trials for stroke. *Neurorehabilitation and Neural Repair, 30*(5), 470–478. https://doi.org/10.1177/1545968315604400

Fox, S., & Duggan, M. (2013). Tracking for health. Washington, DC: Pew Research Center's Internet & American Life Project. Retrieved from http://www.pewinternet.org/2013/01/15/health-online-2013/

Ganz, D. A., Huang, C., Saliba, D., Miake-Lye, I. M., Hempel, S., Ganz, D. A . . . & Detsky, A. S. (2013). Preventing falls in hospitals: A toolkit for improving quality of care. *Annals of Internal Medicine, 158*(5 Pt 2), 390–396.

Gartner Hype Cycle. (2015). Hype Cycle research methodology. Retrieved from http://www.gartner.com/technology/research/methodologies/hype-cycle.jsp

Henly, S. J. (2014). Mother lode and mining tools: Big data for nursing science. *Nursing Research, 63*(3), 155.

IBM. (2015). What is big data? Retrieved from http://www-01.ibm.com/software/data/bigdata/what-is-big-data.html

Institute of Medicine. (2000). *To err is human: Building a safer health system.* Washington, DC: The National Academies Press.

Institute of Medicine. (2010). *Clinical data as the basic staple of health learning: Creating and protecting a public good: Workshop summary.* Washington, DC: The National Academies Press.

Institute of Medicine. (2012). *Health IT and patient safety: Building safer systems for better care.* Washington, DC: The National Academies Press.

Jeskey, M., Card, E., Nelson, D., Mercaldo, N. D., Sanders, N., Higgins, M. S. . . . Miller, A. (2011). Nurse adoption of continuous patient monitoring on acute post-surgical units: Managing technology implementation. *Journal of Nursing Management, 19*(7), 863–875. https://doi .org/10.1111/j.1365-2834.2011.01295.x

Kassam, I., Nagle, L., & Strudwick, G. (2017). Informatics competencies for nurse leaders: Protocol for a scoping review. *BMJ Open, 7*(12).

Keenan, G., Yakel, E., Dunn Lopez, K., Tschannen, D., & Ford, Y. B. (2013). Challenges to nurses' efforts of retrieving, documenting, and communicating patient care information. *Journal of the American Medical Informatics Association, 20*(2), 245–251. https://doi.org/10.1136 /amiajnl-2012-000894

Kossman, S. P., & Scheidenhelm, S. L. (2008). Nurses' perceptions of the impact of electronic health records on work and patient outcomes. *Computers, Informatics, Nursing, 26*(2), 69–77. https://doi .org/10.1097/01.NCN.0000304775.40531.67

Lammintakanen, J., Kivinen, T., Saranto, K., & Kinnunen, J. (2009). Strategic management of health care information systems: Nurse managers' perceptions. *Studies in Health Technology and Informatics, 146*, 86–90.

Lammintakanen, J., Saranto, K., & Kivinen, T. (2010). Use of electronic information systems in nursing management. *International Journal of Medical Informatics, 79*(5), 324–331. https://doi .org/10.1016/j.ijmedinf.2010.01.015

LeSueur, D. (2014). 5 reasons healthcare data is unique and difficult to measure. Retrieved from https://www.healthcatalyst.com/5-reasons-healthcare-data-is-difficult-to-measure

Lin, L. M., Wu, J. H., Huang, I. C., Tseng, K. H., & Lawler, J. J. (2007). Management development: A study of nurse managerial activities and skills. *Journal of Healthcare Management, 52*(3), 156–168.

Marcus, B. (2014). Brainstorming outline: Combining subgroup deliverables. (M0092). Retrieved from http://bigdatawg.nist.gov/show_InputDoc.php

Mayer-Schonberger, V., & Cukier, K. (2013). *Big data.* New York, NY: Houghton-Mifflin Harcourt.

Moody, L. E., Slocumb, E., Berg, B., & Jackson, D. (2004). Electronic health records documentation in nursing: Nurses' perceptions, attitudes, and preferences. *Computers, Informatics, Nursing, 22*(6), 337–344.

Najafi, B., Armstrong, D. G., & Mohler, J. (2013). Novel wearable technology for assessing spontaneous daily physical activity and risk of falling in older adults with diabetes. *Journal of Diabetes Science and Technology, 7*(5), 1147–1160.

National Quality Forum. (2004). National voluntary consensus standards for nursing-sensitive care: An initial performance measure set. Washington, DC: Author.

National Quality Forum. (2014). National Quality Forum. Retrieved from http://www.qualityforum .org/Home.aspx

Ostrovsky, A., Deen, N., Simon, A., & Mate, K. (2014). A framework for selecting digital health technology. *IHI Innovation Report.* Cambridge, MA: Institute for Healthcare Improvement.

Raghupathi, W., & Raghupathi, V. (2014). Big data analytics in healthcare: Promise and potential. *Health Information Science and Systems, 2*, 3. https://doi.org/10.1186/2047-2501-2-3

Shantz, J. A. S., & Veillette, C. J. (2014). The application of wearable technology in surgery: Ensuring the positive impact of the wearable revolution on surgical patients. *Frontiers in surgery, 1.*

Soriano, R. M. (2015). *An examination of how nurse managers access information for nurse-sensitive quality measures* (Unpublished doctoral dissertation). University of California, Davis.

Squires, D. A. (2012). Explaining high health care spending in the United States: An international comparison of supply, utilization, prices, and quality. *Issues in International Health Policy* (Vol. 10). New York, NY: Commonwealth Fund.

Steinhubl, S. R., Muse, E. D., & Topol, E. J. (2015). The emerging field of mobile health. *Science Translational Medicine, 7*(283), 1–6.

Strudwick, G., Hubert, S., & Gehrs, M. (2018). Developing nursing informatics competencies for future nursing leaders: An overview of an internship and learning plan. *Studies in Health Technology and Informatics, 250*, 67.

Swan, M. (2013). The quantified self: Fundamental disruption in big data science and biological discovery. *Big Data, 1*(2), 85–99.

The Joint Commission. (2014). The Joint Commission. Retrieved from http://www.jointcommission.org/

Thorpe, J. H., & Gray, E. A. (2015). Big data and ambulatory care: Breaking down legal barriers to support effective use. *The Journal of Ambulatory Care Management, 38*(1), 29–38.

U.S. Department of Health and Human Services. (2013). Benefits of EHRs. Retrieved from http://www.healthit.gov/providers-professionals/electronic-medical-records-emr

Van Den Bos, J., Rustagi, K., Gray, T., Halford, M., Ziemkiewicz, E., & Shreve, J. (2011). The $17.1 billion problem: The annual cost of measurable medical errors. *Health Affairs (Millwood), 30*(4), 596–603. https://doi.org/10.1377/hlthaff.2011.0084

Wang, T. (2015, January 15). Digital health funding: 2014 year in review [Blog post]. Retrieved from http://rockhealth.com/2015/01/digital-health-funding-tops-4-1b-2014-year-review/

Weberg, D. R. (2013). *Complexity leadership theory and innovation: A new framework for innovation leadership* (Doctoral dissertation). Arizona State University, Tempe, AZ.

Westra, B. L., Clancy, T. R., Sensmeier, J., Warren, J. J., Weaver, C., & Delaney, C. W. (2015). Nursing knowledge: Big data science—implications for nurse leaders. *Nursing Administration Quarterly, 39*(4), 304–310.

Wong, C. A., Recktenwald, A. J., Jones, M. L., Waterman, B. M., Bollini, M. L., & Dunagan, W. C. (2011). The cost of serious fall-related injuries at three Midwestern hospitals. *The Joint Commission Journal on Quality and Patient Safety, 37*(2), 81–87.

Yang, L., Cui, D., Zhu, X., Zhao, Q., Xiao, N., & Shen, X. (2014). Perspectives from nurse managers on informatics competencies. *The Scientific World Journal.* https://doi.org/10.1155/2014/391714

CHAPTER 12

From Patient- to Person-Centered Care: Re-Forming Relationships in Health Care

Daniel Weberg and Sandra Davidson

CHAPTER OBJECTIVES

Upon completion of this chapter, the reader will be able to:

1. Compare and contrast the concepts of patient-centered, person-centered, and relationship-centered care.
2. Describe the consistent themes of person-centered and patient-centered care models.
3. Describe the skills, knowledge, and values that enable relationship-centered care.
4. Discuss ways that leaders can support patient-centered care at different levels, such as the individual, team, and system.
5. Apply evidence-based practice (EBP) and innovation leadership principles that support patient-centered and relationship-centered care.

P atient-centered care is often referenced in healthcare organization missions, visions, and values, yet many organizations struggle to implement the principles necessary for practitioners, teams, and systems to deliver patient-centered care. Even in contemporary health care, patients are often treated as powerless and lacking sufficient knowledge to make decisions about care, and they are assumed to be inherently noncompliant (Levesque, Hovey, & Bedos, 2013). The view of patients as unequal in the system perpetuates a strong power dynamic that influences the behavior of patients, the practitioners, and the system. This traditional practitioner-as-expert power dynamic needs to be reconceptualized and facilitated through leadership behaviors that enable meaningful connections between patients and the healthcare system. This chapter will explore the historical evolution of patient-centered care and related healthcare concepts to provide a context for the current state of practice. Specifically, the influences of EBP, technology, and interprofessional practice will be discussed. The emergence of new language (person-centered and relationship-centered care) and the influence these concepts have on how we organize healthcare delivery will be presented. Case studies that exemplify person-centered care and relationship-centered care at the organizational, team, and individual levels will be presented and discussed.

▶ Origins and Evolution of Patient-Centered Care

The concept of patient-centered care first emerged in the 1960s. Prior to this, health care was steeped in the modern biomedical model, which is very much in alignment with positivism and the age of the machine that are reflected in the broader societal trends of the time. Tremendous breakthroughs were occurring in our knowledge of health and illness in the 1950s (such as the polio vaccine, pacemakers, and organ transplants). Medical research was focused on fixing the body. Physicians were regarded as experts and, in the context of the social conventions of the time, the doctor was always right.

In the 1960s and 1970s, large-scale social movements, such as women's liberation and the fight for equality among marginalized groups in society, moved forward and gained prominence. There was also a growing distrust and questioning of authority (e.g., government, big corporations). Health care was not immune to this trend. Practitioners whose clinical expertise was once beyond contestation now began to be questioned and even challenged at times. An example of this is the growing debate around women's reproductive rights (contraception and abortion) in the 1970s. Health care began to move into the biopsychosocial era. There is a growing acknowledgment of the mind–body connection and research establishing the social determinant of health (Syme, 2005) that began to influence the practice and education of healthcare providers. It is in this climate that the concept of patient-centered care emerged. There was a beginning recognition that patients' unique attributes (e.g., lifestyle, values, socioeconomic status, mental state) influence their health. Healthcare providers began to talk with patients about their health and illness experiences instead of talking at them or down to them.

In the 1970s, the role and scope of nursing in particular were important in the move to patient-centered care. Nurses embraced and formalized their role as patient advocates. Patient advocacy emerged as a concept alongside the development of patient rights in the early 1970s (Mallik, 1997). George Annas, an American attorney, created the Model Bill of Patient Rights in 1974. The formalization of patient rights arose from the larger social context of the time that was imbued with distrust of authority and power, growing consumerism, and the civil rights movement. Annas believed that nurses were poised optimally in healthcare settings to advocate for patients' rights (Annas & Healey, 1974; Mallik, 1997), and, as history has shown, the role of the nurse as a patient advocate became a cornerstone of nursing practice.

The 1980s and early1990s saw the trend toward patient-centered care continue and intensify. McWhinney foreshadowed many of the advances and changes to the patient–provider relationship:

> It will focus on the person and his or her environment and relationships, as strong determinants of health and disease . . . Sometimes the role of the physician will be to prescribe, but always it will be to mobilize, by every means possible, the patient's own healing powers. To do this, physicians will have to be much more than technologists. They will require advanced skills in communication and in understanding the deeper meanings that illness has for patients. (1984, p. 6)

In the1980s and 1990s, there was growth in fields such as medical anthropology and medical ethics. The principles and practices of phenomenology found their way into health care (Suchman, 2011). Thus, there was a greater focus on understanding the patient experience of health and illness, and with this lens patients were viewed as having significant knowledge, and their ability to share with providers and participate in patient–provider collaboration was enhanced. Clinical decisions were no longer the exclusive domain of the clinical expert, but rather shared decision making emerged between patients and providers as the new standard. However, there were still tensions among the long-held identities and traditions of the provider as expert, the movement toward patient empowerment, and shared decision making. This tension still exists today and in recent years, the debate over what we actually mean when we use the term *patient-centered care* has introduced new possibilities for how we might talk about and organize care.

New Lexicons: Person-Centered Care and Relationship-Centered Care

As McWhinney (1984) imagined, by the 1990s the educational preparation of doctors and nurses included an emphasis on therapeutic communication, patient interviewing, and skills for establishing and maintaining relationships with patients. By the mid-1990s, patient-centered care was a widely accepted and practiced model in health care. However, by the early 2000s there was a growing unease with the continued use of the term *patient* in some healthcare circles. Some argued that using this label carried forward the provider/patient power differentials, and the passive connotations seemed more pronounced in light of the knowledge era and consumer access to health information, evidence, and shared-decision-making models (Ekman et al., 2011). Further, the term *patient* reflected the acute illness focus and episodic engagement with the healthcare system, when in fact more and more diseases are chronic in nature, and long-term management of illness occurs in the context of *people* living *with* chronic conditions (Ekman et al., 2011). Hence, the argument to shift from patient- to person-centered care. The term *person-centered care* has been championed in healthcare sectors where engagement in health care is ongoing and sustained over long periods of time, such as complex care (Humowiecki et al., 2018) and cancer care. There is a growing acknowledgment that factors and influences outside the health system must be understood and factored into goals of care and planning if we are to achieve long-term success and improve health outcomes (Humowiecki et al., 2018).

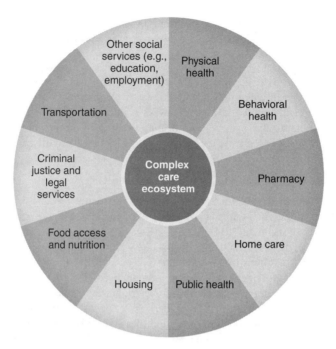

FIGURE 12-1 The complex care ecosystem.

As illustrated in **FIGURE 12-1**, there is also a clear refocusing on the social determinants of health in person-centered care. However, in many cases, providers and health systems continue to treat *person-centered care* and *patient-centered care* as interchangeable terms. Are they really? We will address this query in more detail in a forthcoming section.

On a parallel path of evolution through the 1990s and onward, there was a growing awareness that, although the patient (person) was always central to health care, the *relationships* that care providers formed with patients, communities, and other practitioners had not generally been explored or taught explicitly (Tresolini & Pew-Fetzer Task Force, 1994).

Although the biopsychosocial model that had been embraced since the 1970s helped focus attention on the multidimensional nature of illness, it also invited reductionist thinking and isolation of these elements (specialization, for example), further objectifying the patient and the illness experience (Tresolini & Pew-Fetzer Task Force, 1994). Likewise, although the patient-centered care model promoted a more holistic approach, it did not explicitly embrace the larger constellation of relationships and interactions beyond the provider and patient. As such, the new term *relationship-centered care* was introduced into the healthcare vernacular with the Pew-Fetzer Task Force report in 1994 (Tresolini & Pew-Fetzer Task Force, 1994).

The focus on relationships as a central feature of health care built on many traditions in the nursing profession. However, the new phrase *relationship-centered care* affirmed the centrality of relationships in contemporary health care and their importance in health and healing. Relationship-centered care will be explored more fully in a subsequent section of this chapter. **FIGURE 12-2** is a diagram of the evolution of patient-centered care.

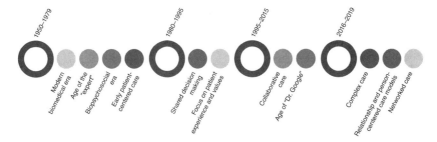

FIGURE 12-2 Evolution of patient-centered care.

From the 1990s to the 2010s there has been an emergence, evolution, and finessing of terminology that relates to the basic concept of collaboration in health care. The terms *multidisciplinarity, interdisciplinarity,* and *transdisciplinarity* are peppered throughout the literature. Often these terms are ambiguously defined and used interchangeably (Choi & Pak, 2006), which contributes to a conceptual fog where we lack clarity about how we should best organize and carry out our work together in health care. Based on an extensive review of the literature and existing definitions, Choi and Pak (2006) proposed the following definitions:

- Multidisciplinarity: Draws on knowledge from different disciplines but stays within the boundaries of those fields.
- Interdisciplinarity: Analyzes, synthesizes and harmonizes links between disciplines into a coordinated and coherent whole.
- Transdisciplinarity: Integrates the natural, social, and health sciences in a humanities context, and in so doing transcends each of their traditional boundaries (Choi & Pak, 2006, p. 359).

Various models and iterations of collaborative care have been a focus in practice and education since the 1990s; however, it often feels like an uphill battle to enact collaborative models that actually achieve intended outcomes (e.g., patient health outcomes, satisfaction and system-level efficiencies). Based on the analysis of interdisciplinary documentation patterns in an electronic health record (EHR), Dow, Zhu, Sewell, Banas, Mishra, and Tu (2017) suggested that the theoretical conception of teamwork might be the issue. Health care has largely adopted models of collaboration that use teamwork as the "operating system" that were adapted from other types of organizations.

In non-healthcare settings, work teams tend to be small, discrete, and fixed; in contrast, healthcare teams (especially in chronic and complex care settings) are typically large, heterogeneous, and dynamic (Dow et al., 2017). Their analysis also suggested that professionals involved in a specific patient's network change frequently and unpredictably, and interactions are characterized as loose associations between professionals and are often indirect collaborations rather than face-to-face interactions. They suggest that *networking* is a more apt description of this way of working. Dow and colleagues propose that networking competencies should be added to existing models of collaborative practice and education. In that spirit, **FIGURE 12-3** builds upon the conceptual analogies proposed by Choi and Pak (2016) to include an additional networking analogy.

In any form of collaborative care, the patient is the raison d'être.

Patient-centered care can be enacted using any of the previous models of collaboration (or a combination of them).

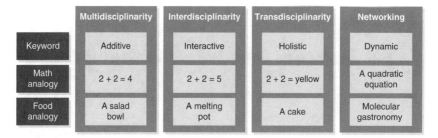

FIGURE 12-3 Comparing perspectives on collaboration.

Data from Choi, B. K., & Pak, A. P. (2006). Multidisciplinarity, interdisciplinarity and transdisciplinarity in health research, services, education and policy: 1. Definitions, objectives, and evidence of effectiveness. *Clinical & Investigative Medicine, 29*(6), 351–364.

▶ Contemporary Patient- and Person-Centered Care—Same or Different?

Foundational literature on patient-centered care has described several common foundations, yet there is no universally accepted definition (Kitson, Marshall, Bassett, & Zeitz, 2013). Likewise, there is no universally accepted definition of person-centered care. Adding to the lack of clarity, terms are often used interchangeably in practice settings. A recent systematic review provides evidence (and relief) that, indeed, we are largely on the "same page" with respect to these two concepts.

Håkansson and colleagues (2019) completed a review of reviews published between the years 2000 and 2017 that addressed the concepts of patient-centered care and person-centered care. Using thematic analysis, the authors concluded that there are nine themes common among the published reviews of each. These themes were present in 100% of both the patient-centered care and person-centered care literature included in the review of reviews (**FIGURE 12-4**).

These findings beg the question: So, what's the difference?

Håkansson and colleagues determined that 91% of the articles on patient-centered care described the goal of care to be to live a *functional life*, whereas 90% of the articles on person-centered care highlighted that the goal of care was to live a *meaningful life* (2019, p. 7). The authors stress that the practice of person-centered care does not mean abandoning the goals of patient-centered care; indeed, a functional life is often very important to the individual and part of living a meaningful life (Håkansson et al., 2019). Ultimately, they conclude that there is no opposition between practicing person-centered or patient-centered care. The term *person-centered care* simply broadens and extends the perspective of patient-centered care by considering the whole life of the patient. Again, the person-centered approach seems more appropriate for individuals that have sustained ongoing interactions with the healthcare system due to complex and chronic illness (Humowiecki et al., 2018).

▶ Tensions in the Practice of Patient-Centered Care

Aside from language about what we claim to be doing (patient- or person-centered care) and the model that we work within (networked, interdisciplinary), there are

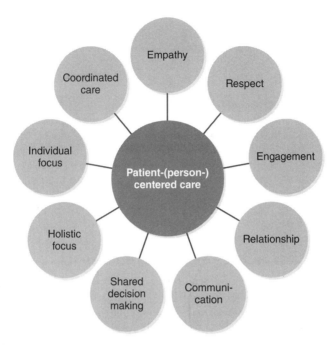

FIGURE 12-4 Common themes in both person- and patient-centered care.

often pragmatic and contextual tensions in our work as health professionals. This section will highlight several as they relate specifically to innovation and evidence-based practice.

SCENARIO

You are the primary care provider for Helen, who you have known for many years. Helen has chronic obstructive pulmonary disease (COPD) that you have both worked hard to manage to keep under control. She has come to see you today for a follow-up appointment after a recent visit to an oncologist (Dr. Chow) who has diagnosed her with colorectal cancer. Suddenly, Dr. Chow and the surgeon (Dr. Halloway) have become members of Helen's care team. You have not worked with either of them before, and they are both located at a regional cancer center that is a two-hour drive away in a large city. You engage in person-centered care in your practice and are relieved to find that the cancer center has a similar model. You also share the same electronic health record (EHR) because your practice is in the same region.

Helen will need to travel to the cancer center for her upcoming surgery and subsequent treatment. Luckily, her daughter Beth lives 20 minutes from the cancer center. Helen has arranged to stay with Beth for the next several months. Helen is also very active in her faith community and frequently has home visits from the faith-based community health nurse (Sue). You have found Sue's input, assessments, and suggestions invaluable over the past several years and work closely with her. There

(continues)

SCENARIO   *(continued)*

is a clear need for networking here and as her longtime primary care provider, you must step up to the challenge.

Questions for Discussion
1. How will you develop relationships with Dr. Chow and Dr. Halloway and ensure that you are in communication with them in the months to come?
2. How might you network to connect Sue with the cancer center care providers?
3. What other changes and additions to Helen's care team might you anticipate over the next year? Is there any networking you might do proactively?
4. What do you see as your unique contribution to Helen's care team and why does it matter?

Tension One: Evidence or Patient Preference

The source of this tension is the result of how practitioners view the distribution of decision-making power between themselves and the patient (Levesque et al., 2013).

Provider content knowledge may overpower patient values and care. The same struggle occurs with the implementation of EBP and innovation. One must sometimes unlearn to adapt, adopt, and evolve. The inability for someone to separate the perceived expertise and individually desired outcomes and submit to a cocreation process in which outcomes, treatments, and decisions are negotiated stands in stark contrast to many medical models of care. In essence, relying solely on individual knowledge and expertise will subvert the ability for organizations to adopt patient-centered care, EBP, and innovation. Additionally, this tension may cause significant and severe cultural conflicts if either the practitioner or the patient has serious objections to care decisions.

Tension Two: Reality versus Patient Expectations

Many times the desired outcome of creating an organization that supports patient-centered care is to achieve better patient satisfaction, better patient outcomes, and improved organizational outcomes (Rathert, Wyrwich, & Boren, 2012). Moderating the journey from patient-centered care to achieving outcomes is patient condition and patient expectations. Mediating the process is patient activation and patient adherence to treatments. These mediating and moderating variables ensure that patient-centered care is not a linear process but requires leaders, practitioners, and patients to find a dynamic equilibrium between what is really achievable and what the expectations of the outcome might be. For example, a patient with type II diabetes might have an expectation to cure him- or herself through exercise and diet changes, but adherence, family support, and financial hurdles may not allow the patient to meet those expectations. In this example, the patient may be less satisfied with the medical treatment, have poorer outcomes, and have an impact on the organization's overall goal of diabetic treatment despite the organization having significant patient-centered care implementation. Frontline care providers who might face similar challenges need to reflect on their ability to work with the patient to create a mutual understanding of the disease, the possible outcomes, and the impacts that life choices may have on expectations. This process is mutual, and patients should be able to set realistic expectations of treatment goals with their provider. Generally, across all studies in a systematic review of patient-centered care, patient-centered care was linked to improving satisfaction and patients' well-being (Rathert et al., 2012).

Tension Three: Care Environment Impacts or Standardized Experiences

Morgan and Yoder (2012) determined that the care setting has a significant impact on how patient-centered care is conceptualized and implemented. For example, patient-centered care behaviors will be much different in a primary care office restricted to 15-minute visits than in a hospital in which the nurse has 12 hours with the patient. Although the core principles will be the same, the behaviors of both the patient and the care team will need to adapt to remain relevant. This also means that standardizing the whole patient-centered care process in a complex organization may be detrimental to implementation. By focusing on standardizing process instead of principles, the organization may remove the ability for the team to adapt behaviors based on contextual factors and deploy less adequate processes instead. On the other hand, allowing for professional autonomy and decision making in regard to patient-centered care according to individual care environments may lead to an inconsistent brand experience and variations in interactions. By using a complexity lens, one can conceptualize these two extremes on the stability to chaos continuum.

The next section explores another element that shapes and defines the nature of the practitioner–patient relationship in health care. The knowledge era and increased accessibility to vast amounts of information via the World Wide Web have forever changed patient-centered care.

▶ Patient-Centered Care in the Knowledge Era

In the past several decades, we have seen the rise of the knowledge era. New knowledge is created at an unprecedented rate, and most of it is widely and easily accessible via the World Wide Web. The Web has democratized knowledge and information. As the old adage goes, knowledge is power. Previously, knowledge was privileged to those who had the means to access it. In the 19th century, this included those with the means to access and read books and/or attend school to access knowledge. This is in alignment with the age of the expert in health care, where health-related knowledge was accessible only to those who entered training programs (physicians, nurses, pharmacists, etc.). This perpetuated the long-held power dynamics in which healthcare experts held power over patients, who had little access to specialized health information.

Today, health-related information is available to anyone with access to an Internet connection. You can access the entirety of medical school content for free, online. This means that patients have access to an ever-expanding amount of health information. From a pure access perspective, the Web has changed the power dynamic by providing patients with access to health-related information. With this access comes new opportunities and challenges.

The concept of health literacy has been a topic of discussion in health care since the 1970s. With the dawn of the knowledge era, *e-health literacy* has emerged as a new form of literacy that forms the basis of informed healthcare decision making and meaningful patient participation in their own health care. E-health literacy is defined as "the ability to seek, find, understand, and appraise health information from electronic sources and apply the knowledge gained to addressing or solving a health problem" (Norman & Skinner, 2006, p. 3). E-health literacy combines components from different literacy skill sets and applies them to e-health promotion and care. Norman and Skinner (2006) described six core skills (or literacies) that are inherent in e-health literacy: traditional literacy, health literacy, information literacy, scientific literacy, media literacy, and computer literacy. From this list, it is easy to see that e-health literacy is a complex competency that requires ongoing engagement and continuous learning on the part of both patients and practitioners.

Dr. Google

The name of the Internet search engine Google has become a verb. It is commonplace that when we have a question to which we do not know the answer, we "google it." In the context of healthcare information and in response to questions such as, "I have (these symptoms), what's wrong with me?" the phenomenon known as Dr. Google has emerged (see **BOX 12-1**).

The Urban Dictionary (2015) defines *Dr. Google* as "a person medically qualified by Google's search engine to diagnose symptoms of sickness."

In an era when information is freely accessible and ubiquitous, patients are able to be more informed about their symptoms and care. Websites such as WebMD, PatientsLikeMe, and Google provide access to detailed, and sometimes inaccurate, information about potential diagnoses, treatments and their risks, and home remedies. This information dynamically changes the patient–provider relationship as patients enter the clinic armed with expectations, treatment recommendations, and potential diagnoses before the care provider even does an assessment. To traditional biomedical care providers, this dynamic may be seen as disrespectful and contrary to the medical expert model of care. In fact, some providers have advocated that patients not discuss their own research until the provider has finished an assessment to avoid inaccuracies in the differential diagnosis.

Instead of rejecting or delaying patient-driven evidence during the encounter, providers and organizations may deploy tactics to facilitate patients in accessing more relevant information to inform their decision making. For example, health systems can set up websites that contain vetted lists of mobile apps, informational content, and tools to facilitate provider–patient discussions. By helping create the context for information gathering, organizations and providers can be better prepared for incorporating patient evidence into the care continuum. By offering

---

BOX 12-1 Dr. Google in Action

Mr. Jones: My son has the plague. I looked up his symptoms on Google.

Dr. McCarthy: Your son has the plague? Well, send him to the emergency room.

Dr. McCarthy: *Note to self—his son is fine, but Mr. Jones has a case of Dr. Google.*

information resources to the patient, the provider or organization is strengthening the relationship with the patient and helping the patient build his or her own external network of support. Even with greater involvement of providers and organizations in developing and providing reputable and evidence-based patient resources, there is still no replacement for high-quality and patient-centered interactions with care providers. **BOX 12-2** reiterates the difficulties and dangers of the Dr. Google phenomenon.

Kemper and Mettler (2002) developed the concept of an *information prescription* as a way to constructively leverage information to enhance the relationship between providers and patients. Practitioners create an information prescription based on the patient's needs and health situation. The care provider is able to ensure that the prescription is filled with evidence-based information that will provide the patient with high-quality resources. In some cases, providers work with informatics specialists or health librarians to fill these prescriptions (Gavgani & Mahami, 2012), and in other settings a practitioner may use a handheld device and the Internet to provide the patient with reputable and high-quality links to resources on the Web (Woolf et al., 2005). The information prescription, or what Kemper and Mettler (2002) described as information therapy, is one example of how providers can leverage technology to engage patients and their families in patient-centered and evidence-based health care.

Many EBP models include patient preference as a core behavior in the evidence and intervention process. Melnyk and Fineout-Overholt's EBP model (**FIGURE 12-5**) is one example of purposefully integrating patient preference and the process of shared decision making between patients and providers. Indeed, the concept of informed choice comes into play here. In light of our conversation about e-health literacy and Dr. Google in the context of patient-centered care, it becomes clear that patients who have access to high-quality evidence and health information, and who also possess e-health literacy skills to make sense of it, can most meaningfully engage in shared decision making about their care.

Patients as Sources of Evidence

Patient-centered care is integral to the evidence and innovation work of organizations. In EBP much of the discussion about sources of evidence focuses on research efforts. Another source of evidence is emerging from patients and goes beyond reported symptoms and diagnostic data. As leaders and practitioners work to build patient-centered care capabilities in their systems and organizations, new sources of data are needed to both facilitate patient-centered care practice and patient-centered care interventions.

Clinical caring context

Research + EBP insights

Clinical expertise + patient assessment

Patient preference and values

Clinical decision making

Improved patient outcomes

FIGURE 12-5 Merging the art and science: EBP in a context of caring.

Data from Melnyk, B., & Fineout-Overholt, E. (2005). *Evidence-based practice in nursing and healthcare.* Philadelphia, PA: Lippincott Williams & Wilkins. (Chapter 1, p. 15).

Patient-centered innovation is founded on the principles of user-centered design, in which solutions are cocreated with the users to build sustainable and relevant iterations. Both patient preference and user-centered design concepts described in EBP and innovation literature are complementary to the patient-centered care research. Patient-centered care is a constant in the healthcare innovation process; together, the patient and practitioner cocreate the interventions to achieve a desired outcome. However, patient-centered care is fraught with unpredictability and is enacted in complex and overlapping contexts. As such, there are no hard-and-fast or one-size-fits-all rules about how to create a patient-centric healthcare environment. Rather, the process can be informed by foundational principles that allow leaders, practitioners, patients, and organizations to have guide rails that help to focus behaviors, structures, and decision making that can result in a cocreated, patient-centered care culture (Kitson et al., 2013).

▶ Tools to Engage Patients in Innovation and EBP

The term *evidence-based innovation* seems counterintuitive. If innovation is something new that drives significant change in the social and economic workings of the organization, and evidence takes 17 years to reach implementation, how can innovation be evidence based (Melnyk, 2014; Weberg, 2013)? Through a linear lens, evidence would appear to limit the ability for organizations to create disruptive patient-centered innovation. In essence, traditional notions of evidence are too slow to support rapid cycle change.

One tool for linking evidence, innovation, and patient-centered care is the user-centered design methodology, which is used to define many different methodologies of engaging the end user in the creation of a product, process, or innovation (Kelly & Litman, 2001). User-centered design is meant to solve difficult problems by extensively studying user habits, presenting users with early product iterations for review, and building processes and products in rapid iteration cycles driven by the feedback loops of users and their needs (Muller & Thoring, 2012). There are many tools to implement user-centered design in practice, including journey mapping, hassle maps, brainstorming, rapid prototyping, and others. Many of these tools can be found online. The key for the healthcare leader who is attempting to implement patient-centered care is that he or she understands that the organization needs to tap the expertise and experiences of the users they serve and reliably incorporate that information back into the creation of their patient-centered care tool kit.

By shifting the lens to view the system as a complex adaptive dynamic, we can conceptualize user-driven evidence to be an essential aspect of the innovation process. According to Porter-O'Grady and Malloch (2018), identifying the problem and understanding the systemic impacts is the first part of any successful innovation framework. Problem identification cannot take place in a leadership silo; studies and practical experience have shown that user-centered design methodologies allow innovation teams to create a link between the best clinical evidence and the needs of the patients or end users (Dykes et al., 2014). From this viewpoint, traditional research provides innovators with evidence to set the foundation of any given problem; however, evidence can also come in the form of real-time data, in-depth process mapping, and data from technologies such as real-time location systems and electronic medical records. By combining these diverse and complex sources of data, innovators can better understand the problem and speed up the innovation process. Additionally, the resulting solution is informed by the end user rather than a separate team trying to anticipate needs.

User-centered design is not as easy as it sounds. One cannot simply ask patients about their experience and label the resulting solution as a patient-centered implementation. User-centered design (**FIGURE 12-6**) is a rigorous process that takes trained experts, ethnographers, and an organizational will to truly inform complex processes with user-generated input. The rigor of user-centered design does not mean, however, that leaders need to hire expensive design firms and consultants to incorporate information into their patient-centered innovation processes. Simple tools exist to aid users in starting the journey. One tool is discovery interviews to gain insights into the user experience and how it might be different from assumptions by those outside the process.

FIGURE 12-6 User-centered design process.

User-Centered Design Tool: Discovery Interviews

Description

Design challenges are often based on real or perceived deficits in service or performance. As previously noted, gap analysis can help clarify where the greatest opportunities for innovation may lie. Equally important, however, is the exploration of the aspects of health care that providers and patients experience in the delivery process, especially those aspects that bring delight and satisfaction to the users. Discovery interviews are rooted in the work of appreciative inquiry. Discovery involves interviews with users of the healthcare system, service, or product and is focused on eliciting their experiences.

Use

1. Identify the users to interview.
2. Construct the interview guide.
3. Conduct the interviews.
4. Analyze the themes that emerge.
5. Group themes into affinity groups.

Users that are chosen should reflect the full spectrum of the experience. They should include patients and families, physicians and nursing staff, and other professional staff.

The interview guide should be a brief, one-page outline of key questions. The questions should be open ended and solicit the users' stories. For example, some questions might be as follows:

- "Tell me what it is like being a [patient, provider]."
- "What do you value most about being a [patient, provider] at this . . ."
- "What do you find unique about being a [patient, provider] at this . . ."
- "Describe your best experience being a [patient, provider] at this . . ."
- "If you had three wishes to make this a better experience as a [patient, provider], what would they be?"
- "If you could redesign one aspect of this experience as a [patient, provider], what would you redesign?"
- "In 5 years, this [name of healthcare setting or service] is being honored for its excellence. Why?"

Arrange for a specific time and place to conduct the discovery interview. Begin by introducing the purpose of the interview and offer an invitation for participants to tell their stories. Ask about their general experience to focus on what brings value and delight. Ask additional deeper questions around themes that are raised, such as "Tell me more about how you get timely and useful information from your doctor." Write down statements as close to verbatim as possible. If you are conducting the interview in the care environment, try to also take notes on the environment and the journey the user is experiencing as you gather information.

After each interview, summarize what you identify as the themes and get feedback from the interviewee. Following completion of the discovery interviews, list all the themes that have emerged across the interviews. The themes, specific problem points, and user insights can be used to design the first prototype of the new process or product. The discovery interviews can also be used as new iterations of the process or product rolled out to elicit new insights and test directional correctness.

User-centered design is a methodology that allows for the incorporation of user-generated evidence into innovation, process design, and product creation within organizations. Leaders should use user-centered design whenever possible, especially when creating patient-centered care practices and processes to ensure that these innovations are built on user need, not on misguided assumptions. Many user-centered design tools exist, but discovery interview is a simple tool to gather user input for an innovative problem-solving effort.

EVIDENCE-BASED INNOVATION IN ACTION

One example of how evidence-based innovation led to significant changes that redefined the social and economic potential of an organization started with a time-in-motion study. In an innovative data collection process, location tags were connected to nurses, the nurses were mapped during a typical shift, and the activities they performed were recorded. The findings provided clarity around several assumptions nursing leaders had made about how nurses spend their time. A significant portion of time was spent on documentation and other care delivery tasks, but more than 30% was spent on finding people, equipment, or supplies to carry out the work. Prior to this study, innovative solutions were sometimes selected based on faulty assumptions about the work or simply by subjective descriptions of problems. Now, innovation was enhanced by evidence. The gap in what nurses could be doing versus what they were actually doing was finally illuminated. This innovative evidence soon catalyzed several innovation projects.

From the Kaiser Permanente Innovation Consultancy, an in-house team trained in human-centered design, came a project called Ready Room. Based on data, experience, and workflow analysis from the time-in-motion study, the team discovered that fragmented and siloed data was causing significant issues in patient throughput from the operating room, through the postanesthesia care unit, to the medical-surgical units. By building on evidence from the study and gathering more real-time evidence through process mapping and interviews, the team created a solution with the frontlines that unlocked data to aid in decision making that ultimately could improve the hospital functions and nursing, housekeeping, and bed management satisfaction. Evidence, in this case, sparked an idea and led to an innovation that was designed by frontline workers to solve a proven need in the organization. The evidence source was a combination of traditional research and contemporary human-centered design processes.

From the design and data elements that came from the project team, it was possible to improve the interaction between previously siloed groups (social change). Prior to this work, teams had easy access only to data in their departments. The operating room managed the operating room, the medical–surgical team managed the medical–surgical unit and the status of rooms; the movement of patients and readiness of staff was fragmented to these groups. By leveraging real-time data and making it easily accessible in meaningful ways, groups could collaborate better, share information faster, and make better decisions. Better efficiency could then have an impact on the financial indicators for the organization. Simply connecting groups with better data to enable better decisions had the potential to decrease wasted time in the expensive operating rooms and improve the patient experience.

Modified from Hendrich, A., Chow, M. P., Skierczynski, B. A., & Lu, Z. (2008). A 36-hospital time and motion study: How do medical-surgical nurses spend their time? *The Permanente Journal, 12*(3), 25.

▶ Patient-Centered Leadership

Patient-centered care is a vehicle for cocreating innovation and EBP within a system and requires leaders to be adaptable, flexible, and collaborative to overcome the tensions described earlier. Leaders must be able to see the complex system as a whole and translate actions and information from the individual, team, and organizational lens.

Patients as Leaders

In the patient-centered care cultures and in complexity leadership principles, leadership is displayed by all agents in the system (Uhl-Bien & Marion, 2008). Therefore, patients are considered leaders in their care and must also practice leadership behaviors. According to Bernabeo and Holmboe (2013), patients should define the relationship with their provider, clearly articulate health goals and problems, share relevant information about their condition, and actively negotiate decision making. The display of these patient leader behaviors will be affected by the organizational culture and the relationship the care teams establish with the patient. To partner with the patient, the care providers, organization, and healthcare system must work together to build relationships, provide evidence, share in decision making, and involve the team.

Build Relationships

In health care, good and sustainable relationships are the foundation for everything (Porter-O'Grady & Malloch, 2018). At the core of patient-centered care are strong relationships among members of the care team, the patient, and the organization. These relationships will provide linkages in the network to share information, understand values and preferences, engage the family and the care team, and support respect. Each part of the network must participate to build strong relationships.

The patient is responsible for defining and communicating his or her desired care relationship. Whether this is done overtly through specific conversations or covertly through behaviors, body language, and other less direct methods, the source of context for relationships in the care starts with the patient. Direct care providers that are interacting with the patient can facilitate the discovery of the patient's desired relationship and be observant for the covert actions that might also provide insight. From these conversations and actions, the care provider can assist in cocreating the relationship with the patient.

Organizations and the healthcare system as a whole also play a role in facilitating care and team–patient relationship building. Organizations can provide time, support, and resources for care teams and patients to interact and build relationships (Bernabeo & Holmboe, 2013). This may be done through less intimidating care environments, supporting longer patient visits, or building a culture that holds care teams and patients accountable for building relationships. Additionally, the healthcare system can be influenced to support stronger relationships. This could be through reimbursement models, care delivery redesign, and supporting cross-functional care teams to interact with the patient.

Provide Evidence

EBP is another foundational function that supports patient-centered care. Patient preference is at the core of EBP practice, and patients are also robust sources of data for evidence-based decisions. Patients provide evidence by articulating their health concerns, goals, and the associated relevant information. Care team members should be astute in translating the information provided by patients into relevant evidence that will inform treatment options that can be used in shared decision making. While patients provide evidence in the process of diagnoses and treatment, the care provider must also provide evidence by reviewing patient preferences and context, and then present relevant information and options that are clear and transparent to the patient (Kitson et al., 2013). This exchange will also help build a trusting relationship between the team and the patient.

To support evidence in decision making, organizations and systems can provide technology tools that enable point-of-care decision making and evidence-based data. This can be done through EMRs supported with clinical decision support tools that link patient information directly to relevant research and treatment options. These systems can speed up and ease the burden of lengthy EBP processes and also catalyze conversations during short patient visits. Additionally, influencing the healthcare system to change reimbursement models to support evidence and patient preference–based interventions and treatments could help in building a culture of patient-centered care.

Foster Shared Decision Making

At the core of shared decision making in patient-centered care is the need to rebalance the power distribution between the patient and the provider or system (Levesque et al., 2013). The patient can help level the power imbalance by being informed about his or her condition and by including family and friends in the decision-making process. Essentially, the patient can help form an individual support network that can better access, interpret, and convey information to the care team. The patient's own network adds power to his or her corner and can help counterbalance the provider experts and intimidating system. Providers can also support the patient network by openly conversing and accepting information from the additional stakeholders. This may mean accepting second opinions and challenges to care plans or facilitating crucial conversations with the patient's network.

Organizations can also provide support for shared decision making. This can be through accountability and culture-building efforts or by creating spaces for the shared decision to occur. For example, allowing unrestricted visiting hours may allow the patient's support network to advocate and participate in care decisions more often. Additionally, organizations can utilize technology solutions, such as video calls, to engage family members in discussions if they are not based locally. Leaders can also influence healthcare system changes to create information that can be linked to family members, shift regulations for more open discussion of critical care decisions, and build care environments that support the patient's network in engaging with the care team easily and openly (Kitson et al., 2013; Morgan & Yoder, 2012).

Involve the Team

Patient-centered care is reliant on team-based care concepts in which the patient's network and the care team can collaborate easily and effectively (Bernabeo & Holmboe, 2013; Morgan & Yoder, 2012). Patients must act as if they are part of the team, and providers must allow patients and their networks to participate in the teamwork. Providers must also work collaboratively with the care team by cooperating with other providers, roles, and organizations to facilitate patient-centered care. This may require reflecting on and eliminating barriers such as ego, professional stigmas, cultural biases, and unnecessary competition among departments. Focusing teams on the desired outcomes of satisfaction, quality patient care, and organizational success may help in removing some barriers (Rathert et al., 2012). Additionally, organizations and systems can support team involvement by integrating systems, building accountability models that reward teams above individuals, and supporting information systems that make team care easy and relevant. **TABLE 12-1** summarizes patient-centered care leadership behaviors.

Patient-centered care is a useful construct for organizing how we go about our work in health care. In patient-centered care, as the name suggests, the focus is on the individual and her or his values, preferences, health outcomes, experiences, and needs. A fitting analogy is how we describe our solar system. Just as the sun is the center of our solar system, the patient is the center of healthcare organizations in this model. Other aspects of health care are described in relation to the patient; in the solar system analogy, planets, meteors, and stars are described based on their position relative to the sun.

Another model that is increasingly applied to health care arises from quantum physics and complexity science: the holographic universe. Holography posits that a complete pattern is represented in any component (a fractal) of a system regardless of the size or location of that component (Porter-O'Grady & Malloch, 2018). From the smallest structure or interaction to the largest and most complex aspects of an organization, the same patterns are present and reflected again and again. *Relationship* is the fractal that we will use in this analogy. In relationship-centered care, the nonreducible unit of service of high-quality care is composed of both technical and *relational* elements (Malloch, Slutyer, & Moore, 2000). The next sections explore relationship-centered care.

There is only one corner of the universe you can be certain of improving, and that's your own self.

—Aldous Huxley

TABLE 12-1 Summary of Patient-Centered Care Leadership Behaviors

Leadership Behavior	Patient	Care Provider	Organization	System
Build relationships	Define and communicate desired relationship	Openly partner with patient in care	Provide time/support for relationship building	Support patient–provider interaction
Provide evidence	Articulate health goals and concerns; share relevant information	Review preferences and present evidence in clear and unbiased way	Ensure access to best evidence for patient and provider	Restructure reimbursement to support patient preference
Shared decision making	Involve family, friends, and informal caregivers as needed and desired	Support family and friends in the decision-making process	Unlimited visiting hours, teleconference support for family meetings, proxy access to medical information	New information systems, redesign care environments
Involve the team	Share information from all sources (multiple providers, Google, family)	Collaborate and network across roles, scopes of practice, and specialties	Facilitate collaboration between providers and team	Support team-based care, top of license scope

▶ Relationship-Centered Care

As introduced in the beginning section of this chapter, relationship-centered care is a more recent development that integrates patient-centered care and multiple disciplinary interactions that take place amid a complex healthcare system. The term *relationship-centered care* is deliberate in that the principles and practices associated with this new movement would not be lumped together with existing practices that seem to perpetuate the linear, mechanistic, and reductionist legacy of the biomedical model. The Pew-Fetzer Task Force report (Tresolini & Pew-Fetzer Task Force, 1994) was the first widely acknowledged monograph about relationship-centered care. In it, the task force acknowledged that health care was on the verge of a new era, and there was reason for optimism. They also suggested that the preferred future of health care would not manifest without attending specifically to the day-to-day work of practitioners and the education required to do that work (Tresolini & Pew-Fetzer Task Force, 1994).

Tresolini and the Pew-Fetzer Task Force warned that

> health care often is based on an individual, disease-oriented, subspecialty-focused model that has led to a focus on cure at all costs, resulting in care that is fragmented, episodic, and often unsatisfying for both patients and practitioners. We are at risk, in a new healthcare system, of reproducing the same attenuated patient-practitioner relationships and professional isolation. (1994, p. 16)

Because the relationship is the central organizing feature of this model of care, three different relationships are highlighted as integral for the development and maintenance in relationship-centered care.

First is the provider–patient relationship. **TABLE 12-2** summarizes the knowledge, skills, and values to be cultivated by the practitioner to sustain patient–provider relationships.

Second is the practitioner–community relationship. Many health concerns that individuals bring to the patient–practitioner relationship also exist in communities and their institutions. By working to solve community problems that are not associated with one particular patient, healthcare practitioners can have a broader positive impact on the health of many and prevent future individual health concerns (Tresolini & Pew-Fetzer Task Force, 1994). To this end, practitioners should seek to understand and interact with communities. Using concepts from sociology and cultural anthropology, along with complexity thinking and the concepts of social justice, practitioners can develop an understanding of community dynamics. Coming to know a community also entails paying attention to demographic, political, economic, and business trends that affect community life.

Third are practitioner–practitioner relationships. The quality of the relationships among members of the practitioner community greatly affects the capacity of all those within it to form effective relationships with patients and communities (Tresolini & Pew-Fetzer Task Force, 1994). Comprehensive care depends on the contributions of multiple healthcare providers from a wide range of professions. Effective and satisfying provider-to-provider relationships begin with the foundational skills of being able to listen openly, communicate effectively, and learn cooperatively. Disciplinary diversity must be acknowledged, valued, and leveraged. Different professional traditions of knowledge, cognitive styles, and ways of perceiving are examples of the diversity that must be embraced. Providers may also vary in their degrees of readiness to learn and function as team members. Remaining open to others' ideas and displaying an attitude of humility, mutual trust, support, and empathy are key attributes of members within a thriving provider community (Soklaridis, Ravitz, Adler Nevo, & Lieff, 2016; Tresolini & Pew-Fetzer Task Force, 1994).

Another useful development in relationship-centered care are the four principles articulated by Beach & Inui (2006, p. S4):

1. *Relationships in health care ought to include the personhood of participants.* "The patient and the practitioner are both unique individuals with their own sets of experiences, values, and perspectives. In RCC [relationship-centered care] practitioners are aware of their own emotions, reactions, and biases, and monitor their own behavior in light of this awareness" (p. S4).

TABLE 12-2 Areas of Knowledge, Skills, and Values for the Patient-Practitioner Relationship

Area	Knowledge	Skills	Values
Self-awareness	Knowledge of self Understanding self as a resource to others	Reflection on self and work	Importance of self-awareness, self-care, self-growth
Patient experience of health and illness	Role of family, culture, community in development Multiple components of health Multiple threats and contributors to health as dimensions of one reality	Recognize patient's life story and its meaning View health and illness as part of human development	Appreciation of the patient as a whole person Appreciation of the patient's life story and the meaning of the health–illness condition
Developing and maintaining caring relationships	Understanding of threats to the integrity of the relationship (e.g., power inequalities) Understanding of potential for conflict and abuse	Attend fully to the patient Accept and respond to distress in patient and self Respond to moral and ethical challenges Facilitate hope, trust, and faith	Respect for patient's dignity, uniqueness, and integrity (mind–body–spirit unity) Resect for self-determination Respect for person's own power and self-healing processes
Effective communication	Elements of effective communication	Listen Impart information Learn Facilitate learning of others Promote and accept patient's emotions	Importance of being open and nonjudgmental

2. *Affect and emotion are important components of relationships in health care.* "In RCC, emotional support is given to patients through the emotional presence of the clinician. Relationship-centered care therefore challenges the notion of detached concern, in which stepping back to maintain affective neutrality breaks the bond that holds people together" (p. S4).

3. *All healthcare relationships occur in the context of reciprocal influence.*
Health-related actions do not occur in isolation but are related to one another in time, space, and content. The smallest unit of measure in RCC is a single person-to-person interaction. Providers undoubtedly benefit from the opportunity to come to know their patients, and RCC encourages clinicians to grow as a result; providers benefit in serving their patients (human to human).

4. *Relationship-centered care has a moral foundation.*
Genuine relationships are morally desirable because it is through these relationships that clinicians are capable of generating the interest and investment that one must possess to serve others and to be renewed from that serving (Beach & Inui 2006). As fully human and authentic participants in care interactions, care providers behave more genuinely than if they were acting out a role. This sort of authenticity is morally desirable as an end in itself.

LEARNING ACTIVITY

1. Read the following case example.
2. Use Table 12-2 to identify elements of relationship-centered care that you see being enacted in the case.
3. Compare your thoughts and ideas with a peer.

🔍 CASE EXAMPLE: PATIENT–PROVIDER

Jon, a patient in a hospital, is dying of cancer. This case study details one interaction that he has with the nurse who is caring for him. The descriptive narrative is told from the nurse's point of view. The interaction is grounded in relationship-centered care. The case study aims to illustrate that by developing self-awareness and purposefully reflecting upon our day-to-day interactions, it is possible to develop our skills in relationship-centered care. This case study also illustrates many aspects of relationship-centered care, such as authentic caring, genuine relationships, importance of affect and emotion, and the power of reciprocal influence.

I enter the room and see him there, in the bed. A man, 68 years old. His face appears peaceful with his eyes closed. I try to turn to leave, but his dark eyes open and meet mine. "I'm sorry," I say. "I did not want to wake you." "That's okay," he replies. "I wasn't sleeping anyway."

"Jon, how is your pain?" I ask. I observe his face and his body as he seemingly processes my question, searching for an acceptable response. His fists clench the cuff of his sheets. His brow forms a furrow of concern, and his mouth flattens into a thin, terse line. There is silence between us. I sense the tension as the silence persists for several moments.

He is not looking at me; rather, his eyes are cast downward. I feel myself wanting to ask another question or make a comment—anything to ease my discomfort. But then I remind myself that I am not concerned with my discomfort—I had asked about his. I stay silent. I stay in the moment with him, even though it is uncomfortable and awkward.

Finally he whispers, "I'm not good." My mind immediately begins to search my internal database of past similar experiences, even back to how I was taught to respond in nursing school. I so badly want to ease my own discomfort, and his. I catch myself searching for a response that has been successful in the past. I stop. I enter again into the moment with Jon. He is looking at me now, his eyes brimming with tears.

I move toward him and sit in the chair beside his bed because this is what feels right at this moment. In a hushed tone I say, "Tell me more." Again we enter into an abyss of silence. I begin to sense that just being there to endure the silence is what I need to do. The awkwardness and discomfort begin to melt away, and we are together in the silence—just being. He sighs, almost in relief, and then speaks. "I saw my daughter today. I haven't seen or spoken to her in 5 years. It is funny how dying of cancer suddenly brings things into perspective."

My mind begins to fire questions. What could have caused this man and his daughter to not speak for 5 years? How would I feel if I were dying of cancer? Did he answer my question about pain? Again, I catch myself. Even though it has been only a nanosecond, I still feel guilty for letting my mind carry me away from the moment. He continues, "I have so much that I wanted to say to her, but she seemed so angry and I . . . I hesitated." "What do you want to tell her?" I ask. "Oh!" he exclaims. "Everything . . . and nothing! I want to tell her that she has grown up into such a confident and beautiful woman—and how proud I am of her. I want to tell her that I am sorry for things that I have done that I know have hurt her. Mostly, I just want to tell her that I love her."

I sense calmness and peace as it begins to fill the room, and Jon once again enters into silence. I am simply there. I focus on just being there as a healing presence, in the moment with him. We are silent for several minutes. Gradually, his brow softens and all the muscles of his face seem to relax. He loosens his grip on the bedsheets and he sighs again. "Thank you," he says. I am startled by his words, and reply "For what?" "For taking the time to be with me," he says. "I think I can go to sleep now." He begins to lower the head of his bed using the control on the side rail. I rise from the chair and he smiles at me. I smile back. I turn off his lights as he turns on his side to face the window.

He sleeps.

Discussion

In life, it is often the case that the small acts or moments have the greatest impact on people. This is perhaps most evident in situations where we have a heightened awareness of life and death. In many clinical settings this heightened awareness exists. Let us not forget that life and death are themselves often viewed as paradox. In this patient–provider case study it is not so much a life-or-death situation but rather the struggle of transition from life into death—a paradox in process. The timescale in the case study is also paradoxical. Although the entire interaction takes place in 10 minutes, the layers of relational caring are deep and rich.

In the transition from life toward death, time takes on new meaning for many. Perhaps it is not so much new meaning as a shift in perspective about the concept of time. Stacey, Griffin, and Shaw (2000) discussed the difference between the macro-temporal and micro-temporal structures of time. Most of us tend to operate in the macro-temporal structure (past to present to future). The micro-temporal structure opens up the here and now and invites us to examine and make meaning of the experience of the present moment (Stacey et al., 2000). These authors further suggest that this focus on the nature of detailed (micro) interactions can result in the potential for transformation. Practitioner–patient interactions from a relationship-centered care perspective can be enhanced when the practitioner strives to be present in the moment with a patient.

In the case study, we see the nurse striving to stay in the here and now with the patient, and in the end the patient is able to express and move past issues of regret related to his interaction with his daughter. Had the nurse been operating in the macro-temporal time frame, she may have been tempted to use a textbook response, or she may have been too busy planning the patient's care to pay attention and respond authentically to the gestures (verbal and nonverbal) of the patient and situation in the here and now (Stacey et al., 2000).

Dimensions of Personhood and Role

In the case study (as told from the nurse's perspective) we can see her engaging her sense of self-awareness in a way that illuminates how she brings her personhood (nurse as person) to the interaction. She is acutely aware of her own emotions and reactions to the situation as she strives to engage with the patient in an authentic way (Beach & Inui, 2006). It is clear that she is not just playing the part of concerned nurse but that she is truly concerned for Jon.

Affect and Emotion

After the nurse chose to be in the here and now with Jon, the experience changed. The nurse was not simply a detached observer, and she consciously resisted the urge to revert to the neutral, detached professional stance that she was taught in her nursing education. She was emotionally present and therefore more attuned to the details of the verbal and nonverbal cueing in the interaction. Instead of implementing a canned response to the patient's cues, she responded in the micro present with a novel approach; she did what she felt was right, based on the present experience (sat down beside the client, used silence). Put simply, emotional support is provided to the patient through the emotional presence of the provider (Beach & Inui, 2006).

Reciprocal Influence

The nurse's intention to be present as a healing presence shaped the transformation of Jon and the nurse herself. Although the nurse did not know at the beginning of the interaction what the outcome would be (unknowable future), she sensed something familiar about how to behave and respond to the patient in the moment. As she entered into the authentic experience of conversation with Jon, the unknown and known future was changed by their chosen coaction toward the future. Beach and Inui (2006) suggested that relationship-centered care creates an opportunity wherein the patient and provider "develop each other's character, and assist in the attainment of moral virtue" (2006, p. S4). In the case study, for example, the nurse's experience of silence changed. It moved from being very uncomfortable and awkward for the nurse to being peaceful and comfortable. For Jon, the nurse's growing comfort with silence created the time and space for him to express and share his emotions in a way that reduced his pain and fear. Another possible change (albeit more gradual) may be the nurse's growing comfort and confidence in her ability to engage in relationship-centered nurse–patient conversations. The nurse's growing sense of self-efficacy may increase the likelihood that the nurse will continue to practice relationship-centered care. In both patient- and relationship-centered health care, the patient's goals and needs are the primary focus. However, relationship-centered care opens the potential for providers to grow and develop in the process of caring for patients.

Moral Foundations

Relationship-centered care challenges the traditional ideal in health care that providers should assume a stance of neutrality and detachment. As Griffin (2002) discussed, the notion of seeing yourself outside an interaction, rather than as a participant in the process of cocreating the interaction, is where the breakdown of the mechanistic biomedical model occurs. Watson concurred: "This totalizing of self and other, this turning away from the mystery of our shared humanity . . . can be an act of cruelty to self and others; an inhumane act" (2003, p. 199). The ethics of caring and intentionality (Watson, 2003) fit well with relationship-centered care. Watson (2003) makes reference to the work of Knud Løgstrup, a Danish philosopher, and she described his work as ethics of hand:

> Holding another person's life in one's hand, endows this metaphor with a certain emotional power . . . that we have the power to determine the direction of something in another person's life . . . we're to a large extent inescapably dependent upon one another . . . we are mutually and in a most immediate sense in one another's power. (Løgstrup, as cited in Watson, 2003, pp. 198–199)

The ethics of caring (Watson, 2003) reminds us that we are dependent on each other and have a duty to choose goodness and caring for ourselves and each other. The case study illustrates this ethics of hand and caring ethic. The nurse chose not to turn away and see herself as separate from Jon's situation. Rather, she entered into the process with him and for him.

▶ Onward to Innovations in Care

In this chapter, we have provided an overview of where we have come from in terms of our thinking and structures of health care over time. We have recounted the evolution from very mechanistic and biomedical models of care toward more holistic and patient-(person-)centered approaches. Relationship-centered care is presented as an additional lens through which providers and patients can cocreate new approaches to care. Information technology, e-health literacy, and collaborative care have also been highlighted as contextual aspects that shape our current (and future) healthcare systems. Throughout the chapter, we have provided examples, case studies, and tools that we hope readers will find useful as they continue to lead innovation and transformation in health care. In terms of EBP, individuals should be engaged in the process of examining evidence and also viewed as sources of evidence themselves. Extending the notion of the care team beyond the clinicians to include the patient and his or her support systems is a critical shift in the structure and process of care. Only then will EBP and innovation intersect to truly transform health care. Without the engagement of individuals and their families, transformation activities and EBP simply fall short of effectiveness.

We encourage you to think big and pose future forming questions to your peers, patients, and communities. "I wonder . . ." and "What would it look like if . . ." are two examples of phrases that can invite others into generative conversations about what we can aspire to create together. Most important, we hope that we have highlighted the critical role of fostering authentic and generative relationships in transforming health care—regardless of setting, model of care, or other contextual factors. Relational competency is essential for leaders at every level.

References

Annas, G., & Healey, J. (1974). The patient rights advocate. *Journal of Nursing Administration, 4*(3), 25–31.

Beach, M. C., & Inui, T. S. (2006). Relationship-centered care: A constructive reframing. *Journal of General Internal Medicine, 21* (Suppl.1), S3–S8.

Bernabeo, E., & Holmboe, E. S. (2013). Patients, providers, and systems need to acquire a specific set of competencies to achieve truly patient-centered care. *Health Affairs, 32*(2), 250–258.

Choi, B. K., & Pak, A. P. (2006). Multidisciplinarity, interdisciplinarity, and transdisciplinarity in health research, services, education, and policy: 1. Definitions, objectives, and evidence of effectiveness. *Clinical & Investigative Medicine, 29*(6), 351–364.

Dow, A. W., Zhu, X., Sewell, D., Banas, C. A., Mishra, V., & Tu, S. (2017). Teamwork on the rocks: Rethinking interprofessional practice as networking, *Journal of Interprofessional Care, 31*(6), 677–678. https://doi.org/10.1080/13561820.2017.1344048

Dykes, P. C., Stade, D., Chang, F., Dalal, A., Getty, G., Kandala, R. . . . Collins, S. (2014). Participatory design and development of a patient-centered toolkit to engage hospitalized patients and care partners in their plan of care. *AMIA Annual Symposium Proceedings* (Vol. 2014, p. 486). American Medical Informatics Association.

Ekman, I., Swedberg, K., Taft, C., Lindseth, A., Norberg, A., Brink, E. . . . Sunnerhagen, K. S. (2011). Person-centered care: Ready for prime time. *European Journal of Cardiovascular Nursing, 10*(4), 248–251. https://doi.org/10.1016/j.ejcnurse.2011.06.008

Gavgani, V. Z., & Mahami, M. (2012). The assessment of information prescription service to patients with heart valve disease: Applying users' satisfaction study. *Library Philosophy and Practice (e-journal)*. Paper 862. Retrieved from http://digitalcommons.unl.edu/libphilprac/862

Griffin, D. (2002). *The emergence of leadership: Linking self-organization and ethics*. London, UK: Routledge.

Håkansson Eklund, J., Holmström, I., Kumlin, T., Kaminsky, E., Skoglund, K., Höglander, J. . . . Summer Meranius, M. (2019). "Same same or different?" A review of reviews of person-centered and patient-centered care. *Patient Education and Counseling, 102*(1), 3–11. https://doi.org /10.1016/j.pec.2018.08.029

Hendrich, A., Chow, M. P., Skierczynski, B. A., & Lu, Z. (2008). A 36-hospital time and motion study: How do medical-surgical nurses spend their time? *The Permanente Journal, 12*(3), 25.

Humowiecki, M., Kuruna, T., Sax, R., Hawthorne, M., Hamblin, A., Turner, S. . . . Cullen, K. (2018). *Blueprint for complex care: Advancing the field of care for individuals with complex health and social needs*. Retrieved from www.nationalcomplex.care/blueprint

Kelly, T., & Littman, J. (2001). *The art of innovation*. New York, NY: Broadway Business.

Kemper, D. W., & Mettler, M. (2002). Information therapy: Prescribing the right information to the right person at the right time. *Managed Care Quarterly, 10*(4), 43–46.

Kitson, A., Marshall, A., Bassett, K., & Zeitz, K. (2013). What are the core elements of patient-centered care? A narrative review and synthesis of the literature from health policy, medicine and nursing. *Journal of Advanced Nursing, 69*(1), 4–15.

Levesque, M., Hovey, R., & Bedos, C. (2013). Advancing patient-centered care through transformative educational leadership: A critical review of health care professional preparation for patient-centered care. *Journal of Healthcare Leadership, 5*, 35–46.

Mallik, M. (1997). Advocacy in nursing—a review of the literature. *Journal of Advanced Nursing, 25*(1), 130–138. https://doi.org/10.1046/j.1365-2648.1997.1997025130.x

Malloch, K., Sluyter, D., & Moore, N. (2000). Relationship-centered care: Achieving true value in healthcare. *Journal of Nursing Administration, 30*(7/8), 379–385.

McWhinney, I. R. (1984). Changing models: The impact of Kuhn's theory on medicine. *Family Practice, 1*(1), 3–8. https://doi.org/10.1093/fampra/1.1.3

Melnyk, B., & Fineout-Overholt, E. (2005). *Evidence-based practice in nursing and healthcare*. Philadelphia, PA: Lippincott, Williams & Wilkins.

Melnyk, B. M. (2014). Speeding the translation of research into evidence-based practice and conducting projects that impact healthcare quality, patient outcomes and costs: The "so what" outcome factors. *Worldviews on Evidence-Based Nursing, 11*(1), 1–4.

Morgan, S., & Yoder, L. H. (2012). A concept analysis of person-centered care. *Journal of Holistic Nursing, 30*(1), 6–15.

Müller, R. M., & Thoring, K. (2012). Design thinking vs. lean startup: A comparison of two user-driven innovation strategies. *Leading Through Design*. Retrieved from http://www .researchgate.net/profile/Erik_Bohemia/publication/233801554_Leading_Innovation_through _Design_Proceedings_of_the_DMI_2012_International_Research_Conference/links/0fcfd50ba 3d8153431000000.pdf#page=181

Norman, C. D., & Skinner, H. A. (2006). eHealth literacy: essential skills for consumer health in a networked world. *Journal of Medical Internet Research, 8*(2), e9. https://doi.org/10.2196 /jmir.8.2.e9

Porter-O'Grady, T., & Malloch, K. (2018). *Quantum leadership: Creating sustainable value in health care* (5th ed.). Sudbury, MA: Jones & Bartlett Publishers.

Rathert, C., Wyrwich, M. D., & Boren, S. A. (2012). Patient-centered care and outcomes: A systematic review of the literature. *Medical Care Research and Review, 70*(4) **351–379.**

Semigran, H. L., Linder, J. A., Gidengil, C., & Mehrotra, A. (2015). Evaluation of symptom checkers for self diagnosis and triage: Audit study. *BMJ, 351*(h3480). Retrieved from http://www.bmj .com/content/351/bmj.h3480.full.pdf+html

Soklaridis, S., Ravitz, P., Adler Nevo, G., & Lieff, S. (2016). Relationship-centered care in health: A 20-year scoping review, *Patient Experience Journal, 3*(16), 130–145. Retrieved from http:// pxjournal.org/journal/vol3/iss1/16

Stacey, R. D., Griffin, D., & Shaw, P. (2000). *Complexity and management: Fad or radical challenge to systems thinking?* London, UK: Routledge.

Suchman, A. L. (2011). Relationship-centered care and administration. In A. L. Suchman, D. J. Sluyter, & P. R. Williamson (Eds.), *Leading change in healthcare: Transforming organizations using complexity, positive psychology and relationship-centered care* (pp. 35–42). London, UK: Radcliffe.

Syme, S. L. (2005). Historical perspective: The social determinants of disease—some roots of the movement. *Epidemiologic Perspectives & Innovations: EP+I, 2*(2). https://doi.org/10.1186 /1742-5573-2-2

Tresolini, C. P., & Pew-Fetzer Task Force. (1994). *Health professions education and relationship-centered care*. San Francisco, CA: Pew Health Professions Commission. Retrieved from http:// www.rccswmi.org/uploads/PewFetzerRCCreport.pdf

Uhl-Bien, M., & Marion, R. (2008). *Complexity leadership part 1: Conceptual foundations*. Charlotte, NC: Information Age.

Urban Dictionary. (2015). Dr. Google. Retrieved from http://www.urbandictionary.com/define .php?term= Dr+Google

Watson, J. (2003). Love and caring: Ethics of face and hand—an invitation to return to the heart and soul of nursing and our deep humanity. *Nursing Administration Quarterly, 27*(3), 197–202.

Weberg, D. R. (2013). *Complexity leadership theory and innovation: A new framework for innovation leadership* (Doctoral dissertation). Arizona State University, Tempe, AZ.

Woolf, S. H., Chan, E. Y., Harris, R., Sheridan, S. L., Braddock, I. H. Kaplan, R. M. . . . Tunis, S. (2005). Promoting informed choice: Transforming health care to dispense knowledge for decision making. *Annals of Internal Medicine, 143*(4), 293–300.

CHAPTER 13

Toxic Leadership: Leadership Behaviors That Kill Innovation and How to Avoid Them

Daniel Weberg and Courtnay Caufield

"When a toxic person can no longer control you, they will try to control how others see you. The misinformation will feel unfair, but stay above it, trusting that other people will eventually see the truth, just like you did."

—Courtesy of **Dr. Jill Blakeway**, DACM, L.Ac

CHAPTER OBJECTIVES

Upon completion of this chapter, the reader will be able to:

1. Identify at least three behaviors of toxic teams.
2. Discuss the impact of toxic leadership on innovation outcomes.
3. Compare and contrast toxic leadership behaviors and learn how to address them in practice.

The creativity, support, and competence to lead change and innovation in healthcare organizations is an essential skill for leaders. Everyone has or will experience leaders or teams whose behaviors undermine the essential work of collaborative change. These undermining behaviors can be intentional or unintentional, but they do create massive disruptions in an organization's work. Toxic leaders and teams are those whose behaviors become so distracting, awkward, and time-consuming to others that they completely derail daily work.

While there are many examples of toxic people who disrupt teams in a gusto of ego and attention, most toxicity in teams builds over time by one or more people. Small, repetitious daily interactions between leaders and team members can manifest over time to create toxic cultures. Leaders need to be aware that toxicity is a slow and iterative process just like innovation. Toxicity builds over time and leaders, including innovation leaders, need to recognize these smaller interactions and patterns that signal issues and respond properly. Toxicity kills innovation! Leaders must recognize, stop, and prevent toxic behaviors before they infest entire organizations and lead to the destruction of individuals and the patients and staff they care for. Leaders must also look inward to understand when their own behaviors may be facilitating a toxic response in their teams. This self-reflection may seem like an impossible feat to some; however, it is possible by self-checking and reflecting on your behaviors.

In the struggle to move the status quo forward, using the best evidence and disruptive innovation, teams can experience significant resistance. Sometimes this resistance is normal and originates from the stress caused by people giving up the known to do something new and discomfort with the unknown. Normal resistance is healthy; it keeps the team's energy balanced on the edge of chaos, far from stagnation but not in the swirl of complete ambiguity, frustration, and fragmentation. Normal resistance is not toxic; it is a sign that the organization is evolving. These behaviors can be managed through information sharing; relationship building; transparency in goals; and clear, consistent outcome communication (Weberg, 2013).

Toxic leadership and toxic team members are different. In nature, toxicity primarily occurs in two ways. One, a foreign organism invades its host, rapidly spreading throughout. The toxin either changes the normal function of the host system by making it dysfunctional and leading to death, or the toxin drains the energy and debilitates the host system until it finally can no longer sustain life. Second, toxic substances can be ingested or created by the body and disrupt the body's cellular function, destroying energy production and cell life, ultimately resulting in organ shutdown and eventually death. Without an immune response or direct intervention from a curing agent, toxins and toxic leaders have fatal outcomes. Similarly, in human organizations, toxic leadership behaviors and toxic team members can infect the organization and kill the functioning of a team, much like how a toxin destroys a cell.

Toxic leadership creates burnout, stress, confusion, and chaos, and ultimately leads to the death of teams (Weberg, 2010). Resistance in toxic teams stems from ego, personality issues, poor communication and listening skills, individual grudges, alternative motives, and poor relationships between team members. This chapter will discuss the origins of toxicity in leadership and its impact on complex organizations and teams. We will also identify ways leaders can be the antibiotic, curative agent, or immune response to stop toxicity in its tracks.

▶ Complex Systems and Toxicity: Origins of the Infection

As discussed, toxicity in human beings occurs when too much of a substance builds up and cannot be processed out by the body, thus removing the ability for the human to sustain life. Sometimes toxicity occurs because of ingesting too much of a chemical or because the body cannot rid the toxins from itself. Sometimes toxicity occurs when the body begins to break itself down (i.e., rhabdomyolysis) and its own elements build up. These analogies give us insight into how healthcare organizations can become toxic as well. As leaders and teams work to continually adapt to the people and interactions around them, sometimes dysfunctional behaviors can build up over time and lead to toxic systems. Complex systems stay adaptable and healthy when their energy is focused on growth, change, and adaptation. If this energy is redirected to distractions or to building stagnant structures, toxicity can begin.

Complexity science describes the concept of chaotic systems (Stacey, 2016). These are systems that are sensitive to the initial conditions that they grow from and, while they are chaotic, have recognizable patterns. This means that small changes to a chaotic system can have disproportionate impacts to that systems behavior, but even with the disproportionate changes, the pattern of movement is not random. Think about a highly stressed and burned-out team you may have interacted with. When a new request is made of this team's members, their reactions can be very disproportionate to the actual work needed to accomplish the task. You cannot predict how this team will react when under stress, but you can make a good guess as to the pattern of behavior you might see (frustration, anger, anxiety, etc.). You may also anticipate that the team reacts in this way to support or follow its toxic leader. The team may be made up of innovative and subdued leaders who have given up the fight against the toxic leader. However, the toxic leader will represent the whole team, and those who follow will either abort the team or assimilate and assume a passive follower role to the toxic leader and their team. As a leader of innovation, you must be very good at recognizing patterns of behavior in teams and systems because this is the closest you will ever come to predicting change or the ability for teams to adapt to change. Patterns also help you understand how to find toxicity within systems.

REFLECTION ACTIVITY

Have you ever participated in or observed toxic team behaviors? Share the patterns of behavior you witnessed. What feelings did you notice? What interaction patterns were there? How did people respond to new work? How did others view that team? How would a high-performing team look different?

Pattern recognition will allow the innovative leader to make decisions on where to positively disrupt the pathway of the toxic team and will inspire others to do so as well, challenging the system and the broken status quo with confidence.

Evolutionary biological sciences (one of the sciences that inform complexity theory) frequently suggest that living systems require the following features (Goldstein, Hazy, & Lichtenstein, 2010):

1. Autonomy: able to function and survive on its own
2. Self-reproduction: able to reproduce copies of itself
3. Self-repair: ability for the system to determine the issue and repair itself to functioning
4. Survival instinct: inherent drive to be alive and stay alive
5. Adaptation: able to adjust to immediate changes in the systems environment
6. Evolution: able to change over time to adapt to environmental changes

Autonomy

Toxic leaders disrupt or remove these requisites for a system to sustain life. Toxic leaders remove autonomy by creating requirements (intentionally or unintentionally) that require team members to act with the approval, with the supervision, or by the command of the leader. For example, a nursing unit that has excellent care outcomes has a new physician attending. This attending physician requires the nurses to get approval for all care interventions, including those that are covered by standard orders or a nursing practice act. Quickly, the team can only follow protocols built by the physician's own practice, and the resulting care outcomes decline. Additionally, the team is afraid to change practice without approval and, over time, does not change practice. They only follow the physician leader's instruction.

The impact of a controlling leader created a toxic environment that resulted in a loss of autonomy and created fear for those who thought about going against the norm. The team may discuss its loss of autonomy, but over time and with poor repercussion, it will assimilate despite the ability to make independent decisions.

CHALLENGE

Think of a time you or a team you were on was in a similar situation. How did you feel as a clinician or leader? How did this affect your personal feelings about yourself? How did you react or, retrospectively, how would you have wanted to react? What would you tell the toxic leader if you could recap the feelings and the impact to your practice and/or patient care? What would you have done differently and how would that have made you feel? Can you describe the value of autonomy to a toxic leader or to a new leader?

Reproduction

Toxic leaders are unable to reproduce, or they stop the team from reproducing. This may sound awkward but it is very true. Leaders fail to reproduce themselves by failing to create quality succession plans or by reducing high-performing team members' contributions. When the leader is absent, moves to another role, is on vacation, decides to retire, or otherwise leaves the organization, there is no person or group that can quickly take on the work. Thus, the team enters chaos, loses organization, and can become unproductive.

A toxic leader usually has talented staff members who can assume the work or who are ready for the challenge, but they are not provided training opportunities, allowed to take more complex work, and are purposefully excluded from opportunities to develop due to the perceived threat to the toxic leader. Toxic leaders can also stop teams from successfully reproducing themselves by reducing staffing levels without good rationale, hiring poor-performing teammates, adding non-value-added tasks, limiting the exposure to new groups or ideas, and limiting who can attend meetings by rank or title. By restricting team members from sharing their skills with the rest of the organization, the leader limits knowledge growth for the individual and the organization. Thus, when the team or an individual who possess knowledge decides to leave the organization, their understanding, impact, skills, and historical knowledge and information are lost. Another possibility is that the toxic team actually becomes very good at reproducing toxicity, assimilating to the leadership style, and losing their individual personas. This may be the worst outcome, and the infection spreads across the system like cancer and quickly overcomes the organization's healthy functioning, leading to death.

Self-Repair

Toxic leaders limit the ability for teams to self-repair and thus recover from stress and injury. Healthy teams can resolve conflict, replace lost team members, and fill gaps in information by learning and adapting their behaviors quickly. Toxic leaders can stop self-repairing functions through various policy, personality, and conflict avoidance behaviors. For example, a team that has experienced significant turnover may be told they now must "do more with less," without any further discussion of adaptation. In another example, a team may be given a mandate to implement a new workflow without direction and consistency, leading to inefficient variation, including inconsistent outcomes and varied practice. When these directives are challenged, a toxic leader simply minimizes the team's concerns and pushes forward.

Another example of limited self-repair is when a leader restricts (intentionally or unintentionally through poor communication) the ability of a team to access information needed for decision making and the team adapts poorly. In the absence of information, human-based systems will attempt to fill those gaps through assumptions, fragments of information, and rumors (Kapferer, 2017). The fragmented information leads to maladaptive and misinformed behavior changes.

Survival Instinct

Toxic leaders disrupt teams' survival instincts. High-performing teams create an attractive energy that keeps them together and continues the generation of high-performance behaviors. In toxic teams, the survival instinct shifts to individual self-preservation while team bonds begin to weaken and break. In toxic teams, individual team members begin to show their worth to the leader hoping they will not be removed or disregarded. The team might also focus on pleasing the toxic leader instead of keeping work outputs relevant with the needs of the larger system. For example, a toxic team might change practice to meet the desires of its new manager even though the evidence suggests differently. Over time, practice does not change, and the team's work becomes irrelevant to the system. Other consequences involve team members maintaining self-preservation by leaving the team for more hopeful activities. Toxic disruption of team survival instincts can also result in team members producing just enough work to keep from being terminated from employment.

Adaptation and Evolution

Finally, toxic leaders reduce the team members' ability to adapt and evolve their relationships and work to sustain relevancy in the larger organization. Toxic leaders reduce the information flow, connections, and relationships in their teams, which in turn affects the team's ability to process change, think about ways to work differently, and then share those practices throughout their network. Without the ability to process and effect change, the team is not able to respond to threats, stressors, or new ways of work in a meaningful way. Team members either maladapt as we discussed, or they do not adapt at all. Without adaptation to immediate shifts in the environment, the team cannot evolve to longer-term shifts in the environment. Without adaptation, the team's work becomes antiquated and cannot support the work or the trajectory of the larger system.

Innovation leaders are susceptible to toxic behaviors, and innovation leaders require frequent reflection and feedback to avoid the toxic trap. Additionally, innovation leaders can be food from which toxic leaders feed. The leadership of creating innovation requires significant energy. Energy to overcome resistance, energy to build relationships, energy to push teams forward, and energy to redirect chaotic movement into focused innovation processes. Innovation leaders are balls of energy and facilitators of energy management for teams. They help focus and redirect the work of innovation to stay on the edge of chaos, far from the status quo. Innovation leaders can become the focus of toxic leaders because toxic leaders are hungry for that energy to fill their own egos, gaps, or insecurities. Toxic leaders can kill innovation by removing connections, destroying relationships, and limiting momentum of innovation leaders while focusing the innovation leader's attention, stress, and work toward the toxic leader. Toxic entities suck the energy from the team and system around them and redirect it toward their individual needs, work, and vision. This creates a void in which innovators and teams can fall.

Given the living systems framework, toxic leaders reduce the ability for teams to reflect the requisites of living systems. If teams are unable to meet these requisites, they begin to die, just like living beings. Complex systems are also required to be interdependent, meaning that teams in an organization are dependent on each other to gather information, adapt, and evolve over time. Toxic leaders can also affect how teams interact with other teams, which results in system impacts. Specifically, toxic leaders have an impact on how people connect, develop relationships, and share information, all of which are functions of an adaptable and innovative system (Uhl-Bien, Marion, & McKelvey, 2008).

Connections, Relationships, and Information Flow

The origins of toxicity in healthcare teams are complex because often toxic teams arise unintentionally. Similar to the concept of the "butterfly effect" in which the right initial conditions can catalyze small inputs to a system that build to create massive unpredictable change, toxicity in teams builds from small interactions that eventually become normalized and infect the system (Watt, Javidi, & Normore, 2016). While there are many hypotheses that try to explain how leadership and teams can turn toxic, this section will focus on using some easy-to-understand complexity science principles to help leaders understand the origins of toxicity as it relates to innovation and evidence-based practice. By understanding the theoretical origins of toxicity in teams and leaders, leaders of innovation can be better prepared to recognize and address issues.

High-performing teams that are good at innovation have built nimble processes that build three things: connections and relationships between people; conflict resolution leadership skills; and information sharing that is transparent, constant, and consistent. When each of these three processes are interrupted, deleted, or manipulated, the team has the initial conditions to build dysfunctional and toxic behaviors. Often, the disruption to these innovation processes are a result of teams and leaders overreacting or using dysfunctional behaviors to attempt to meet their basic needs—certainty, purpose, and relationships/connections. For example, when uncertainty is high, leaders may create more controlling structures that limit the team's creativity and innovation. In the absence of purpose, leaders may remove the team's connections to the system so the team focuses on the leader's needs and importance. Finally, if the leader lacks in relationships throughout the system, he or she may force more focus from the team on the leader's immediate issues to fill the gap.

Fragmentation Causes Toxicity

Connections are defined as the ability for a leader or team to access other parts of the organization (Weberg, 2013). Leaders can build connections through personal interaction, electronic communication, social media, and individual networks. While connections represent the ability to simply contact others in a network, relationships represent the ability for people who have a connection to share meaningful information among themselves. To have relationships, you must have connections, and just because you are connected does not mean that you have a relationship.

Complex systems thrive when they are highly networked (many connections and strong relationships for information sharing), emergent (flexible structure as work changes), and interdependent (depend significantly on each other for success; Uhl-Bien, Marion, McKelvey, 2007; Kahn et al., 2018). If high-performing leaders are built on numerous and adaptable connections to the rest of the system and environment, then toxic leaders are created when connections and relationships with the system are flawed or absent. When a system is fragmented and there are limited connections to other teams/groups inside and outside the organization, information is limited, and dysfunction ensues because the team is unable to adapt to new demands.

Toxic leaders emerge in the shadows of the system where time, structure, understanding, and information are absent. System shadows are developed when complex systems become less adaptable, become overwhelmed, and lack sufficient energy to keep relationships with all the various teams. In the absence of this energy, the chaotic toxic leader becomes attractive and rises to influence. For example, a team experiences the retirement of a longtime supervisor. The executive leadership teams take several months to gather, interview, and select a viable candidate. While the time frame seems long, the process is actually very rushed as the executives do not have bandwidth or energy to devote to the selection of the new leader, thus creating a vacuum of oversight and an urgency in the team to fill the leadership void. The interviews are superficial, the team is not allowed to interview the candidates, and finally a unilateral selection is made. The result: a disconnected leader who is set up for failure.

With limited connections to the system, the leader receives limited information with which to make decisions or inform the team. In the absence of information, teams and leaders will use rumors, assumptions, personal agendas, and fragmented information to fill in the gaps, which will lead to dysfunctional decision making and, over time, toxicity (Kapferer, 2017). For example, an executive leader might only want to communicate with his or her peers at an executive level while limiting connections to other levels in the organization. This only provides the leader with access to a limited amount of information and a homogenic view of the system. Over time, unresolved fragmentation will lead to toxicity as teams stay inwardly focused and direct their chaotic energy toward themselves and not dissipate it throughout the system for resolution.

Chaos and Stability as Sources of Toxicity

In every organization there are pockets of uncertainty and ambiguity. These are inherent to complex systems, and you have learned throughout this text that leaders of innovation should be comfortable with these characteristics (Weberg, 2013). When leaders accept ambiguity, chaos, and uncertainty as normal, they can harness energy that these characteristics attract to catalyze innovation. Using the example of the leaderless team mentioned previously, an innovative team can harness the chaos caused by the departure and work diligently to reimagine processes, policy, structure, and work. While the team may not be able to select the incoming leader, it can create the conditions that are more attractive to innovative leaders over toxic ones. Additionally, teams could also create comprehensive onboarding plans to help the leader connect with the right parts of the system rather than leaving the onboarding up to the unfocused executive search team. However, these same characteristics of chaos and uncertainty can be a source of toxicity as well.

Chaos as a Source of Toxicity. In the frame of complex systems, chaos is simply the existence of extreme unpredictability. Contrary to many views, chaos in complex systems may be unpredictable, but chaotic systems have distinct patterns and are usually governed by simple rules (Stacey, 2016). One example is a school of fish. It is impossible to track or predict where any individual fish will be as the school moves together through the ocean, but you can see the highly coordinated and distinct shape and shimmer of the school as it moves along. Even when predators attack the school, the fish fluidly shift and move to avoid death but again regain their recognizable shimmering ball when the threat passes. This is an example of an adaptable, complex, and chaotic system that is not entirely predictable but demonstrates recognizable patterns of action.

High-performing teams move back and forth across the edge of chaos (the line between stability and ultimate predictability and chaos and ultimate unpredictability) in a pattern that resembles a dynamic equilibrium. When there is too much stability, a team is unable to adapt to stressors, and if there is too much chaos, the team's energy is not focused to accomplish the needed work. If the school of fish did not move, the shark would eat them instantly, and if they were uncoordinated, the shark could hunt down any one of them individually. In teams, chaos can be recognized by the breakdown of normal patterns of behavior and predictability (Hayles, 2018). When a team is on the edge of chaos, this frequent yet small move into chaotic behavior allows the team to continually challenge and shift behaviors, thus not overstructuring routines to the detriment of evolving practice. For example, when teams are faced with new leadership (a new supervisor), behavior is disrupted, norms are shifted, and for a short period the team may be in chaos as the team members question which norms to keep and which will change with the new input (leader) to the system. Chaos allows for adaptation to changes in the environment.

When teams are stuck in chaos, their cultural norms and behaviors change rapidly. Small inputs into the system cause unpredictable changes in team dynamics. For example, a team in chaos might get a request for a deliverable from the new leader. Without some semblance of structure, the team might overreact and spend hours trying to impress the leader when the request was of a routine nature.

On the other hand, the team may react by ignoring the request in an attempt to establish new power dynamics. More than likely, in practice, both situations occur. Because there are no clear operating norms for the team, individuals become disconnected and act more like individuals than reflecting the highly coordinated efforts of a high-performing team. As a result, teams in chaos may have some individuals that try to please the leader and others who ignore and establish dominance, and the interaction between both extremes creates unclear connections and relationships among teammates, thus leading to even more chaos. Toxic leaders are unaware or unable to intervene when teams turn more chaotic because they lack the connections, information, and relationships to interpret the behavior. They simply cannot or will not recognize the patterns of dysfunction that a chaotic team displays. High-performing teams and leaders are able to reestablish expectations, boundaries, norms, and relationships in chaotic teams through communication and information sharing, thus restoring some recognizable patterns back to the team's behavior.

See **FIGURE 13-1** for a visual of a high-performing team that resembles dynamic equilibrium. A core concept of innovative systems is that they best function on the

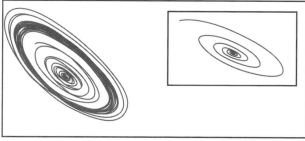

FIGURE 13-1 High- and low-performing team dynamics.

edge of chaos and far away from stability. These high-performing innovative teams continually challenge the status quo to stay far from stability but have processes in place that keep the team from moving over the edge of chaos for significant lengths of time. To stay on the edge of chaos, teams need to establish what is negotiable and changeable in their culture and what is not. Also, clear and concise communication of expectations and impact of change will help teams evolve their behaviors to meet new needs. Without either of these structures in place, teams catapult into chaos, and it takes an equal amount of energy from the system to restore order to a chaotic system. For example, think about how much energy it takes to terminate an employee who is disruptive and dysfunctional.

Stability. In complex systems, the concept of stability refers to a lack of movement and energy (Stacey, 2016). In nature, the only things that are stable are rocks and things very near death. Teams that reside on the stable side of the stability/chaos continuum are not able to adapt to change. Quite literally, teams that are stable, in terms of relationships, information, and connections, lack the features and required energy of a living system. These stable teams either are unable to change based on pressures that are placed on the system, or they are unaware of the pressures on the system and therefore do not adapt. When teams are not able to adapt or are uninformed about the need to adapt, the work they do becomes irrelevant. Teams producing work that does not match the needs of the organization infect the system so that the system becomes slightly more stagnant and thus increases the irrelevance of the entire organization. Not addressing stagnant toxic teams can kill your organization.

Stagnant systems are locked in rigid order and incapable of evolution. Examples include rigid bureaucracies, monopolies, dictatorships, and teams that resist any new advancement—aka laggards—(Rogers, 2010). Stagnant systems are predictable, overly structured, and inflexible (see low-performing teams in Figure 13-1). These low-performing teams are so focused on working within the status quo that they are unable to change their interpersonal dialogue and thus cannot solve even the simplest problems that arise. Often, these structures were an overcorrective response to times when the organization was too chaotic.

On the other end of the energy spectrum is chaos. Teams that move into and stay in a chaotic state will have problems focusing their work, and the excess energy can lead to deviant and disruptive behaviors that create toxicity. A healthcare example that highlights the consequences of chaotic energy is a heart in ventricular fibrillation. In ventricular fibrillation the energy of cardiac conduction is not focused, and the heart muscle responds in unpredictable twitches rather than blood-pumping contraction. The energy, while chaotic, has a recognizable pattern, the classic fibrillation jostling, but it is sending mixed and inefficient signals to the muscle. The energy is no longer coordinated by the electrical nodes of the heart, but each individual cell is producing excitation without coordination. The muscle is confused by the information it's receiving and unable to function properly, resulting in the death of the entire complex system: the body.

Chaotic teams create similar results in organizations. Teams that lack any patterns of interaction that can be interpreted by the system create confusion, and the system stops responding to the chaos. Confused systems can either work to remove the chaos by removing the team or isolate the team so that the chaos does not spread. When chaotic teams become more isolated from the system, they turn that energy inward and self-destruct by becoming stuck in a cycle of negativity or becoming so unstructured that work is no longer accomplished. In toxic organizations, the chaos is allowed to spread and creates organizations that can no longer focus and adapt, and eventually dissipate that energy by disbanding, reorganizing, or imploding all together.

"The problem for the innovative leader is that chaotic teams can be extremely high functioning in the short term."

Think about a hypothetical start-up company as an example. Teams spend days on end working, hyperfocused on building their passion-filled product. They adapt quickly and respond to market changes. They create changes in structure and, in the beginning, have very few predictable or interpretable operating structures. They are making it up as they go. While this type of work and interaction is a catalyst for their innovation, over time they are not able to sustain this work. They must control the chaotic work by fitting it into more organized patterns to shift from innovation to adaptable operations. Similarly, healthcare teams that focus only on solving the problems of the day, fighting the latest drama, and taking pride in how many hours they put in at the office will soon burn out and create toxic by-products.

Stagnant or chaotic teams create the conditions that lead to toxicity over time. Leaders should be aware of where their teams fit on the spectrum from stable to chaotic and work hard to keep their teams far from stagnation and close to the edge of chaos without staying in chaos for long periods of time. Chaotic teams perpetuate

DISCUSSION

Think about teams you may have been on or worked with. Can you identify three behaviors that signal stagnation in a team? Can you list three behaviors that signal a team is in chaos? What did the leader do to promote or resolve those behaviors?

POINT TO CONSIDER

The entire healthcare industry is at a tipping point. It is wrestling with a generational shift from industrial models of production and restructuring into dispersed models of care. This is evidenced by the shift from large hospital buildings to smaller community-based clinics, the move from in-person visits to virtual visits, and the move from physical exams by a clinician to exams conducted by technology.

The industry is also struggling to adapt its organizational structure to meet a new generation of workers—those who see value in outcomes and not a physical presence in an office, and where loyalty is to the professions (nursing, medicine, etc.) and not to the organizations where they work. This is in stark contrast to the beliefs of previous working generations.

These tensions of delivery of care and philosophy of work, left unaddressed, can be a severe source of toxic leadership because the divides reflect uncertainty to one group and stagnation to another. For example, teams that require physical presence 5 days a week can be seen as archaic by millennial workers. On the other side, millennial workers who continually work from remote locations can provide a sense of uncertainty to other generational leaders. These exact tensions must be addressed and clarified in teams or toxic reactions might occur. Innovation leaders are usually in the center of these tensions.

uncertainty and ambiguity in systems. Uncertainty and ambiguity, if left unresolved, cause teams to make misinformed decisions, increase team stress levels, and eventually create extreme structures to remove chaos, which rapidly move them toward stagnation.

Recognizing Toxicity

The ability for leaders to understand and identify toxic behavior patterns is an essential skill. Because teams and organizations are hyperconnected through electronic means, including social media and e-mail, toxic behaviors can spread rapidly and undermine gains made toward change. While it might be easy to find overtly toxic behaviors such as loud and disruptive behaviors, it is also important for the leader to look for the beginning interactions that might signal toxicity early, before they become infestations or worse. Even though the behaviors and impacts of toxicity are complex and hard to measure individually (chaotic), the patterns of behavior over time are easier to observe and address. This section will discuss ways leaders can use daily interactions with the team to gather data that might root out toxic beginnings.

Using complexity science concepts as an assessment framework for identifying toxic patterns can help innovation leaders find and address the beginnings of toxic behaviors. These patterns can be assessed in candidate interviews, interactions in team meetings, presentations, and other venues in which you can observe leaders in action. **TABLE 13-1** links the complexity concepts described earlier in the chapter to toxic leadership behaviors found in the evidence. These behaviors are then linked to some specific daily examples that might signal patterns of toxicity.

DISCUSSION

Can you identify other behaviors that might create stagnation and/or chaos or diminish relationships, connections, and information sharing? What are the consequences to the team, the organization, and the system?

The behaviors in Table 13-1 are small interactions that can build over time to create a toxic work environment. There are also other ways to identify toxicity in teams. Just by examining the way and intent by which teams interact, leaders can assess if those teams are high-performing or spiraling toward toxic stagnation.

Recognizing Toxicity through Conversation

Adaptability and flexibility are essential skills for high-performing teams in complex systems (Uhl-Bien, Marion, & McKelvey, 2008). In complex systems, each system is a reflection of the smaller systems that comprise it. This is seen in science in the form of fractals like crystals—each large structure is made up of other smaller and smaller identical structures. Teams operate in a similar way. High-performing teams are made up of high-performing individuals, who display high-performing behaviors and have strong high-performing relationships. One of the smallest structures a leader can examine in teams is the conversation and communication patterns among team members as they conduct work and forge relationships. These patterns can lend insight into healthy tensions or toxic tendencies.

TABLE 13-1 Complexity and Toxic Leadership Behaviors

Complexity Science Concept	Toxic Leader Behavior Pattern	Daily Action Examples
Disrupting Connections	<ul><li>Poor management of people networks (peer and superiors)</li><li>Absence from operations</li><li>Too busy to meet with direct reports</li></ul>	<ul><li>Cancels staff meetings</li><li>Does not receive or read updates on progress</li><li>Frequently in meetings with door closed</li><li>Inaccessible by e-mail, by phone, in person</li></ul>
Disrupting Relationships	<ul><li>Unconventional behaviors that alienate people</li><li>Alternates between idealizing and devaluing others</li><li>Attention to the superficial</li></ul>	<ul><li>Focuses on own successes (personal or professional)</li><li>Carrot-and-stick (transactional) leadership</li><li>Focuses on numbers and not people or system impacts</li></ul>
Creating Chaos	<ul><li>Creates cliques and rivalries</li><li>Informal and impulsive style that creates dysfunction</li><li>Unable to manage details</li><li>Unable to act as an administrator</li></ul>	<ul><li>Exclusion of team members from meetings</li><li>"Need to know" only style of communication</li><li>Cancels staff meetings to address arbitrary deadlines instead</li><li>Unaware of feedback, employee skills, or review processes—writes them off as overly bureaucratic</li></ul>
Structuring Stagnation	<ul><li>Autocratic or controlling style creates excessive dependence on others</li><li>Unable to listen to or understand new ideas</li></ul>	<ul><li>Titles matter more than influence</li><li>Years of service count more than employee value/impact</li><li>Frequently confused or dismissive of ideas or suggestions</li><li>Relies on team for direction or blames team for own inadequacies</li></ul>

Data from Conger, J. (1999). Charismatic and transformational leadership in organizations: An insider's perspective on these developing streams of research. *Leadership Quarterly, 10,* 145–169.

TABLE 13-2 Conversation Impact on Team Movement	
Moves toward Stagnation	**Moves toward Possibilities**
Self	Others
Advocacy	Inquiry

The reason conversations are good data points for teams in complex systems is because conversations are inherently nonlinear. It is not very often that people converse according to a script; instead, their language flows naturally and provides insights into the team members' beliefs, values, and actions. There are patterns in communication between teams that can lend great insights into their working culture. Leaders need to listen with different ears when assessing team interactions.

Losada (1999) conducted research that examined the conversations of teams while those teams conducted work on an innovation project. The research team examined the sentiment of the conversations teams had while problem solving. Specifically, the team looked at whether the conversation was focused on others versus self and inquiry versus advocacy. **TABLE 13-2** shows how the conversation focus affected the outcomes of the team. For example, if a team conversation focused mostly on self (individual accomplishments) and advocating for individual points of view, the team momentum toward innovation stopped. However, the opposite was not true. Teams that focused mostly on others (team skills and contributions) and inquiry (possibilities and appreciative questions) were not automatically high performing. This is because it represents the other extreme of the scale. While self and advocacy represent stagnation, others versus inquiry represents blue-sky unstructured (chaos) thinking. Neither is helpful when examining innovation because teams that are good at innovation live on the edge of chaos.

Based on their performance on the innovation project, Losada was able to identify the teams as "High Performing" and "Low Performing" teams. Figure 13-1 shows the output of the data for high-performing and low-performing teams after the data were run through a nonlinear mathematical algorithm. The figure on the right demonstrates the visual of the conversation for a low-performing team. The picture demonstrates the rapid movement of the team toward stagnation and dysfunction. The conversation starts with a focus on self and advocacy and quickly spirals toward a point. The conversation was so one-sided that the team was unable to explore possibilities and became paralyzed in regard to problem solving.

The picture on the left shows the high-performing team's conversation. The conversation is in constant oscillation between self and others, advocacy and inquiry. This means that team members were able to explore possibilities and challenge themselves on their thinking. Individuals could express ideas and have them challenged in a healthy way. The dynamic equilibrium like movement of this conversation was reflective of the team's energy and innovation capacity. Innovation requires movement and adaptability, and the high-performing conversation data demonstrate the ability for the team to adapt and move the conversation accordingly. The low-performing team shows that the team could not adapt and thus spun to failure. Leaders can use these pictures and descriptions to better assess and recognize which direction their own team conversations are taking and intervene before they become low performing, thus killing innovation.

CHALLENGE

The next time you are in a team meeting, pay special attention to the conversation in the room. This might be in a staff meeting, a huddle, or a class session. What is the dialogue in the room? Are people pushing personal agendas or team ideas? Can you determine the performance of the team by the conversation?

Draw the conversation on a piece of paper using similar data points as Losada did. What do you see? What other communication patterns emerge?

Tips for Recognizing Toxic Conversations in Practice. While it would be great to replicate this study in every team across every organization, we know that is not possible. Instead, we can use the insights from Losada to identify patterns in the leaders' own daily work with teams to help quickly assess if teams are trending high performing or low performing. Leaders do not have to overcomplicate their observations. Simply read the energy and intent in the room. Is the conversation inquisitive and gathering more information or judgmental and defending a position? Is the conversation flowing or stuck on a single issue without resolution? Are there individuals that disrupt when the status quo is challenged? How do influencers in the meeting interact? All of these questions can serve as the start for a leader to assess teams. Remember that toxicity and pleasant demeanor are not mutually exclusive. Later, I will provide tips for addressing toxic behaviors.

The hardest part about finding toxicity is that leaders can be blinded by the infrequent "good times" that occur. Stay focused; if the pattern shows significant negativity, it's a toxic team, no matter how many "good times" might be interspersed between.

🔎 CASE EXAMPLE: TOXIC VOICES

In a healthcare team made up of several senior leaders and several support staff members, toxicity was brewing. While most of the team was discussing inquiry and others were in their work-around forming a new strategy, two members of the team continued to resist. The two team members continually challenged the team's agreements and spoke in place of others. For example, one toxic team member evoked the absent executives' "voice" when challenging the agreements with little data to support such claims. The team leaders did little to stop these outbursts, and eventually many team members stopped bringing up ideas or speaking in meetings entirely. The two team members would often suggest that they had a good sense of humor but when challenged by any member of the team, these two quickly perceived these challenges as personal attacks. This created an apprehension by the leaders to openly address concerns or facilitate further dialogue. After several meetings the team members' body language changed: shoulders were hunched, meetings were quiet, and passing glances and eye rolling became normal. The team began to "just get through" the meeting rather than actively participate, and the two toxic team members were often the only input on topics. This quickly skewed the meetings toward their agenda while the team spiraled in frustration and stagnation.

In this case we can see patterns of toxicity that might be familiar to you. You can see the low-performing spiral take shape. The team, over the course of several meetings, began to move back toward stagnation. Barriers to conversation were set in place, toxic team members dominated the conversation, and you can see the focus on self and advocacy rather than a healthy tension of others and inquiry.

Identifying Individual Toxic Behavior

Toxic behaviors that individuals can display in team settings that create chaos and uncertainty are illustrated in **TABLE 13-3**.

TABLE 13-3 Toxic Behaviors That Individuals Can Display in Team Settings That Create Chaos and Uncertainty

Pattern	Example	Rationale
Verbal communication	Dismissing comments by others either verbally or nonverbally	Shows lack of respect, discourages conversation, closes doors to team-think Sign of need for attention, low self-esteem, putting up a "front"
Body language	Sighing, eye rolling, verbal outbursts, immediate contrary remarks directed at individuals, elitism, belittling	Outward display of uncontrolled emotion, lack of empathy, lack of awareness
Gossip, rumors, and assumptions	The meeting after the meeting	Insights are not brought up in a meeting but small clique meets afterward informally
Cliques, friendships, and access to the leader	Individuals with access to leader or documents influence without informing team	Limits those who are "in the know" Creates control for the toxic leader
Disruptive outbursts	Frequently disrupting meetings in disagreement Inappropriately challenging ideas without evidence	Attention seeking, looking for attention, lack of self-awareness, trying to be "right"
Poor emotional intelligence	Venting, blaming, scapegoating, victimizing	Focus is on retaliation, who is "out to get them" and or how to "win" Task at hand is a vehicle to demonstrate these behaviors

TABLE 13-4 Toxic Team Behaviors	
Clique formation	Small subgroups form dominating conversations, excluding others and/or undermining work
	Hegemony
Lateral violence	Mutual passive-aggressive behavior
	Consistent and frequent feuds
Elitism	Team members see themselves as better than others in the system
	Disregarding feedback from non-team members
	Verbal belittling of other teams in the organization

Recognizing Toxic Team Behavior

While it might be easier for a leader to find toxic individuals, leaders must also be able to assess the interactions between team members as well. Toxic teams are rarely created overnight. Team cultures are created by the frequent interactions that occur on a minute-by-minute and day-by-day basis. If you are observing the the toxic behaviors shown in **TABLE 13-4**, you know that inappropriate and deviant behavior has started to spread and normalize.

Toxic teams require significant work to correct because toxic team energy is attractive and contagious to teams that lack vision and purpose. This means that when a team begins to trend toward toxicity, the energy to move away from these toxic behaviors requires a significant catalyst. While sometimes external coaching can help team members recognize their deviant behaviors and work to correct them, often leaders must find and remove the source of toxicity. This may be a person, a stressor, or cultural norms that feed the behavior. Later in this chapter, I will discuss further the ways to kill off toxicity.

▶ The Toxic and Failing Leader

There are scenarios where high-performing teams can become toxic because of the behaviors and practice of the team's formal leaders. The business literature is rife with contemporary examples of failed and toxic leadership, including the stories of Enron's collapse, Blockbuster's death, Polaroid's demise, and DeLorean's failures. We see fewer extreme examples from health care, but we are seeing the patterns that let us know that toxicity in leadership exists. These patterns include provider burnout, expensive yet subpar care, slow rates of change, and poor team performance. It is important to note that deficiencies in a leader's skill set do not automatically qualify that leader as toxic. The difference is that leaders who are toxic either never adapt their leadership practice (stability) or never establish any normal leadership pattern (chaos).

Nurse, physician, and caregiver burnout and suicide is one example of the consequences of toxic leadership and teams. If you are a member of a healthcare team with a toxic leader, it is essential that you are able to identify the behaviors specifically and work to correct them. Rankin, Russell, Matthews, and Pollard (2017) showed that leaders displaying toxic tendencies had worsening patient outcomes, and team members reported higher stress levels than normal. If toxicity is left unaddressed in a team, it will eventually lead to catastrophic loss. This loss could be financial, personal, patient, or team. In any of these cases, toxicity is not acceptable.

If toxicity is left unaddressed in a team, it will eventually lead to catastrophic loss.

▶ Organizational Sources of Toxicity

The goal of this chapter is not to blame or stigmatize leaders or their growth and practice but to help leaders understand how to recognize behaviors that lead to poor team performance. Complex organizations have complex sources that feed toxic behavior and allow it to flourish. Toxic behaviors are not always individually sourced but a consequence of the boundaries, policies, norms, and acceptance by the organization as a whole. Much like the individual causes of toxicity, the organizational toxicity sources also have an impact on the connections, relationships, and information flow of teams in the organization.

Organizational Connection, Relationship, and Information Fragmentation

Organizational structure has a significant impact on the way toxicity can grow and remain. Organizations that limit the ability of their teams to connect with each other will be more likely to cause toxic behaviors to emerge and allow them to remain unaddressed. For example, teams that are overly reliant on hierarchal position and strict communication lines limit the ability for teams to make connections outside that hierarchy. This creates conditions so that the teams near the frontline cannot easily connect with those teams near the administration without going through layers of hierarchy levels.

In this example, a unit-based team (UBT) working on implementing a new evidence protocol would have to first ask its manager for permission to do the change. That manager would then have to ask the director; further, that director would have to ask the executive team, who then would have to ask the physician team. This creates multiple opportunities for the change to be killed by a single individual, thus removing the UBT's flexibility, adaptability, and decision-making ability. The UBT then is restricted from adapting (adopting new evidence or change) and it becomes stagnant over time. This causes the team to maintain old practices, which perpetuate frustration and conflict over time. Unaddressed frustration and conflict then lead to toxicity. In a more networked and innovative organization, the relevant stakeholders are brought to the table together to work through the idea, create a collaborative solution, and implement based on the requirements of the entire subsystem.

Organizations can also limit connections and information flow by restricting boundary spanning. Boundary spanning occurs when teams connect with systems outside their own (Weberg, 2013). For example, attending education sessions, conferences, and site visits would be examples of how healthcare teams might expand their networks. Often, organizations are under operational stressors (financial, quality, staffing, etc.) and they begin removing nonoperational processes. For example, a hospital under financial stress may reduce this stress by removing clinical educators because they are seen as nonessential to operations and care delivery. Another example is that the same organization might remove all travel and external conference attendance from the teams as well.

When organizations limit the ability for teams to connect, gather, and consume information from beyond their own system, they will, again, restrict movement of the organization. When information and connections are restricted, the teams will have limited information by which to make decisions. When information is limited, teams will begin to fill in the gaps with fragments, assumptions, and rumors. When inaccurate or misinterpreted information is allowed to continue, misaligned decision making occurs, and the teams cannot adequately adapt and move forward with their work. They then lose momentum and begin to either stagnate in their work or leap into chaos in which decisions become random, further frustrating the organization as a whole. Remember, chaotic systems are not random; they are simply unpredictable. Chaotic systems actually have metapatterns, and in the case discussed here, teams without connections and information will display patterns of decisions that reflect fragmentation and immediate stressor reduction. This means they are not deciding in the context of the system, thus limiting the ability for the system to adapt as well. The reduction in adaptability leads to stagnation. You can recognize these types of decision-making processes when leaders use their own personal agendas, limited information, and misguided connections in communicating with their teams.

Leaders of evidence-based innovation need to seriously assess their organizational structure, policies, and communication patterns to see if there is a risk for stagnation. There are always trade-offs here. It may not be possible to retain the education team, but completely eliminating the associated information flow from the educators does not allow for continued adaptability by the teams. Leaders must creatively think about ways to adapt the changing system when parts are lost to facilitate adaptation of the team. In the educator example, information flow might be maintained with the use of more team huddles, the creation of a journal club, using technology to facilitate evidence sharing, or leveraging other educators in the system to temporarily support the lost teams. Leader-facilitated adaptation will be much more successful than if the system is left to adapt on its own, with limited context and information, as we discussed previously.

It is the obligation of the leader to continue to monitor for structures that might facilitate and trap toxicity in the system. There is no algorithm or list of exact patterns to watch for because complex systems are nearly impossible to fully assess (their complexity limits how much one can measure). Leaders need to look for

ACTIVITY

There are many ways that organizational structures can have an impact on connections, relationships, and information flow. With your team, list behavior patterns, policies, or structures in your experience that might facilitate the creation of toxic behavior.

Make a list with your classmates and discuss how you might recognize and address these behaviors.

patterns that reflect the removal of connections between people, a decrease in the building of relationships between teams, and restrictions in the way information enters and is consumed by the system and reference that with how these patterns are afffecting the interactions and work of those teams.

▶ How to Address Toxicity

Now that we have discussed the origins of toxicity and how to recognize the behaviors of toxic teams and leaders, we now need to share tools that leaders can use to address behavior. The impact of toxic leaders is greater for those who find their jobs meaningful and have a strong sense of commitment (Harris, Kacmar, & Zivuska, 2007). Translating this to healthcare organizations, healthcare professionals are more susceptible to toxic cultures and the impact of those cultures because they are bound by a moral and ethical standard. Additionally, leaders of innovation and evidence are potentially more affected by toxic teams because they represent an irrational resistance to the change they are trying to implement, or toxicity diverts energy needed for meaningful change to other, less important foci.

The need for innovation leaders to learn how to address and remove toxicity from their team's environment is a critical skill. Toxicity erodes cohesion (connections and relationships) and reduces the team spirit (energy), and under the worst-case scenarios, toxic leadership could even lead to mutiny and death. There are several interventions that individuals and teams can employ to reduce and remove toxicity from their system.

Framing the Interventions

Much of the evidence related to removing toxic people or leaders is focused on individual skills. They range from leaving the team to having tough conversations to addressing the toxic behaviors in various ways. While these are important skills, it is more important to address the underlying system issues that allow toxicity to occur. Remember that toxicity stems from removal or dysfunction in connections, relationships, and information sharing in teams. To address toxicity, leaders must regenerate the system while addressing the individual behaviors. Innovation leaders have an obligation to the system to help it regenerate because innovation leaders are charged with keeping organizations alive and thriving.

Intervention 1: Stop the Toxic Energy Source

The most important, and most difficult, intervention to carry out is stopping the toxic energy source. Teams must have energy inputs to continue to move, and this is true for toxic teams as well. Toxic energy feeds toxic behaviors. Individuals working in a toxic environment can easily become attracted to the energy and behave as a conduit to spread that toxic energy forward. Behaviors like rumor creation, complaining, disrespecting the leader, and gathering negative experiences from others to validate personal concerns are all ways individuals spread toxicity. The evidence-based innovation leader is able to rise above this energy, recognize the patterns, and begin to shift his or her behavior to counteract the toxicity. Calling out incorrect information sharing, keeping teams focused on the work instead of the drama, and not tolerating bullying activities in the workplace are a few ways individuals can stop the toxic energy flow.

Schein (2010) suggested three ways that people can change culture in organizations. They can change the way people interact, the norms of communication, and even the pictures on the office walls. All of these are called "artifacts" and provide day-to-day representations of what is valued, allowed, and communicated. People use these artifacts to develop team norms. One of the easiest ways leaders can change culture is by changing the artifacts. For example, instead of having the manager lead a meeting from the front of the room with the staff listening in a classroom-style setup, move the meetings to standing huddles; place the chairs in a circle to reduce the appearance of formal hierarchy; and allow the staff, instead of only the formal leader, to facilitate. These small changes can shift the perception of power unconsciously and overturn some of the sources of toxic energy flow.

Another example of changing artifacts is simply shifting how the team members interact and communicate with each other. For example, if a toxic team has a few more vocal negative voices that continually speak up in meetings or daily interactions, shift the focus from those few to the voice of the many. This can be done by stopping the negative energy in its tracks and respectfully interrupting the outburst and addressing it outside the view of the larger group. Additionally, asking for specific input from the rest of the team when a single voice is dominating can help validate the information flow or help you see that there is little relevancy in the negativity.

These interactions are tools you can enact tomorrow in the conversations you have with your teammates and require little to no training. Although they are simple in concept, the courage to stand up to the chaotic and toxic energy of a dysfunctional team member is one of the most difficult things a leader must do.

Intervention 2: Building a Network of Support

Toxic leaders thrive when the energy of the team is focused on them, whether that energy is devotion to the leader's word or the chaotic energy that forces teams to rely on the leader for even the smallest direction. One reason this energy and attention focuses on the leader is because the toxic team is disconnected from the system and environment. This means that the chaotic energy that is churning in the system has no outlet to dissipate into the system and trigger signaling for intervention or support.

One way individuals in toxic environments can address toxic behaviors is to build their professional networks inside the organization. By maintaining strong relationships with other teams, other leaders, and the work of the organization, individuals can accomplish a few things: (1) they have a source for validating concerns with other objective viewpoints, (2) they have a personal outlet to professionally signal distress (not venting) to the other parts of the organization, and (3) they can build a critical mass to help resist or create movement to eliminate the toxic energy sources.

A frequent issue that arises from individuals in toxic situations is the perception that they do not have the permission to talk or reach out to others. It is important to remember that in the age of technology and social media, reaching out to build a network does not rely on permissions. Many leaders have even leveraged professional social media sites to solicit insights on how to build and maintain positive work cultures. Build your network around the barriers but ensure that when your network has critical mass, you must address and remove the barrier, not simply work around it.

Intervention 3: Leave the Toxicity

Although this may seem like an extreme intervention, it may be required to maintain health, happiness, and ethical congruence. Leaving the toxic organization is a difficult choice, but there is increasing evidence that remaining in one can lead to burnout, stress, depression, exiting from the profession, and even death (of clinicians and patients). These are not acceptable outcomes in the 21st-century organization. If you have tried the first two interventions but continually see the toxic patterns reemerge, it may be time to simply find a new place to be creative and thrive.

▶ What to Do If You Are Stuck in Toxicity

Our journey in leadership and professional life will cause us to be in situations that are very toxic. While the interventions mentioned previously are great tools to address toxicity, it is still entirely possible that toxicity might remain. There is no magic bullet. This creates a tension that individuals must deal with: stay in the team or leave. The latter is not always an option. It is not easy to leave a position, a group of colleagues, or financial security of having a job. It is important to note that even if you cannot leave the toxic environment, there are ways to maintain and grow professionally and personally and stay healthy. This section will explore options for those innovators who cannot remove themselves if toxicity remains unsolved.

Continuous Learning

In our experience, toxicity thrives in the uninformed. One way to combat the effects of toxic leadership is to continue your education on leadership practices, team dynamics, and organizational culture. If you are reading this text in a class, you have made that decision! Understanding leadership better allows you to rise above, call out the dysfunction from a base of evidence, and develop skills to help you grow out of your current role. Continuous learning allows you to adapt your behavior while others stay stagnant, and that alone can provide resiliency and hope in the face of a toxic workplace.

Be a Positive Deviant

"Positive deviants" are those who thrive in a system that is failing. There are many good success stories about how individuals and teams were able to challenge the status quo to develop positive changes. Positive deviance behaviors are those that you undertake to create a positive outcome despite a toxic environment. Maybe you have found a way to find joy in the work you do when the rest of the team seems unhappy. A positive deviant would help share the joy with others to help them adapt to new behaviors that help the team thrive as well. Positive deviants challenge organizational and team norms to create better working conditions, outcomes, and interactions. These are key skills to have as a leader of innovation.

Have a Difficult Conversation

When faced with a tough working environment, it is always better to confront the conflict in an open and transparent manner. In toxic teams, rumors, assumptions, and stories drive the decision making and stress of the team members. The quickest intervention to reduce these faulty decisions is to elicit fact. If you are frustrated with a leader, it is essential that you address the behaviors, actions, and decisions with the leader directly. There are several texts on the skills needed to have these difficult conversations. By addressing issues directly, you are reducing the toxic energy creation by limiting the chaotic movement of yourself and your team. Transparency and vulnerability as a leader creates a safe environment that allows you to release built-up anxieties in a constructive manner and may open the door for others to share concerns as well.

It may also be helpful to have a conversation with the leader's supervisor. This action takes some courage, but for the innovation leader, stopping toxicity is essential for future success, and calculated risk taking is an essential leadership skill. Approaching a leader's supervisor should only be done after attempting to address the situation with the source of the toxicity or if the environment is physically or psychologically unsafe. Be prepared to provide examples, documentation, and a description of the impact the behaviors have had on the team and be prepared to discuss and implement the resulting solution. It is not effective to simply make others aware of your frustrations; you must be prepared to act and fix them.

▶ Conclusion

Toxic leadership and toxic teams will ultimately lead to the death of an organization and system. Burnout, stress, poor outcomes, and lack of innovation are results of allowing toxicity to continue in any setting. Leaders of evidence-based innovation can combat toxic environments with several interventions and must continue to see the system through the chaos. By working deliberately to address toxic behaviors, leaders can create culture change that supports innovation and evidence. If the toxicity is too rampant, leaders must also know when to move on. Innovation will not work in toxic environments, and our patients, families, colleagues, and system will suffer. Leaders must stomp out toxicity in every situation.

References

Comaford, C. (2018). Safety belonging and mattering index. *Forbes.* Retrieved from https://www.forbes.com/sites/christinecomaford/2016/02/21/surrounded-by-toxic-jerks-at-work-do-this-and-soar-above-the-conflict/#4c04c58c543b

Goldstein, J., Hazy, J., & Lichtenstein, B. (2010). *Complexity and the nexus of leadership: Leveraging nonlinear science to create ecologies of innovation.* New York, NY: Springer.

Harris, K. J., Kacmar, K. M., & Zivnuska, S. (2007). An investigation of abusive supervision as a predictor of performance and the meaning of work as a moderator of the relationship. *The Leadership Quarterly, 18*(3), 252–263.

Hayles, N. K. (2018). *Chaos bound: Orderly disorder in contemporary literature and science.* Ithaca, NY: Cornell University Press.

Kapferer, J. N. (2017). *Rumors: Uses, interpretation and necessity.* New York, NY: Routledge.

Khan, S., Vandermorris, A., Shepherd, J., Begun, J. W., Lanham, H. J., Uhl-Bien, M., & Berta, W. (2018). Embracing uncertainty, managing complexity: Applying complexity thinking principles to transformation efforts in healthcare systems. *BMC Health Services Research, 18*(1), 192.

Losada, M. (1999). The complex dynamics of high performance teams. *Mathematical and Computer Modelling, 30*(9–10), 179–192.

Rankin, J., Russell, M., Matthews, A., & Pollard, M. (2017). Clinical leadership and effective nursing teams. *GSTF Journal of Nursing and Health Care (JNHC)*, *4*(1).

Rogers, E. M. (2010). *Diffusion of innovations*. New York, NY: Simon & Schuster.

Schein, E. H. (2010). *Organizational culture and leadership* (Vol. 2). Hoboken, NJ: John Wiley & Sons.

Stacey, R. D. (2016). *The chaos frontier: Creative strategic control for business*. Oxford, UK: Butterworth-Heinemann.

Uhl-Bien, M., Marion, R., & McKelvey, B. (2007). Complexity leadership theory: Shifting leadership from the industrial age to the knowledge era. *The Leadership Quarterly*, *18*(4), 298–318.

Uhl-Bien, M., Marion, R., & McKelvey, B. (2008). Complexity leadership theory. *Complexity Leadership: Part, 1,* 185–224.

Watt, S. R., Javidi, M., & Normore, A. H. (2016), Increasing darkness: Combining toxic leadership and volatility, uncertainty, complexity, and ambiguity (VUCA). In A. H. Normore & J. S. Brooks (Eds.), *The dark side of leadership: Identifying and overcoming unethical practice in organizations* (Vol. 26, pp. 195–206). Bingley, UK: Emerald Group Publishing Limited.

Weberg, D. (2010). Transformational leadership and staff retention: An evidence review with implications for healthcare systems. *Nursing Administration Quarterly*, *34*(3), 246–258.

Weberg, D. R. (2013). *Complexity leadership theory and innovation: A new framework for innovation leadership* (Unpublished doctoral dissertation). Arizona State University, Tempe, AZ.

APPENDIX 13A

Are You Resolved to Reduce Friction in Your Workplace?

Telling the truth about where you and your culture stand in terms of safety, belonging, and mattering is a great place to start.

Truth matters, safety matters, and belonging matters. According to a *Forbes* commentary titled "Safety Belonging and Mattering Index" (Comaford, 2018), these are three key things that people crave, and almost every behavior can be linked to times when people feel a lack of one or all of these three. These feelings are primal in nature and when they are missing, people can take toxic measures to meet these needs. **BOX 13A-1** provides three sample questions to get you started. Rate yourself from 0 to 10, where 0 = never, 2.5 = rarely, 5 = somewhat consistently, 7.5 = consistently, and 10 = always.

Now that you have a sense of whether you feel like you have safety, belonging, and mattering, go back and answer the same questions from the point of view of your team. If your scores continue to reflect an environment that is toxic, try using the interventions in this chapter to make changes in yourself or your team.

BOX 13A-1 Before You Solve a Problem, You Need to Assess It

Answer the questions first from your personal point of view *(be honest)*:

1. When I make a mistake, I am corrected with respect and the desire to help me improve.
2. I trust my team members and colleagues to support my and the company's success.
3. I receive acknowledgment and appreciation at work.

SECTION 4

Exemplars

© Everything Possible/Shutterstock

CHAPTER 14

Organizing Systems for Successful Innovation: Examples from the Field

Cheryl Hoying

CHAPTER OBJECTIVES

Upon completion of this chapter, the reader will be able to:

1. Describe the infrastructure of a patient services department that allows for continuity of care across the organization's healthcare system.
2. Understand the importance of reliability in a healthcare organization and the importance of a resilient staff in achieving reliability.
3. Discuss the role that healthcare systems play in fostering community health and decreasing utilization of the emergency department and hospital services.
4. Recognize the move toward interdisciplinary practice and the benefits to consumers.

▶ Introduction

In 2001, Cincinnati Children's became one of seven healthcare centers to join Robert Wood Johnson Foundation's Pursuing Perfection initiative. The purpose of the initiative was not just to improve the performance of the seven participating healthcare institutions but also to demonstrate to the broader provider community that ideal care is attainable (Kabcenell, Nolan, Martin, & Gill, 2010).

That step became a pivotal point in Cincinnati Children's innovative pursuits, spurring leaders to set the strategic objective of transforming health care through organization-wide quality improvement. It was a commitment that quickly spread across the many departments and programs. Subsequent innovative efforts were designed to support the medical center's clinical, teaching, research, and advocacy mission.

Four years later I became Cincinnati Children's new senior vice president of the Patient Services Division. I had come from the Ohio State University Medical Center, where I was responsible for nursing. In my new role at Cincinnati Children's, I also was accountable for nursing and the allied health professions. The added span is now becoming more commonplace—the scope of authority for 60% of chief nursing officers includes areas outside nursing (Boston-Fleischhauer, 2014b). With this broader role came a new perspective. Not only did I want to determine how we could improve processes, I also wanted to launch the medical center into a new way of thinking interprofessionally.

DISCUSSION

The role of chief nursing officer is expanding to include oversight for allied health and other disciplines. In the future, do you also see the role of nurse manager or director expanding? How? What are the advantages? How might other disciplines react if asked to report to a nurse manager or director? Would a matrix reporting structure be better? Why or why not?

In his book *Leading the Life You Want*, Stewart Friedman states, "Being innovative is to act with creativity and courage in continually experimenting with how things get done, bringing others along with you as you progress toward goals that matter" (2014, p. 14). With this sentiment in mind, I will explore and discuss some of the innovative thoughts and changes that have taken place at Cincinnati Children's over the past 10 years.

Grow Leaders, Not Managers

Managers are an integral part of organizations. They make sure everyone is doing as they should and that tasks are accomplished as planned. An effective leader, however, should focus on finding and developing more leaders, not managers. Leaders are visionaries. They seek to make changes based on cutting-edge research. Leaders help an organization move forward.

In his book *Joy, Inc.*, Richard Sheridan encourages the elimination of hierarchy: "It's not easy, and some team members grapple with the freedom and responsibility of this leadership style . . . look at every moment, whether difficult or important, as an opportunity to see whether a new leader is ready to step up and exercise his or her leadership skills" (2013, p. 144). Sheridan's overarching advice for growing leaders, not bosses, is this:

- "Let your team lead without you" (2013, p. 144). When meetings are unproductive, express your confidence, give your team the authority to make the needed decisions, and then exit.
- "Be vulnerable" (2013, p. 146). Admit that you are not perfect and do not have all the answers, but say that you will keep trying until you get where you want to be.
- "Encourage new leaders" (2013, p. 148). Do this by being supportive and encouraging your team to develop its own ideas.

The best way to support leadership development in your staff, Sheridan suggests, is to "feed their dream and encourage them as they pursue it" (2013, p. 149).

Leaders must be action oriented. Leaders cannot theorize on an idea forever. Instead, effective leaders must push forward, remembering that change is good! At Cincinnati Children's, the effectiveness of new approaches is verified with small tests of change. Implementation takes place in test mode. If it works, roll with it. If it does not work, tweak it and try again. The point is to continue pushing forward for new and better outcomes. Impress this upon staff and shared governance councils. Ask yourself, How can I encourage staff to always be thinking of the next great idea?

Encourage Breakthrough Thinking

Breakthrough thinking is necessary to move forward, but it does not happen without a culture of openness to new ideas and willingness to take risks. Leaders are wise to encourage staff to engage in renewal activities as often as possible. Alison-Napolitano and Pesut, authors of *Bounce Forward: The Extraordinary Resilience of Nurse Leadership*, state that "personal renewal is important for your health and well-being—it allows you to show up for your life, and it gives you energy to do meaningful work . . . Renewal provides you with the interludes you need to solve complex problems with creativity" (2015, p. 42).

Interludes that lead to breakthrough thinking are built into work advances at Cincinnati Children's. During quarterly advances for assistant vice presidents and vice presidents of the Patient Services Division, fun activities pull thinking away from the task of creating strategy or budgets. Cooking healthy meals and repairing a playground for developmentally disabled children provide mental breaks and the opportunity to develop camaraderie and forge personal relationships.

Unlearning May Be Needed

A report published in *The Lancet* reviews strategies for transforming education to strengthen health systems in an interdependent world. The authors indicate that competencies to be developed include patient-centered care, interdisciplinary teams, evidence-based practice (EBP), continuous quality improvement, use of new informatics, and integration of public health. In short, undergraduate education needs to provide students with a foundation for lifelong learning (Frenk et al., 2010).

Part of the learning process is unlearning, which is necessary to enhance quality and safety. Unlearning is letting go of old knowledge or old ways of doing business. As difficult as unlearning may be, it is a skill that prepares you for a better way of doing something (Uldrich, 2011). The inability to unlearn can be detrimental to moving forward. As leaders, we can become victims of our own insights and past successes. This can cause us to cling to outdated recipes for success (Porter-O'Grady & Malloch, 2011). They add that "moving into a new age does not mean leaving everything behind. It does mean thinking about what needs to be left behind and reflecting on what does go with us as we move into an age with a different set of parameters" (Porter-O'Grady & Malloch, 2011, p. 10).

Every mile you go in the wrong direction is really a two-mile error. Unlearning is twice as hard as learning.

—Anonymous

Unlearning and breakthrough thinking can be supported by how our workplace and workflow is organized. Often, new structures and processes can help us to see different, more innovative possibilities that can be implemented.

▶ Innovative Organizational Structure

An innovative change in the way the Cincinnati Children's Patient Services Division is organized is making an important impact on patient care and on staff practice. The reorganization gives leaders responsibility for both inpatient and outpatient areas of the medical center. The concept was implemented first with a restructuring of responsibilities for vice presidents in the Patient Services Division. After a year, the division's assistant vice president roles were realigned to include inpatient and outpatient oversight in the patient care areas they managed. Later, the realignment cascaded to directors and managers. This departure from the silo structure of limiting patient care to strictly inpatient or outpatient broadened their perspective while also giving patients the opportunity to see the same caregivers in various healthcare settings.

Most hospital-based staff nursing roles are traditionally designated as either inpatient or outpatient, limiting the nurse's view of practice in other phases of the healthcare continuum. To expand that view, Cincinnati Children's nurse directors are collaborating to design caregiver roles that include work in both inpatient and outpatient settings. It is a major shift in how a person thinks about staffing and in how staff members think about their work. The newly designed roles place nursing and allied health staff in rotations between inpatient and outpatient settings. The anticipated aim is to do the following:

- Observe the patients' progress along the care continuum.
- Decrease burnout by providing nurses with a break from a highly intense or acute area (such as the cardiac intensive care unit) to a lesser acute area (such as the cardiology clinic).
- Increase job satisfaction (fewer weekend, holiday, and night shifts in the outpatient setting).
- Maintain skills and technical competence with frequent practice.

After piloting the research study with six nurses in three specialties, which was approved by the institutional review board (Mason & Fiorini, 2013), the study was expanded to 21 nurses in 10 specialties. The end goal is for the nurses to permanently rotate between settings within the same service line and spend half of their workweek in each setting. The aim is to determine the impact of the cross-setting role on the nurses' perspective of practice and on job satisfaction and engagement. Preliminary findings show promise in achieving the established aim of the research study.

Preliminary Findings

One nurse who had worked 6 years on the inpatient units found her knowledge broadened in numerous ways when she transitioned to working in the outpatient orthopedic clinics. In the outpatient setting, she learned a patient's entire history, she explained. She saw patients before they had surgery and understood why it was needed. Because of her inpatient experience, she was able to explain to patients and parents exactly what they could expect at the hospital. Then she would see them in the clinic for follow-up visits after surgery. She reported significant learning from being able to observe the entire continuum of care. The experience of interacting with a higher volume of patients and families each day, and the diverse ways of working with families (such as via telephone follow-up calls), has improved her communication skills. The outpatient setting nursing role has an enhanced focus on building relationships, which does not always happen in the hospital where nurses may see patients with short lengths of stay. For nurses who primarily worked in out-patient settings, the foray back into inpatient settings helped them to sharpen their skills, such as using IV pumps, and experience more invasive procedures that are not typically seen in outpatient settings. Another nurse said that rotating helped her understand what happens after the inpatient stay so she can better prepare patients for care beyond the hospital.

Challenges

Rotating nurses through both settings comes with challenges that leaders are work-ing to overcome:

- Scheduling is done differently in inpatient and outpatient settings. If rotating nurses are working a schedule that includes both inpatient and outpatient, the schedules need to accommodate both.
- Inpatient shifts are typically routine hours in the same location. Outpatient shifts often involve different locations and hours in the course of a week. This means that nurses who cannot travel to different locations or work different hours each day due to family obligations may not be suited to rotating schedules.

The best way to fill these blended roles is to have two inpatient nurses from the same service line jointly fill an outpatient job opening. After orientation to the outpatient setting, one nurse works inpatient while the other works outpatient, then they switch.

To further broaden the staff's perspective and to maintain staff competencies, a new organizational model is being implemented at Cincinnati Children's newly expanded Liberty campus, which is located 20 miles north of the hospital's main campus. Many of the operating room staff members at Liberty are the same care providers who work at the base hospital, giving them the experience of urban and suburban settings. As new inpatient staff are hired for the Liberty campus, they are asked to rotate to the main hospital location to enrich their perspective. The pediat-ric intensive care unit, oncology, and medical–surgical staff also rotate between lo-cations. Doing so allows staff to provide care for two different populations—Liberty is more of a community facility, and the hospital is quaternary (highly specialized care). With the cross-trained staff, greater coverage is enabled because the nurses can provide care where the patient need dictates.

Learning From Diverse Settings: Home Visits

Other organizational changes at Cincinnati Children's are having a positive impact on population health. One significant change resulted from a 2012 visit to Cuba. As an educational endeavor, 11 nurse leaders from across the United States visited the country; the visit included an overview of the Cuban health system. In Cuba, the space and cost of hospitalization is problematic, and home visits to patients are prevalent. These home visits are so effective in Cuba that they were pilot-tested and subsequently implemented at Cincinnati Children's with a goal to reduce readmissions for at-risk postacute populations. The program is designed to meet the transition of care needs for patients and families who are not eligible for traditional home health. Families receive a nurse home visit within 48 hours of discharge with this new home-visit program.

After 2 years of the Cincinnati Children's home-care program, which was funded with a grant from Patient-Centered Outcomes Research Institute (2013), nearly 375 patients were visited in their homes. Within 30 days of each visit, only 6.4% of patients were readmitted. At the same time, an additional 365 patients were referred for home visits, but the patients either refused the visit or the caregiver deemed that a visit was not necessary. Of this second group, 12.3% were readmitted or visited the emergency department. These results demonstrate a significant statistical difference and evidence that in-home assessments provide a valuable service that may reduce readmission for at-risk patient populations. Assessments show multiple examples of patient harm that was averted, improved coordination of care, and an overwhelmingly positive family experience.

Cincinnati Children's decided to initiate a home-visit program because it was deemed the right thing to do, regardless of reimbursement. The administrators believed that if patient care could be streamlined with home visits, the finances would follow. The same line of thinking resulted in Cincinnati Children's leadership developing a home-visit program for psychiatric patients; nurses provide patients with once-a-month injections to ensure compliance with medication regimes.

Increasing Role of Advanced-Practice Registered Nurses

In 4 years, the number of advanced-practice registered nurses (APRNs) at Cincinnati Children's has increased by 58%, to 348. The number is projected to continue to increase. Their value to the organization and to population health is evident in the number of requests and hires each year. The literature also supports their value. A systematic review (Newhouse et al., 2011) supports a high level of evidence that APRNs provide safe, effective, quality care to a number of specific populations in a variety of settings. Researchers concluded that "APRNs, in partnership with physicians and other providers, have a significant role in the promotion of health" (2011, p. 19). At Cincinnati Children's, APRNs currently work in inpatient and outpatient settings, including the following

- Outpatient clinics in more than 30 subspecialties
- School-based health centers
- Emergency rooms and urgent care settings
- Psychiatry
- Telehealth (pilot program for bariatric surgery patients)

APRNs also provide around-the-clock coverage in numerous inpatient units, including neonatal intensive care, cardiac intensive care, cardiology, neurosurgery, and general/colorectal surgery.

Playing the Role of Disruptor

Innovative organizational structures are designed and led by innovative leaders. One of the roles of an innovative leader is to be a disruptor. If there is an idea that is worth trying, disruptors push to test the implementation of the idea, even if it means treading into new territories. The view that we have never done it that way before is not a reason to shelve a new idea. One former Cincinnati Children's chief executive officer (CEO) instilled this thinking in his leadership staff: it is possible to move in two directions simultaneously.

As Ralph Nader so aptly stated, "I start with the premise that the function of leadership is to produce more leaders, not more followers" (Nader, n.d.). Being a disruptive leader may not be easy, and sometimes it can be uncomfortable, but many believe it is necessary for innovation.

▶ Innovative Practice Model

Health systems have renewed their focus on strengthening interdisciplinary collaboration for at least three reasons (Virkstis, 2012): "First, as the level of collaboration rises, the likelihood of negative outcomes diminishes" (2012, p. 2). Second, "interdisciplinary collaboration enhances the patient experience" (2012, p. 3). Third, "interdisciplinary communication can improve efficiency and reduce costs of patient care" (2012, p. 3).

In its report titled *The Future of Nursing: Leading Change, Advancing Health*, the Institute of Medicine (2011) states that "those involved in the healthcare system— nurses, physicians, patients, and others—play increasingly interdependent roles. Problems arise every day that do not have easy or singular solutions . . . What is needed is a style of leadership that involves working with others as full partners in a context of mutual respect and collaboration" (2011, pp. 222–223). The authors indicated that leadership should flow in all directions at all levels.

In 2002, Cincinnati Children's move to adopt a new multidisciplinary approach to patient care prompted leaders to rethink its practice model and to begin developing a new model based on interprofessional collaboration. In 2011, the medical center sought to transform the way the organization cares for its patients by building a model that focused on accountable care across the continuum (Hoying et al., 2014). As an academic medical center, Cincinnati Children's already had a history of embracing staff empowerment and shared decision making (Hoying & Allen, 2011). Shared governance for nursing was implemented at Cincinnati Children's in 1989, and a separate allied health structure was created in 1999. However, the two bodies operated in parallel with few occasions to interact and with little collaboration.

By 2005, this increase in collaborative practice precipitated discussions that questioned the purpose and efficiency of two separate structures (one for nursing, the other for allied health). The Patient Care Governance Council (PCGC) was formed in 2006, bringing professional staff together in a patient services shared governance structure. Organized around initiatives, the PCGC's goal was, and continues to be, to deliver better patient care through interprofessional collaboration.

To further enhance collaboration, the immediate past chairs of the Nursing Profession Coordinating Council (NPCC) and the PCGC began attending the Patient Care Committee meetings of the medical center's board of trustees. Also added to the meeting's list of attendees were representatives from pastoral care, physicians, and patients and their families. By 2012, council chairs were named to the medical center's Safety Operations Committee; the chairs of the Interprofessional Management Council and the Nursing Professional Practice Council (NPPC) joined leadership meetings as well. This structure ensures that all voices are heard by senior leadership.

Development of Interprofessional Practice Model

"The articulation of a professional practice model provides a framework for . . . the achievement of exemplary clinical outcomes" (Erickson, 2011, p. 35). Until 2006, the Patient Services Division at Cincinnati Children's had two separate practice models: one for nursing and one for allied health professionals. The two practice models ran parallel to each other and duplicated efforts, yet leaders agreed that achieving exemplary clinical outcomes requires input from all professions. It required new intra- and interprofessional practice behaviors for working together in new ways. To remedy the situation, leaders sought to develop a new practice model that would support the new vision of exemplary interprofessional care.

To allow true collaboration, leadership did not rush the process to develop, adopt, and implement a new practice model. Instead, because the medical center works within a shared governance structure, developing an interprofessional practice model could take shape only after careful analysis, consideration, and feedback from nursing and allied health staff. Development of the new model began in September 2012 when the NPPC initiated the process of reviewing and recommending changes to the nursing practice model. A review group was formed. In November 2012, the group recommended increased nursing participation in developing a revised practice model. Thirteen interdisciplinary focus groups were held to provide feedback and recommendations.

Next, the PCGC reviewed the focus group feedback and revised the practice model. In February 2013, the review group confidently agreed that the new Interprofessional Practice Model (IPM) provided a more succinct yet comprehensive representation of the expectations for nursing practice; the review group recommended that NPPC adopt the IPM as the only practice model for the nursing profession at Cincinnati Children's.

The NPPC agreed. The consensus was that the IPM was considered easier to understand than the current nursing practice model, and the opportunities for the broader interdisciplinary partnership through shared values and expectations outweighed the risks associated with maintaining a discipline-specific model.

Today, the resultant model (**FIGURE 14-1**) is the overarching conceptual framework for nursing and interdisciplinary patient care at Cincinnati Children's. The figure depicts how all parties collaborate, communicate, and develop professionally to provide patients the highest quality of care. It incorporates these six facets:

- Safety
- Professionalism
- Best practice
- Collaborative relationships
- Comprehensive coordinated care
- Innovation and research

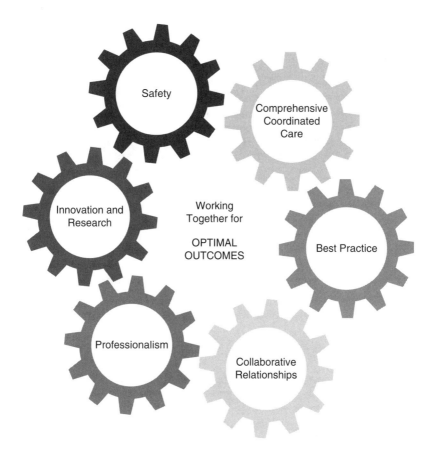

FIGURE 14-1 Working together for optimal outcomes.

Reproduced from Cincinnati Children's Hospital Medical Center (2013).

Since implementation, feedback from frontline nurses about the impact of this new practice model has included the following:

- "It requires mutual respect from the entire care team . . . it is getting us to a new way of practice for the future."
- "It truly is a team-based approach to patient care with the patient's optimal outcome in the center."

The timeline of the IPM's formation, which included allied health, is outlined in **FIGURE 14-2**.

The implementation of the new practice model was not without challenges. More than 2 years after the practice model was launched, the level of understanding and implementation varies across the organization. To improve recognition and promote day-to-day usage of the IPM, practice councils continually discuss and review the benefits of using it in problem solving and decision making. For example, clinicians were unable to reach a decision about chlorhexidine baths for patients, so they looked to the gears of the IPM to determine the sticking point. The gears in the model clarify how it works, unlike the former model, which had a lot of words but was not easy to digest.

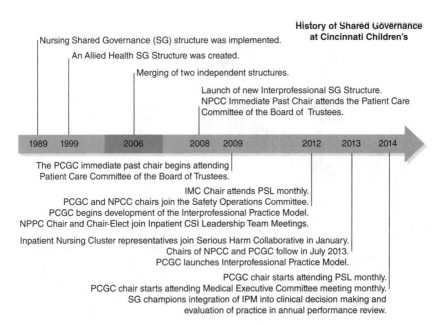

FIGURE 14-2 Timeline.
Property of Cincinnati Children's Hospital Medical Center.

FIGURE 14-3 Decision-making worksheet.
Property of Cincinnati Children's Hospital Medical Center.

To help staff effectively use the practice model for decision making and problem solving, a worksheet (**FIGURE 14-3**) is available on the Cincinnati Children's intranet in the shared governance pages. Staff members are encouraged to use the worksheet to help make decisions and find solutions.

All patient services staff members can submit a problem or idea to the NPCC. This is indicative of the highly collaborative nature of Cincinnati Children's shared governance structure. Accessed online via the shared governance web page, the submission process gives everyone a voice. After submissions are received, they are reviewed by the NPCC, who then assigns them to the appropriate council for review. An online database charts the progress of each submission; 70 to 80 submissions are received each year.

> … [I]nnovation excellence is often built in a multiyear effort that touches most, if not all, parts of the organization. (de Jong, Marston, & Roth, 2015, p. 47)

Since 1989, this staff-driven structure of governance has been at the core of Cincinnati Children's Patient Services Division. Additionally, the inpatient, hospital-wide, management-driven Operational Excellence initiative was implemented in 2014. The focus of Operational Excellence is to improve safety, the patient and family experience, and the flow in inpatient areas through empowered and accountable unit leaders. Each unit's clinical director and medical director manage the operations of their units and work together to improve the unit culture and clinical results. These leaders are responsible for a partnered approach to unit-level strategic thinking and planning, communication, and improvement, all with the goal of creating focus, defining priorities, and building a culture of engagement and ownership. Across the unit leadership, teams apply safety, leadership, and staffing principles, processes, advanced situation awareness, and risk prediction tools.

Shared governance and Operational Excellence share the same passionate intent: to dramatically improve patient care and safety while delivering better outcomes and patient and employee experiences. This intent is also prominent in the medical center's strategic plan.

The challenge for the future at Cincinnati Children's is to develop a model where all staff, in every division and profession, work within the same model and by the same agreed-upon tenets. A step in that direction is still in development.

Interprofessional Education

To fully ingrain the idea of interprofessional practice into the minds of clinicians, you should look upstream to the educational process. This is where clinicians can first learn about the value of an interdisciplinary approach to patient care. The work of the Institute of Medicine (2011) and others has clearly shown that healthcare professionals who understand each others' roles and are able to communicate and work effectively as a team are more likely to provide safe and effective patient care.

> Continuing to function in the educational silos of current educational institutions limits formalized exposure to interdisciplinary opportunities, compromises the ability to function in future team based practice and research environments, and contributes to the lack of skill portability required by students and faculty in diverse and constantly changing facility and community-based service environments. (Jansen, 2008, p. 222)

Jansen believes that multiple barriers exist in the development and teaching of teamwork in healthcare students: "Thus, the emphasis on business values of cost-effective operations means that resources are not readily directed to support the education and development of interdisciplinary teams, a factor that may affect the ability of health professionals to participate in a team context" (Jansen, 2008, p. 220).

Additional barriers include reluctance to alter curricula to include interprofessional education and logistics of scheduling common times for students to engage in interdisciplinary education.

In an unpublished study of the effectiveness of interprofessional teamwork at Cincinnati Children's, 26 nursing and medical students worked together in three pediatric simulation training exercises over an 8-month period. The results indicated that their learned scores were higher than control groups who did not train in an interprofessional setting. Nursing students demonstrated a higher score on teamwork, collaboration, and positive professional identification compared to medical students in both groups. Plans to continue simulation training in an interprofessional environment are underway, with a goal to boost teamwork among all hospital professions.

When representatives from the Robert Wood Johnson Foundation visited Cincinnati Children's in preparation for writing a white paper about interprofessional collaboration, they witnessed the simulation training previously described and the importance of training people in the manner in which they work. "At Cincinnati Children's we were able to see the powerful effects of reflection on a simulation, and how the realizations that occur during reflection can translate to improving interprofessional collaboration and patient care" (Robert Wood Johnson Foundation, 2015, p. 44). Instead of nurses practicing with nurses and doctors practicing with doctors, they witnessed the benefit of training in multidisciplinary teams—physicians, nurses, respiratory therapists—just as in the clinical environment. "At the end of the day, interprofessional collaboration is more than a philosophy—it is about getting real work done through teams" (Robert Wood Johnson Foundation, 2015, p. 45).

DISCUSSION

If you were in a healthcare system, what would be an ideal organizational structure to blend both inpatient and outpatient care delivery? What changes would you make to ensure that caregivers provide services where the need exists instead of expecting patients to come to caregivers? As you contemplate settings, consider community centers, homes, and schools.

▶ Innovative Employee Engagement

Employees are the cornerstone of a successful organization. They are often the "face" of a healthcare system and can be the best resource for ideas that improve processes. Employees who feel empowered and appreciated will contribute in immeasurable ways. The topics described next can result in an engaged workforce, satisfied patients, and a safer environment.

You Cannot Be Innovative Unless You Have an Engaged Staff

Effective organizations should have a culture that encourages employee satisfaction. "When employees believe in and trust their management it motivates and encourages employees' participation in decision making which improves employees' efforts, benefits their job satisfaction and commitment to work" (Appelbaum et al., 2013, p. 222).

Yet, as indicated by General Electric in its report *Strategies for Success: Managing Complexity in Health Care* (2015), in the United States less than 43% of the healthcare workforce is happy. That is down from 61% in 1983 and 55% in 2005. It is an even worse situation in Europe, where only 11–23% of the workforce feels engaged. As the authors point out, the constant decline in satisfaction at work is "despite all of the leadership development programs and other initiatives to help managers engage and motivate their teams" (2015, p. 13).

Worse, according to a Gallup report, "30% of U.S. workers are engaged" (2013, p. 8), "52% are not engaged" (2013, p. 12), and "18% are actively disengaged" (2013, p. 13). In a separate study of one hospital system, Gallup found that engagement translates to revenue (Kamins, 2015). The study results indicated that fully engaged physicians were 26% more productive than their less-engaged counterparts, which amounts to an additional $460,000 on average in patient revenue per physician per year.

The authors of the General Electric report (2015) attribute disengagement trends to overcomplicated workplaces. Managers spend about 40% of their time writing reports (matrices, scorecards, etc.) and 30% of their time in meetings, which does not leave much time to work with their teams. As a result, teams do not get the support they need, and consequently they become overworked and disengaged.

The answer, the report states (General Electric, 2015), is not to bring in psychologists to create soft initiatives (a common response). Rather, it suggests the following:

- Simplifying
- Making sure management adds value
- Cooperating
- Giving staff the power to take risks
- Creating feedback loops that expose staff to the consequences of their actions
- Removing layers that do not add value
- Rewarding those who cooperate

The American College of Healthcare Executives (2015) indicates that the most engaged employees are those who are able to make daily progress on meaningful work. They recognize meaningful work as that which helps the organization move forward and achieve its goals. This can be achieved only if the organization's goals are clear, attainable, and broadly communicated.

DISCUSSION

Imagine you are assigned the role of chief nursing officer in a system with poor employee engagement. What ideas would you implement to boost engagement? How would you ensure that long-term engagement remained?

Positioning Nurses to Lead Change

The Institute of Medicine (2011), in response to objectives set forth in the Patient Protection and Affordable Care Act of 2010, states that nurses should be well positioned to lead change and advance health in an evolving healthcare system. The institute's recommendations include the following:

- Remove the scope of practice barriers; nurses should be able to practice to the full extent of their education and training.

- Nurses should achieve higher levels of education and training through an improved education system that promotes seamless academic progression.
- Nurses should be full partners, with physicians and other healthcare professionals, in redesigning health care.
- Effective workforce planning and policy making requires better data collection and an improved information infrastructure.
- Ensure that nurses engage in lifelong learning. (Institute of Medicine, 2011, pp. 29–34)

Shared governance and empowerment go hand in hand; in one study, researchers found that in a hospital setting there was a statistically significant positive relationship between perceptions of shared governance and empowerment (Barden, Griffin, Donahue, & Fitzpatrick, 2011).

Popular author and speaker Matthew Kelly (2011) states, "One of the major issues plaguing human potential in the corporate world today is work-life balance . . . The future of an organization and the potential of its employees are intertwined; their destinies are linked?. . . An organization can only become the-best-version-of-itself to the extent that the people who drive that organization are becoming better-versions-of-themselves" (p. vii).

Broadening the Scope

An innovative way to encourage staff members to think beyond their own care setting is being implemented by Intermountain Healthcare based in Salt Lake City (Boston-Fleischhauer, 2014a). Leaders there have begun a nurse shadowing program, enabling nurses to spend 24 hours over the course of 3 months shadowing a nurse in another care setting within the health system.

For example, a nurse in the pediatric intensive care unit can shadow a nurse in the emergency department. Or a nurse working in an inpatient setting can shadow a nurse in an outpatient clinic, and vice versa. To ensure nurses participating in the program have a meaningful shadowing experience, leaders set clear learning objectives and ask shadowing nurses to write clinical narratives about their experience. **BOX 14-1** summarizes the objectives and focus of the shadowing experience.

At Cincinnati Children's, nurses are offered a different shadowing opportunity. For 7 years the Nurse Exchange Program has provided the opportunity for nurses to share their expertise with colleagues from eight pediatric hospitals around the nation. The goal is for experienced nurses to seek, learn, and share best nursing practices. This can be accomplished by adoption of a best practice, improvement science project, or further investigation of research at the unit or organizational level. At Cincinnati Children's, participation is open to RNII-level nurses with a minimum of 2 years of employment.

Employee Engagement and Patient Satisfaction

When their accreditation agency served Midland Memorial Hospital in Midland, Texas, with a leadership deficiency notice, they were faced with an urgent need to boost patient satisfaction scores. The low scores were caused, in part, by low levels of employee engagement. Although leaders had assumed that employee engagement and patient satisfaction would improve substantially with the opening of a new tower in late 2012, in reality the reverse occurred. After a year they found that their beautiful new facility raised patient expectations but did not alter the care experience.

BOX 14-1 Summary of Shadow Experience

The objectives and focus of the shadowing experience are as follows:

- To understand:
  - The role of the RN
  - The care process
  - Challenges in the setting
  - The patient care operation
  - Clinical goals
  - Compliance and regulatory issues pertaining to nursing practice
  - Role of the patient and family in the care process
  - Patient access to the setting and movement through the setting
- To hear about satisfiers in the setting
- To dialogue:
  - Related to what is important to know about learning to practice here
  - Ideas for nursing practice evolution to meet future patient care needs

Leaders committed to change, and, with assistance from consulting firm Values Coach Inc., they spent 2014 implementing new ideas. Information gleaned from a culture assessment survey of employees confirmed low employee engagement and a perception of an overly negative workplace environment. The results were shared with staff members, who were asked to pledge that they would no longer participate in complaining, gossiping, and other negative attitudes. Staff members also were asked to recite a daily self-empowerment pledge. Ultimately, the hospital's values statement was rewritten, and all staff members were enrolled in a series of courses on personal values.

In a case study on values and cultural initiative (Tye, 2014), Midland Memorial president and CEO Russell Meyers reported, "As a result of our commitment to a culture of ownership, we have documented record-high patient satisfaction and clinical quality indicators and have calculated a cultural productivity benefit of more than $7 million annually" (2014, p. 2).

To create and maintain a healthy work environment, three structures must be in place: leadership, design, and staffing (Dent, Armstead, & Evans, 2014). Evidence and scientific data can build a road map to ideal nurse staffing. This road map could lead to higher quality and efficiency in the delivery of care, according to Baggett and colleagues (2014). With these findings in mind, Midland Memorial incorporated evidence and scientific data into the complex process of nurse staffing. Midland Memorial's Robert Dent, senior vice president and chief operating and chief nursing officer, said the following:

> Each unit is unique particular to patient populations, acuities of the patients, skill mix of nurses, education and competency of the nurses among other variables to consider in making assignments. Understanding these variables, the clinical managers, staffed mostly 24-hours per day, seven days per week, have the power and autonomy to make appropriate nurse staffing assignments. Nursing leaders must understand data-driven nurse staffing plans to clearly communicate and budget appropriately for nursing resources. (Dent, 2015, p. 44)

Empowered Employees Reduce Injury Rate

Cincinnati Children's robust psychiatric program includes 125 beds (acute and long-term care) at three facilities and offers daytime hospitalization for an additional 30-plus patients. Many patients have behavioral challenges. Injuries to mental health specialists and other caregivers unfortunately did occur. Periodic injuries to staff were thought to be part of the job. Asked to make recommendations regarding ways to reduce (ideally to eliminate) staff injuries, the team took a situation awareness approach. Situation awareness is recognized as a way to reduce serious safety breaches in patients, according to a Cincinnati Children's study (Brady et al., 2013).

Empowered with a different mind-set (injuries will no longer be considered a routine consequence of the job), the staff developed a situation awareness planning tool (**FIGURE 14-4**) and an algorithm (**FIGURE 14-5**) that includes steps for predicting patients at risk, mitigation planning, communication, and next steps if aggression results in staff injury or patient restraint. In the 2 years since the tool was implemented, the baseline days between Occupational Safety and Health Administration (OSHA) injuries more than doubled, and the baseline days between patient injuries that required treatment beyond first aid increased more than sixfold.

DISCUSSION

Although much focus has been placed on patient injury rates, how much focus should be placed on staff injury rates? What are your ideas for boosting resiliency and decreasing stress and injuries among staff? How often should employee injury rates be conveyed? Should employee injury rates be as readily available as patient injury rates? Should they be made public or kept internally?

Unit: Date: Shift: Outgoing Staff Name: Incoming Staff Name:
SA Triggers: FR = Flight Risk WH = Watch Hot WC = Watch Cold A = Aggressor ST = Self Threat MC = Medical Concern FC = Family Visitor
                                                             Concern

Name, Room Number			
SA Trigger			
S/R High Risk			
Aggression/ Escalation Signs			
Plan			
PRN Medication			
Expected Outcome Must Be Yes/No Criteria			
Outcome Deadline (specific time)			
Escalation/ Contingency Plan			

FIGURE 14-4 Situation awareness planning tool.

Property of Cincinnati Children's Hospital Medical Center.

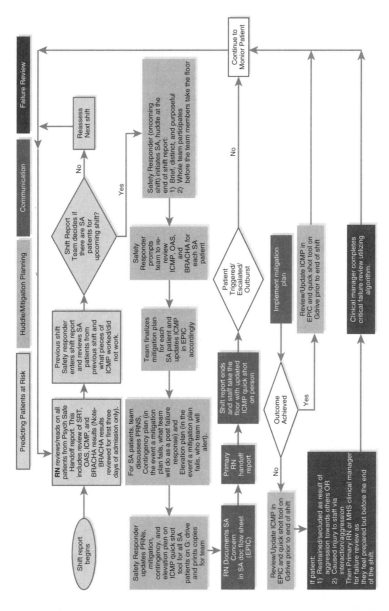

FIGURE 14-5 Situational awareness algorithm.

Property of Cincinnati Children's Hospital Medical Center.

Empowerment, Engagement, and Recognition

Staff should be encouraged to suggest new ideas to improve outcomes, then be willing to test their implementation. They will not always be successful, but improvement comes only with the willingness to try. It is important to applaud the efforts of staff who are eager to test new ideas. Recognizing and celebrating achievements can go a long way in boosting engagement, even if those achievements are small. Harvard Business School researchers found that when it comes to change, recognizing small wins serves to regularly confirm for staff members that they are making progress on meaningful work (Amabile & Kramer, 2011).

▶ Innovative Thinking

Empowering employees not only results in engagement, it also can generate innovative ideas. The following are examples of innovative thinking that are having an impact on patients at Cincinnati Children's. Ideas can originate from expected (and sometimes unexpected) sources, such as leaders, staff members, patients, and families.

Collaborating for Patient Safety

> . . . [T]here's no proven formula for success, particularly when it comes to innovation. (de Jong, Marston, & Roth, 2015, p. 37)

Sometimes a good idea evolves into a great idea. Children's Hospitals Solutions for Patient Safety (www.solutionsforpatientsafety.org) is one such example. Here is how the idea got its start.

In the 1980s, pediatric hospitals in Ohio formed the Ohio Children's Hospital Association (OCHA) to advocate for legislative and regulatory issues that affect children's health. Over time the group's aim broadened to emphasize quality and safety. As Ohio state officials became more aware of OCHA and its success in improving quality and safety, they asked for OCHA's involvement on quality improvement projects. The results were impressive and included reducing surgical site infections, adverse drug events, and serious harm events.

After achieving significant results in the state, Ohio's children's hospitals were asked in 2011 to lead a national effort to implement their strategies in children's hospitals throughout the country. In 2012, 25 hospitals from across the nation joined the Ohio hospitals, forming the Children's Hospital's Solutions for Patient Safety (SPS) network.

By 2015 the SPS network—funded in part by the Cardinal Health Foundation—had grown to more than 80 children's hospitals nationwide. Their shared visions are as follows:

- No child will ever experience serious harm while we are trying to heal them.
- By putting aside competition and sharing our safety successes and failures, we can achieve our goals faster.
- We all learn from and all teach each other to ensure every child is safe in our care, every day.

The network members support each other on their journey toward zero harm by providing frequent training and learning opportunities, tools, data collection and analysis, and opportunities to collaborate. Together they committed to these shared network goals of harm reduction:

- 40% reduction in hospital-acquired conditions
- 10% reduction in readmissions
- 25% reduction in serious safety events

To achieve these goals, CEOs, hospital boards of trustees, and clinical leaders are aligning their organizational goals with the network harm reduction goals in a way that is transforming the safety and quality of care delivered in children's hospitals in the United States.

DISCUSSION

How can hospitals be more transparent with patients on their quality scores? What role can partnerships among hospitals play in boosting quality and safety? Using SPS as an example, how would you initiate such a partnership?

Daily Briefs Focus on Quality and Safety

Huddles can lead to improved efficiencies and quality of information sharing, as well as increased levels of accountability, empowerment, and sense of community, according to researchers Goldenhar, Brady, Sutcliffe, and Muething (2013). Together these create a culture of collaboration and collegiality that increases the staff's quality of collective awareness and enhanced capacity for eliminating patient harm.

Although small huddles take place frequently throughout all Cincinnati Children's locations, a house-wide daily safety brief, held each morning at 8:35, recaps the previous day and plans for the current day. Key leaders from the following areas attend in person or via phone:

- Employee safety
- Family relations
- Emergency department
- Inpatient services
- Perioperative area
- Outpatient services
- Psychiatry
- Home health
- Pharmacy
- Radiology
- Laboratory
- Infection prevention and control
- Supply chain
- Information services
- Protective services
- Facilities

The briefing puts real-time knowledge into the hands of those who can predict and solve problems. The following occurs at each daily safety brief:

1. A review of safety and quality issues from the past 24 hours
2. Discussion of quality and safety issues that may occur in the next 24 hours so they can be anticipated, predicted, and planned for
3. Follow-up report on issues identified today or on previous days and what is being done to resolve them (e.g., repair plan for malfunctioning equipment, update on manufacturer back order on equipment, update on pharmaceutical shortage)

These morning gatherings have plenty of benefits, including the following: (1) help the journey to high reliability by making sure staff members are preoccupied with quality and safety, (2) keep staff at all sites on the same page, (3) identify and fix problems while they are small, and (4) provide a distinct determination of who is responsible for an issue and when the fix will occur.

Each day, units and departments have their own safety briefs. The information that is compiled and shared at these smaller briefs are fed to the house-wide brief.

Three Daily Huddles for Perioperative Safety

As previously mentioned, huddles can create a culture of collaboration and collegiality that increases the staff's quality of collective awareness and enhances the capacity for eliminating patient harm. Cincinnati Children's perioperative team is aiming to accomplish each of these objectives with three daily huddles (**TABLE 14-1**).

TABLE 14-1 Huddle Summary

Time of Huddle	Who Attends	Reason for Huddle
6:45 a.m.	▪ Charge nurse for same-day surgery, OR, and PACU ▪ Anesthesiologist ▪ Perioperative coordinators ▪ SPD manager ▪ VAT, MRI	▪ Review the status of every patient ▪ Change a patient's risk level if appropriate
2:15 p.m.	▪ Charge nurse for same-day surgery, OR, and PACU ▪ Anesthesiologist ▪ Perioperative coordinators ▪ SPD manager ▪ VAT, MRI	The charge nurse runs the huddle ▪ Every patient's risk level is determined based on health condition, procedure, or both ▪ Patients arriving the next day are reviewed
9:00 p.m.	▪ OR and PACU charge nurse ▪ Anesthesia board runner	Patient status is reviewed with input from staff members and perioperative coordinators, who have been updated by surgeon and anesthesia

TABLE 14-2 Patient Status Color Tracking

Color	Description
Green	All clear, patient prepared and verified that there are no threats to patient safety through the perioperative area.
Yellow	Keep close watch; elevated risk factors for patient safety identified (e.g., another patient has same last name, patient has behavioral issues or comorbidities). Proceed with caution. Communicate additional needs to charge nurse.
Orange	High-alert risk for patient vulnerability during the perioperative process (e.g., transplant patient). Requires additional resources and/or support from perioperative expert.
Red	The highest indicator, which requires stopping the line until the perioperative safety communication system has resolved the identified threat (e.g., equipment is malfunctioning).

At each huddle, the patient status (**TABLE 14-2**) is recorded and tracked throughout the patient's stay. This status is reported at Cincinnati Children's daily operations brief, previously mentioned.

At any time, any staff member is eligible to throw in the red card. Doing so stops activity until the concern is resolved. Convincing nurses to feel comfortable stopping a procedure can be challenging, yet nurses have an important voice that must be heard.

The following excerpt from an article published by the Robert Wood Johnson Foundation speaks to the need for all voices to be heard (Robert Wood Johnson Foundation, 2011):[1]

> Mary Jean Schumann DNP, MBA, RN, CPNP, executive director of the Nursing Alliance for Quality Care, a Foundation-funded partnership among the nation's leading nursing organizations and consumer groups, touts shared decision-making and better communication as effective strategies, and says it "comes down to the culture. Everyone needs to be heard." Too often, she notes, nurses are not in the room when solutions are devised and are brought in only when it's time to talk about implementation. Even when nurses are included in problem-solving, "a single nursing voice is not enough," she cautions.
>
> Aline Holmes MSN, RN, director of the New Jersey Hospital Association's Institute for Quality and Patient Safety, says nurses need to push themselves as well. "We need to get out there, develop more leadership

---

[1] Copyright 2011. Robert Wood Johnson Foundation. Used with permission from the Robert Wood Johnson Foundation.

skills—but top leadership needs to support that too. They need to focus on quality and safety, and bring nurses into those conversations." (Robert Wood Johnson Foundation, 2011, para. 13–14)

The Robert Wood Johnson Foundation (2010) commissioned a poll that found that large majorities of opinion leaders would like to see nurses exert more influence in a number of areas. Reducing medical errors and improving patient safety (90%) and improving quality of care (89%) topped the list.

Reuniting Patients and Their Pets

Often great ideas come from patients. At Cincinnati Children's, one such idea came from a teenage cancer patient. She spent so much time in the hospital, she knew the pain of not being able to spend time with her beloved dogs, so she set a goal to see that other kids would not feel that pain.

We have known that animal-assisted interventions, which include both animal-assisted activities and therapies, have historically been beneficial to human health. When the animal is the patient's beloved pet, the benefits might be even greater. "Animal-facilitated therapy has shown to decrease pain, change vital signs, provide distraction, decrease fear, increase socialization, increase pleasure and decrease emotional distress in hospitalized pediatric patients" (Urbanski & Lazenby, 2012, p. 272).

In 2013, thanks to efforts by the teenage cancer patient and others, a grant was secured and the Pet Center at Cincinnati Children's opened, enabling reunions between sick children and their beloved pets. Since then, reunions are commonplace, including patients who, after weeks in isolation due to a bone marrow transplant, are wheeled to the Pet Center for what they describe as the best day they had during their month in the hospital. Since the Pet Center opened, dogs, cats, a guinea pig, and a rabbit have enjoyed visits with their owners. Many families indicate the reunion is the first time things felt normal since their child was admitted.

The Pet Center, believed to be one of the few of its kind in the country, is mostly indoors. Radiant heat makes it comfortable except during Cincinnati's coldest winter days. Pet visits are available to children who have been hospitalized 5 or more days, pending approval of their medical team. Many children have not seen their pets in months. Their emotional reunions are exactly what the teenage cancer patient had in mind, says her mother. Sadly, the patient lost her battle with cancer at age 19, shortly after the Pet Center opened. However, this young woman's dream to reunite patients with their pets has resulted in an enduring legacy.

One-of-a-Kind Program Has Worldwide Impact

A frustrated emergency department nurse manager at Cincinnati Children's came up with an idea that has had worldwide impact (Riehle, Daston, Rutkowski, & Wehman, 2012). Erin Riehle, MSN, RN, had a difficult time keeping the emergency department supply room stocked, and she eventually hired a young woman with Down syndrome for the job. This was the beginning of Project SEARCH, a one-of-a-kind program that helps young people with intellectual and developmental disabilities make successful transitions from school or sheltered workshops to integrated, competitive employment.

Since that day in 1996 when the program began, Project SEARCH has grown to more than 400 sites in a variety of businesses across the United States and in Canada, England, Scotland, Ireland, and Australia. In the near future, programs are likely in Germany, Gibraltar, Holland, India, Israel, and Wales.

Project SEARCH programs serve nearly 3,500 young adults each year, totaling nearly 30,000 young adults with disabilities since its inception. The rate of employment is 69.5%, which means that 20,850 young adults with significant disabilities have found jobs that translate to more fulfilling lives, work in inclusive settings, access to employer-paid benefits, and the potential to live independently.

Project SEARCH is an impressive example of the results that can be attained not only by empowering staff but by having the willingness to test new ideas.

Partnering to Improve Outcomes

Cincinnati Children's 2015 strategic plan called all staff to lead, advocate, and collaborate to improve the health of local children with asthma, the most common childhood chronic illness affecting children. Asthma is especially prevalent among Cincinnati's African American children from low socioeconomic and inner-city backgrounds. Within Hamilton County, where Cincinnati is located, one child in every six has been diagnosed with asthma. One of the most common barriers that impedes positive health outcomes for this population is medication adherence (Burgess, Sly, & Devadason, 2012).

Obtaining a child's corticosteroid inhaler in a timely manner was often hampered by logistical problems (Crosby, 2012). To alleviate the obstacle and to help prevent visits to the emergency department, Cincinnati Children's formed innovative partnerships with local pharmacies. Tapping into recent advancements in technology for prescription refill automation, affected patients now are provided automated refills and home delivery of medications. Initially the goal was to increase the inhaled corticosteroid refill rate from 20% to 50% through these partnerships. After the intervention, the monthly fill rate now is 80%, and the program has spread to a second county near Cincinnati.

Partnering with school nurses has further improved outcomes for children with asthma, as reported by Kimberly Toole (2013). What began in 2006 in eight schools now has spread to the entire Cincinnati public school district. The partnership provides school nurses with additional training about asthma and access to a student's asthma action plan and medication records via access to the electronic health record. The goal of these interventions, although not yet determined, includes increased school attendance for the students living with asthma and increased work time for parents.

Providing a Service: The Right Thing to Do

According to the American Hospital Association (2012), annually one in four Americans experiences a behavioral health-related illness. Nearly half of all Americans will develop a mental illness during their lifetime, and 27% will suffer from a substance abuse disorder. Although chronic behavioral health disorders primarily affect adults, half of all chronic mental illness begins by the age of 14 years, and three-quarters begin by the age of 24 years. Of the adults with mental illness, the majority also have a comorbid physical condition. One of every four admissions to a general hospital has a behavioral health disorder.

A FUN TWEAK TO DISCHARGE INSTRUCTIONS

It is common to send an asthmatic child home from the hospital with written discharge instructions. It can be more effective to demonstrate the proper use of an inhaler with an instructional video starring the patient.

Discussion

Think of a time that you proposed a new idea to a colleague or supervisor, and answer the following questions:

- How did you make your case for your suggestion?
- Did it encompass both art and science?
- How was your suggestion received?
- Did it get implemented?
- If it was deployed, what were the results?
- If not acted upon, would your suggestion work today?

To help address the need for highly specialized hospital-based behavioral health services, Cincinnati Children's has devoted a total of 125 beds (acute and long-term care) at three facilities to patients with behavioral issues. The decision to do so, in spite of a lack of financial reimbursement, was made because it was necessary and important. The medical center's former CEO believed that, when faced with a dilemma, people should ask themselves three times, "Is it the right thing to do?" If the answer is always yes, then it must be done, no matter how hard it is to pursue. Although caring for psychiatric patients is costly and challenging, it is best for the community according to this line of thinking.

Sam, an adolescent female, is a perfect example of how facing the challenges of caring for psychiatric patients can have far-reaching benefits. "After losing her father, Rob, to suicide in 2008, Sam struggled with depression and post-traumatic stress disorder. More than two years after his death, Sam thought about suicide herself and on two different occasions spent time at [Cincinnati] Children's Hospital" (Salmons, 2014).

Because she does not want children in similar situations to feel as helpless and alone as she once did, Sam founded Rob's Kids, "an organization 'passionately committed to making a difference in the lives of children who struggle with depression or post-traumatic stress disorder'" (Salmons, 2014).

Benefits Patient and Pharmacist

Traditionally, Cincinnati Children's lung transplant clinical pharmacist and cystic fibrosis clinical pharmacist have visited only the hospital's inpatients. By expanding their reach to the hospital clinics, the pharmacists have provided continuity of care for their patients (previously, clinic patients did not see a pharmacist during visits). The change has also provided pharmacists with a broader perspective of their work.

During a trial period, in addition to inpatient visits, the lung transplant clinical pharmacist saw four patients in the clinic for a total of 10 separate encounters. The average time spent during each encounter was 1 hour. Follow-up comments from the pharmacist indicate significant benefits to the patient. The pharmacist's notes include the following:

- Identified inappropriate medication list and updated with the coordinator
- Identified inappropriate dosages of medications due to patient's weight gain
- Numerous recommendations for antibiotics, weaning of sedation medications, immunizations, switching from liquid to tablet form (patient could not tolerate liquid, but care team was not aware of this)
- Patient counseling occurs at every visit; many patients are on more than 15 medications with multiple drug–drug and drug–nutrient interactions

In this same period of time, the cystic fibrosis clinical pharmacist saw 30 individual patients during clinic visits. Learnings from this pharmacist include the following:

- During visits, discrepancies on the patients' medication lists were caught
- Medication education is helping to increase adherence and understanding
- Involvement in two patient admissions from clinic to hospital. They are able to assist the physician with the choice of antibiotics and any medication changes that should be made during hospitalization

Because visiting clinic patients is in addition to the pharmacists' already crowded workload, a challenge moving forward will be to find the time and resources to accommodate the expanded appointment schedule. Pharmacists and staff members who go the extra mile and are willing to try innovative new ideas that improve patient care also need to be encouraged to care for themselves. Innovators need resiliency!

▶ Innovative Ways to Build Resilience

Resilience is defined as the ability to become strong, healthy, or successful again after something bad happens. In the healthcare arena, resilient staff can more quickly recover from the frequent disruptions, stressful situations, and turbulence of our constantly changing environment. A person with a high level of resilience tends "to be skilled in preparing for emotional emergencies (as can happen frequently in patient care settings) and adept at accepting what comes at them with flexibility rather than rigidity—times are tough but I know they will get better" (Waters, 2013, para. 5).

Authors Zolli and Healy indicate that personal resilience is a habit: "Whether cultivated through wise mentors, vigorous exercise, access to green space, or a particularly rich relationship with faith, the habits of personal resilience are habits of mind—making them habits we can cultivate and change when armed with the right resources" (2012, p. 130).

A 2012 Gallup poll (Bass & McGeeney, 2012) found that nurses, along with the general adult population, are more likely to smoke and less likely to eat healthy and exercise than physicians. Obesity is more prevalent among nurses than physicians. Armed with the knowledge that resilience can be developed over time and that nurses lag behind their physician colleagues in healthy behaviors, Cincinnati Children's has implemented numerous programs aimed at improving staff resilience, health, and wellness.

Walking Desks

Staff members who spend most days sitting at a desk can get a boost of energy and improve their mood with a quick exercise break. To make those breaks easier to take, walking desks were installed in areas of Cincinnati Children's where staff members are less likely to be on their feet at work, including the administrative area in the Specialty Resource Unit. The desks provide the opportunity to walk in place while working on a laptop or taking a break. In an interview in *Nursing Administration Quarterly* (Sanford, 2015), Senior Vice President of Patient Services Cheryl Hoying indicates, "I have a walking desk in my office so I can get 10,000 steps a day in while I work" (2015, p. 100).

Another frequent walker at Cincinnati Children's states, "The desk in my area is a great way to boost my energy level and decrease my stress after long periods sitting. I love that I can be active at work while still completing my job responsibilities." With a walking desk, leaders are able to model good behavior by exercising while answering e-mails and other seated tasks.

Healthy Challenge

Regular exercise can help prevent the impact of stress on the body. There are "substantial and highly statistically significant associations between the frequency of moderate to vigorous physical activity (MVPA) and different indicators of psychological distress. Frequent participation in MVPA reduces psychological distress and decreases the likelihood of falling into a high-risk category" (Perales, Pozo-Cruz, & Pozo-Cruz, 2014, p. 91).

Encouraging a healthier lifestyle through regular exercise, proper nutrition, and healthier habits as a way to improve staff resilience is the goal of a quarterly healthy challenge for the Patient Services Division at Cincinnati Children's. Each challenge enables staff to earn points in the workplace wellness program that supports employees as they adopt and sustain behaviors that reduce health risks and improve quality of life.

More than 1,000 staff members routinely accept the challenge each quarter. Some challenges are suggested by staff members who are eager to engage their co-workers in the typically fun activities. Challenges have included the following:

- Trying a new vegetable each week for 4 weeks
- Doing one new thing each week for 4 weeks that will result in less stress and a calmer holiday season
- Completing a triathlon over a 4-week period
- Kicking a bad habit

Schwartz Center Rounds

Could the stresses of today's healthcare system threaten the delivery of compassionate care? Schwartz Center Rounds, implemented at Cincinnati Children's in 2014, provides an outlet to openly and honestly discuss the social and emotional issues caregivers face in working with patients and families. Each monthly session begins with panelists from diverse disciplines, including physicians, nurses, social workers, psychologists, and allied health professionals, who share an experience on an identified case or topic. Afterward, caregivers in the audience are invited to share their own perspectives on the case and broader related issues. The premise is that caregivers are better able to make personal connections with patients and colleagues when they have greater insight into their own responses and feelings.

This national program is now in place at more than 400 healthcare facilities. The Schwartz Center website (www.theschwartzcenter.org) reports these benefits as expressed by participants:

- Increased insight into the social and emotional aspects of patient care, increased feelings of compassion toward patients, and increased readiness to respond to patients' and families' needs.
- Improved teamwork, interdisciplinary communication, and appreciation for the roles and contributions of colleagues from different disciplines.
- Decreased feelings of stress and isolation and more openness to giving and receiving support.

Topics discussed at Cincinnati Children's Schwartz Center Rounds have included experiencing the death of a patient, running on empty, and compassionate care for international patients.

The Schwartz Center was begun by healthcare attorney Ken Schwartz, a nonsmoker and health advocate who was diagnosed with advanced lung cancer at age 40 years. During his 10-month ordeal, Ken came to realize that what matters most during an illness is the human connection between patients and their caregivers. He wrote movingly about his experience in an article for the *Boston Globe Magazine*. At the end of his life, Ken outlined the organization he wanted to create and founded the Schwartz Center in 1995—just days before his death—to ensure that all patients receive compassionate and humane care.

▶ Other Resiliency Builders and Stress Relievers at Cincinnati Children's

It can be physically and emotionally difficult for healthcare providers to care for fragile patients on a daily basis. Even the most resilient staff members struggle when a patient's health suddenly deteriorates or a patient dies. The ideas on the following pages describe stress-relieving processes available to staff in the Patient Services Division of Cincinnati Children's. The staff members' ability to effectively deal with the inevitable stress of their jobs helps them to be more resilient.

Emotional Support Team

When two or more individuals experience a sudden, unanticipated event, such as an employee or patient death, situation, or injury, Cincinnati Children's Emotional Support Team (EST) will establish a confidential support session. The EST is intended to facilitate the processing of emotions. The team helps employees handle the distress, pain, confusion, and fear that can result from crisis situations. The EST also helps employees continue to deliver safe patient care by providing a timely and appropriate outlet for their emotions.

Time to Grieve

Staff members in the pediatric intensive care unit experience the death of a patient more often than other areas of the hospital. Should a death occur, the unit's policy is to allow the caregiver to take the rest of the day off to privately deal with the grief.

Assistance from Police Psychologist

The hospital environment is focused on providing the best possible medical and quality of life outcomes. When a serious safety event occurs, the effect on staff can be devastating. To improve resiliency during these difficult times, Cincinnati Children's has enlisted the help of a local police psychologist who routinely assists law enforcement staff in stress management and counsels police officers and families. While the two disciplines are different, both involve stress while providing service to the public.

"An important aspect of critical incident is the feeling of helplessness when facing a life or death situation," explains James M. Daum (2015). In his work with police, Daum has learned that after an incident, a police officer typically will try to "recollect and sequence what was experienced, and determine whether there was any alternative to firing shots or taking the action they chose. Emotional reactions can include guilt, anger, depression, anxiety or numbness. Physical symptoms such as nausea, gastro-intestinal disturbance, headaches, fatigue and sleep disturbance are common" (2015).

During a mandatory psychological debriefing, which is strictly confidential, the police officer is given support in his or her efforts to regain a sense of self-control and well-being. Similar debriefings are under consideration for Cincinnati Children's staff who are involved in a serious safety event. The goal is a return to work feeling healthy and emotionally ready.

Gauging Stress

The noise of hospital construction can be difficult for parents of sick children to handle, especially when those children are critically ill. During months of construction in Cincinnati Children's neonatal intensive care unit, leaders wanted to be certain that parents were getting the support they needed. As a gauge, parents were asked to place a yellow, orange, or red fuzzy ball into a fishbowl (**FIGURE 14-6**) at the unit's reception desk to indicate if they were getting the support they needed. When orange or red balls made their way to the fishbowl, it was time for a staff huddle to determine why.

Construction noise can also adversely affect caregivers, so the neonatal intensive care unit staff members have their own fishbowl. Four times each day, team leaders and charge nurses use colored balls to gauge stress. The results are charted. When stress is high, it is time to find out why and make adjustments.

Lowering the Noise

The potentially dangerous effects of noise fatigue have been made apparent by The Joint Commission. In April 2013, The Joint Commission (2013) issued a sentinel event alert warning of the dangers of alarm desensitization and urging hospitals

FIGURE 14-6 Fuzzy ball stress gauge.

to improve alarm management protocols and alarm-setting guidelines. The Joint Commission followed up by requiring hospitals to demonstrate that they have made alarms an organizational priority and identify the types of alarms they plan to target. By 2016, hospitals will need to develop and implement specific protocols aimed at curbing unnecessary alarms.

Excessive cardiac monitor alarms lead to desensitization and alarm fatigue. Researchers at Cincinnati Children's created and implemented a standardized cardiac monitor care process (CMCP) on a 24-bed pediatric bone marrow transplant unit. The aim of the project was to decrease monitor alarms through the use of team-based standardized care and processes.

Using small tests of change, researchers developed and implemented a standardized CMCP that included four components:

- A process for initial ordering of monitor parameters based on age-appropriate standards
- Pain-free daily replacement of electrodes
- Daily individualized assessment of cardiac monitor parameters
- A reliable method for appropriate discontinuation of the monitor

By implementing these standardized CMCP processes, Cincinnati Children's researchers (Dandoy et al., 2014) found that cardiac monitor alarms significantly decreased per patient day from 180 to 40. Overall compliance with the CMCP increased from a median of 38% to 95%.

Alarms are not the only source of disruptive noise in hospitals. After identifying the sources of noise on one unit at Cincinnati Children's, the following changes were made:

- Repaired noisy carts/ice machines
- Hung reminder signs to minimize noise

- Lowered volume on pagers
- Replaced phone ringers with lights
- Closed doors during rounding
- Asked that new trash bags be shaken outside patient rooms

Taking Fun Seriously

Cincinnati Children's Patient Services Division routinely incorporates exercise and fun into the workday to relieve stress. Activities include a monthly dress-up day, when staff are invited to do things like celebrate the start of a sports season by wearing a favorite team's jersey or be a twin for the day by dressing exactly like a coworker. The medical center's annual fitness on the field event lets staff members and their families participate in fun activities on the turf at the Cincinnati Bengals' stadium. After-work neighborhood walks and weekend hikes led by hospital leadership demonstrate a commitment to staff health and wellness.

Ideas for maintaining a healthy mind and body are a regular part of new staff orientation. Maintaining financial stability also is discussed during orientation. It is recognized that personal finances can be a persistent source of stress that affects staff. For example, new graduates may be burdened with student loans. Addressing financial stability in orientation is an important support. Advice on how to systematically reduce debt and save for retirement are examples of topics discussed.

▶ Other Ideas for Boosting Resiliency

Mindfulness

Mindfulness practice holds promise for increasing individual and workplace resilience (Goldstein, 2013). The research team sought to evaluate the effectiveness of a mindfulness-based program for increasing health and a sense of coherence and decreasing depression, anxiety, and stress in nurses and midwives. Mindfulness is described as paying attention on purpose, in the present moment, and nonjudgmentally to the unfolding of experience from moment to moment. Learning to become more present frees us to be more flexible and creative—and ultimately, more resilient, enjoying better health and well-being.

In his book *The Equanimous Mind* (2011), Manish Chopra, PhD, recommends one of India's most ancient techniques of meditation to reach the highest happiness. Called *vipassana*, this meditative practice helps you learn more about your thoughts, feelings, and judgments. Vipassana focuses on the deep interconnection between mind and body. "It is this observation-based, self-exploratory journey to the common root of mind and body that dissolves mental impurity, resulting in a balanced mind full of love and compassion" (Chopra, 2011, p. xi).

Modeling Healthy Behavior

Physical activity is a key factor in resilient behavior, suggests molecular biologist John Medina, PhD (2014). "When combined with the health benefits exercise offers, we have as close to a magic bullet as exists in modern medicine" (2014, p. 22).

Referring to physical activity as cognitive candy, Medina reports that research has consistently shown that exercisers outperform couch potatoes in tests that measure long-term memory, reasoning, attention, problem solving, and fluid intelligence. Nurse leaders would do well to model physical activity at every opportunity (e.g., walking desks, participating in fund-raising walks, and taking the steps instead of the elevator).

Alone Time

Nurses and other care providers should not deny the pressures and stresses they are experiencing in their life—at home and at work (Wicks, 2014). "That is the first piece of what makes a resilient organization and leader: facing the issues directly" (2014, p. 11). To boost resiliency, Wicks encourages people to

> find crumbs of alone time in their day and look for places where they can have some kind of silence and solitude for reflection so they can process things . . . Because with the right perspective, it's not the amount of darkness in the healthcare system or in our family or ourselves that matters; it's how we stand in that darkness. And that requires patience, perseverance and courage if we are going to be a leader, which requires a period of debriefing. (2014, p. 14)

Reduce Nurse Workload

Reducing nurse workload may be one way to avoid burnout and boost resiliency. Nurse workload, such as nurse-to-patient staffing ratios, can influence nursing care quality and lead to adverse patient outcomes. A growing body of research in pediatrics demonstrates this relationship. Tubbs-Cooley, Cimiotti, Silber, Sloane, and Aiken (2013) from the University of Pennsylvania demonstrated a significant increase in the odds of pediatric readmission in hospitals with leaner pediatric nurse-to-patient ratios, leading the team to speculate that higher workloads may result in rushed or incomplete discharge preparation. Since 2013, Tubbs-Cooley has been leading a team of researchers at Cincinnati Children's Hospital Medical Center to study relationships among nurse workloads, missed nursing care, and patient outcomes to better understand how shift-to-shift variation in bedside nurse workload causally affects nursing care quality and patient outcomes. This work, focused primarily in neonatal intensive care, has established preliminary linkages among nurse workloads, missed care, and outcomes:

- In a pilot study of 230 certified neonatal intensive care nurses, the nurses reported missing oral care for vented babies, missing discharge preparation, and missing oral feedings on their last shift worked. Nurses cited workload-related factors as the most significant reasons for missed care.
- Missed oral feeding opportunities led to significant prolongation of feeding milestones and neonatal intensive care hospitalization among preterm infants.
- Intubated infants whose nurses report missed adherence to ventilator-associated pneumonia guidelines during a shift are up to four times more likely to experience an unplanned extubation on the same shift.

Prioritizing

Leaders should recognize that they cannot do everything. They should engage in true prioritization to determine what should be done first. Kraemer (2011) describes true prioritization as a list of all items to be accomplished, from most important to least important. This process enables leaders to "commit your time, attention, and resources to what matters most" (2011, p. 18). This may seem simple, but often the most straightforward and effective strategies can be overlooked. Modeling good prioritization practices is a powerful opportunity for leaders that can result in a ripple effect of better prioritization throughout the organization. Simultaneously, another valuable practice is *exnovation*, the purging of non-value-added practices to allow the organization to adopt different and fresh thinking to new activities.

Microsystem Stress Reduction

> Remember that if you don't prioritize your life someone else will. (McKeown, G., 2014, p. 235)

Nurse fatigue and information overload can result in patient care error (Sitterding & Broome, 2015). The inability to control attention can result in the failure to notice something about the current situation or the failure to notice that something is different. This possibility of patient harm is what has spurred nurse leaders at Cincinnati Children's to investigate.

Believing that unexpected increases in patient volume may be causing stress to staff, and concerned that this stress correlates with levels of patient harm, Cincinnati Children's nurse leaders have initiated a study to validate and mitigate this hypothesis. Nursing hours per patient day and qualitative stress (a four-point scale) are under review on a shift-by-shift basis by microsystem (unit-level) charge nurses and clinical supervisors. They also are being reviewed on a weekly basis, along with other measures, including operational vacancy rate, percentage of float staff used, 13-hour shifts, and shifts that reported high levels of stress. Data is currently being analyzed, and mitigation strategies are being developed.

Short-Termism

Even the most resilient staff members today may find themselves lacking in the long run, particularly those who practice short-termism—that is, tuning out everything except the most immediate outcomes. Laurence Fink (2015), chair and CEO of BlackRock, believes this craving for immediate gratification prevents leaders from "grappl[ing] effectively with complex, long-term challenges . . . There seems to be a great deal more upside to placing a simple bet for a quick win than for staying the course through difficult times to create sustainable gains that are more widely shared" (2015, para. 3).

Other Ideas for Building Resiliency

An American Psychological Association web page called Road to Resilience recommends implementing the following ideas to build resiliency:

1. **Look for opportunities for self-discovery**. You can learn something about yourself and might even experience growth as a result of

challenging times. Often, those that experience hardships report that their relationships become stronger and they themselves have a greater sense of personal strength.

2. **Accept that change is a part of living**. Goals that you once held may no longer be attainable as a result of adverse contextual changes. Accept circumstances that are not within your control and focus instead on those things that are within your control – such as your actions and attitude.

3. **Move toward your goals**. Develop realistic goals. Even things that seems like a small accomplishments can enable you to move forward. Setting small achievable goals daily that move you in the direction of your overall goal can be an effective and manageable way forward.

4. **Make connections**. Good relationships with family members and friends are important. Accepting help from those who care about you strengthens resilience; reciprocally, the act of helping others in their time of need also can benefit you as the helper.

5. **Take care of yourself**. Pay attention to your own needs and emotions. Make time to do things that energize you and/or that you find relaxing. Taking care of yourself will help you to deal with situations that require resilience and endurance. (Comas-Diaz et al., 2015, page 4 of website, para. 1–10)

Staff resiliency is vital to healthcare organizations. It enables staff to refresh, move forward, develop new ideas, and implement change.

▶ Conclusion

Any conversation about innovation should include the importance of change. Change is constant, and it waits for no one. To keep innovating, you must be open, enthusiastic, and continually asking questions. Without it, stagnancy sets in. By coproducing creative solutions with patients and staff members, better health and value will be achieved.

References

Advisory Board. (2014). *Intermountain Health System nurse shadowing program*. Washington, DC.

Alison-Napolitano, E., & Pesut, D. (2015). *Bounce forward: The extraordinary resilience of nurse leadership*. Silver Spring, MD: American Nurses Association.

Amabile, T. M., & Kramer, S. J. (2011, May). The power of small wins. *Harvard Business Review, 89*(5). Retrieved from https://hbr.org/2011/05/the-power-of-small-wins

American College of Healthcare Executives. (2015). *Congress on healthcare leadership. COO bootcamp*. Presented by R. Brace & W. Riley. Retrieved from https://www.ache.org/Congress/bootcamps.cfm

American Hospital Association. (2012). *Bringing behavioral health into the care continuum: Opportunities to improve quality, costs and outcomes, 48*(3). Retrieved from http://www.aha.org/research/reports/tw/12jan-tw-behavhealth.pdf

Appelbaum, S., Louis, D., Makarenko, D., Saluja, J., Meleshko, O., & Kulbashian, S. (2013). Participation in decision making: A case study of job satisfaction and commitment. *Industrial and Commercial Training, 45*(4). https://doi.org/10.1108/00197851311323510

Baggett, M., Batcheller, J., Blouin, A. S., Behrens, E., Bradley, C., Brown, J. J. . . . Yendro, S. (2014). Excellence and evidence in staffing: A data-driven model for excellence in staffing. *Nursing Economics, 32*(Suppl. 3), 3–35.

Barden, A. M., Griffin, M. T., Donahue, M., & Fitzpatrick, J. J. (2011). Shared governance and empowerment in registered nurses working in a hospital setting. *Nursing Administration Quarterly, 35*(3), 212–218. https://doi.org/10.1097/NAQ.0b013e3181ff3845

Bass, K., & McGeeney, K. (2012). U.S. physicians set good health example. Retrieved from http://www.gallup.com/poll/157859/physicians-set-good-health-example.aspx

Boston-Fleischhauer, C. (2014a). Aiming for care continuity? Help staff see beyond their own care setting. Retrieved from http://www.advisory.com/research/nursing-executive-center/expert-insights/2014/help-staff-see-beyond-their-immediate-care-setting

Boston-Fleischhauer, C. (2014b). The changing CNO role (and how to succeed within it). Retrieved from http://www.advisory.com/research/nursing-executive-center/events/meetings/2014/2014-2015-nursing-executive-center-national-meeting-cno-roundtables/locations/dc/120814/the-changing-cno-role/presentation#slide/2

Brady, P. W., Muething, S., Kotagal, U., Ashby, M., Gallagher, R., Hall, D. . . . Wheeler, D. S. (2013). Improving situation awareness to reduce unrecognized clinical deterioration and serious safety events. *Pediatrics, 131*(1), e298–e308. https://doi.org/10.1542/peds.2012-1364

Burgess, S., Sly, P., & Devadason, S. (2012). Adherence with preventive medication in childhood asthma. *Pulmonary Medicine.* https://doi.org/10.1155/2011/973849

Chopra, M. (2011). *The equanimous mind.* Singapore: Author.

Comas-Diaz, L., Luthar, S., Maddi, S., O'Neill, H., Saakvitne, K., & Tedeschi, R. (2015). The road to resilience: 10 ways to build resilience. Retrieved from http://apa.org/helpcenter/road-resilience.aspx

Crosby, L. K. (2012). *Exploration of Cincinnati Children's Hospital Medical Center* (Unpublished doctoral dissertation). Wright State University, Dayton, OH.

Dandoy, C. E., Davies, S. M., Flesch, L., Hayward, M., Koons, C., Coleman, K. . . . Weiss, B. (2014). A team-based approach to reducing cardiac monitor alarms. *Pediatrics, 134*(5). https://doi.org/10.1542/peds.2014-1162

Daum, J. M. (2015). [Biographical information presented at a meeting with Cincinnati Children's]. Copy in possession of Cheryl Hoying.

de Jong, M., Marston, N., & Roth, E. (2015). The eight essentials of innovation, *McKinsey Quarterly, 2015,* 2, 37, 47.

Dent, R. L. (2015). Nine principles for improved nurse staffing. *Nursing Economics, 33*(1), 44.

Dent, R. L., Armstead, C., & Evans, B. (2014). Three structures for a healthy work environment. *American Association of Critical-Care Nurses Advanced Critical Care, 25*(2), 94–100.

Erickson, D. (2011). Professional practice model: Strategies for translating models into practice. *Nursing Clinics of North America, 46*(1), 35.

Fink, L. (2015). Our gambling culture. Retrieved from http://www.mckinsey.com/insights/strategy/our_gambling_culture

Frenk, J., Chen, L., Bhutta, Z.A., Cohen, J., Crisp, N., Evans, T. . . . Zurayk, H. (2010). Health professionals for a new century: Transforming education to strengthen health systems in an interdependent world. *The Lancet, 376,* 22.

Friedman, S. (2014). *Leading the life you want: Skills for integrating work and life.* Boston, MA: Harvard Business Review Press.

Gallup. (2013). State of the American workplace. Retrieved from http://www.gallup.com/services/178514/state- american-workplace.aspx

General Electric. (2015). Strategies for success: Managing complexity in health care, p. 13. Retrieved from http://www3.gehealthcare.com/en/insights/forward_thinking/forward_thinking/strategies_for_success_managing_the_complexity_in_health_care

Goldenhar, L., Brady, P., Sutcliffe, K., & Muething, S. (2013). Huddling for high reliability and situation awareness. *BMJ Quality and Safety, 22*(11), 899–906. https://doi.org/10.1136/bmjqs-2012-001467

Goldstein, E. (2013). *The now effect: How a mindful moment can change the rest of your life.* New York, NY: Atria Books.

Hoying, C., & Allen, S. (2011). Enhancing shared governance for interdisciplinary practice. *Nursing Administration Quarterly, 35*(3), 252–259.

Hoying, C., Lecher, W. T., Mosko, D. D., Roberto, N., Mason, C., Murphy, S. W. . . . Britto, M. T. (2014). On the scene: Cincinnati. *Nursing Administration Quarterly, 38*(1), 27–54.

Institute of Medicine. (2011). *The future of nursing: Leading change, advancing health.* Washington, DC: National Academies Press.

Jansen, L. (2008). Collaborative and interdisciplinary health care teams: Ready or not? *Journal of Professional Nursing, 24*(4), 220, 222.

Kabcenell, A., Nolan, T. W., Martin, L. A., & Gill, Y. (2010). *The pursuing perfection initiative: Lessons on transforming health care* (IHI Innovation Series white paper). Cambridge, MA: Institute for Healthcare Improvement.

Kamins, C. (2015). What too many hospitals are overlooking. Retrieved from www.gallup.com /businessjournal/181658/hospitals-overlooking.aspx

Kelly, M. (2011). *Off balance.* New York, NY: Hudson Street Press.

Kraemer, H. M. J. (2011). *From values to action.* San Francisco, CA: Jossey-Bass.

Mason, C., & Fiorini, P. (2013, September 27). *Nurses' practice, experiences, and satisfaction with the inpatient outpatient role at Cincinnati Children's Hospital Medical Center* (IRB approved unpublished research). Cincinnati, OH.

McKeown, G. (2014). *Essentialism: The disciplined pursuit of less.* New York, NY: Crown Business.

Medina, J. (2014). *Brain rules.* Seattle, WA: Pear Press.

Nader, R. (n.d.). BrainyQuote.com. Retrieved from http://www.brainyquote.com/quotes/quotes/r /ralphnader110188.html, para. 1.

Newhouse, R., Stanik-Hutt, J., White, K. M., Johantgen, M., Bass, E. B., Zangaro, G. . . . Weiner, J. P. (2011). Advanced practice nurse outcomes: A systemic review. *Nursing Economics, 29*(5), 19.

Patient-Centered Outcomes Research Institute. (2013). Improving post-discharge outcomes by facilitating family-centered transitions from hospital to home. Retrieved from http://www.pcori.org /research-results/2013/improving-post-discharge-outcomes-facilitating-family-centered-transitions

Perales, F., Pozo-Cruz, J., & Pozo-Cruz, B. (2014). Impact of physical activity on psychological distress: A prospective analysis of an Australian national sample. *American Journal of Public Health, 104*(12), 91.

Porter-O'Grady, T., & Malloch, K. (2011). *Quantum leadership.* Sudbury, MA: Jones & Bartlett Learning.

Riehle, E., Daston, M., Rutkowski, S., & Wehman, P. (2012). *High school transition that works: Lessons learned from Project SEARCH.* Baltimore, MD: Brookes.

Robert Wood Johnson Foundation. (2010). Groundbreaking new survey finds that diverse opinion leaders say nurses should have more influence on health systems and services. Retrieved from http://www.rwjf.org/en/library/articles-and-news/2010/01/groundbreaking-new-survey -finds-that-diverse-opinion-leaders-say.html

Robert Wood Johnson Foundation. (2011). Nurses are key to improving patient safety. Retrieved from http://www.rwjf.org/en/library/articles-and-news/2011/04/nurses-are-key-to-improving -patient-safety.html

Robert Wood Johnson Foundation. (2015). Lessons from the field: Promising interprofessional collaboration practices. Retrieved from http://www.rwjf.org/en/library/research/2015/03/lessons -from-the-field.html

Salmons, S. (2014). Burlington teen is "making a difference." *Cincinnati Enquirer.* Retrieved from http://www.cincinnati.com/story/news/local/burlington/2014/05/03/burlington-teen-making -difference/8682341/

Sanford, K. (2015). The resilient nurse leader. *Nursing Administration Quarterly, 39*(2), 100.

Sheridan, R. (2013). *Joy, Inc.: How we built a workplace people love.* New York, NY: Portfolio/Penguin.

Sitterding, M., & Broome, M. (2015). *Information overload: Framework, tips and tools to manage in complex healthcare environments.* Silver Spring, MD: American Nurses Association.

The Joint Commission. (2013, April 8). *Sentinel event alert: Medical device alarm safety in hospitals.* Retrieved from http://www.jointcommission.org/assets/1/18/SEA_50_alarms_4_5_13_ FINAL1 .PDF

The Schwartz Center for Compassionate Healthcare. (2016). Schwartz Center Rounds. Retrieved from http://www.theschwartzcenter.org/supporting-caregivers/schwartz-center-rounds

Toole, K. (2013). Helping children gain asthma control: Bundled school-based interventions. *Pediatric Nursing, 39*(3), 115–120

Tubbs-Cooley, H., Cimiotti, J., Silber, J., Sloane, D., & Aiken, L. (2013). An observational study of nurse staffing ratios and hospital readmission among children admitted for common conditions. *BMJ Quality Safety, 22*(9), 735–742.

Tye, J. (2014). *Midland Memorial Hospital case study on values and culture initiative.* Solon, IA: Values Coach.

Uldrich, J. (2011). *Higher unlearning: 39 post-requisite lessons for achieving a successful future.* Edina, MN: Beavers Pond Press.

Urbanski, B., & Lazenby, M. (2012). Distress among hospitalized pediatric cancer patients modified by pet-therapy intervention to improve quality of life. *Journal of Pediatric Oncology Nursing, 29*(5), 272–282. https://doi.org/10.1177/1043454212455697

Virkstis, K. (2012). Strengthening interdisciplinary collaboration: Best practices for enhancing partnership and communication. Retrieved from http://www.advisory.com/research/nursing-executive-center/studies/2012/strengthening-interdisciplinary-collaboration

Waters, B. (2013). 10 traits of emotionally resilient people. Retrieved from https://www.psychologytoday.com/blog/design-your-path/201305/10-traits-emotionally-resilient-people

Wicks, R. (2014). The resilient leader: Mind, body and soul. *Healthcare Executive, 29*(6), 11.

Zolli, A., & Healy, A. (2012). *Resilience: Why things bounce back.* New York, NY: Simon & Schuster Paperbacks.

CHAPTER 15

Building Diverse Partnerships in Health Care and Industry: How Organizations Must Partner to Build Disruptive Futures

Denise Duncan, Joshua Rutkoff, and Jerry E. Spicer

CHAPTER OBJECTIVES

Upon completion of this chapter, the reader will be able to:

1. Describe the nature of successful labor and management partnership behaviors in healthcare organizations.
2. Define the three paradoxes of labor–management innovation.
3. Discuss examples of innovative partnerships and how they inform healthcare change.

Author Note: For the second edition, the editors have decided to make this a legacy chapter. We believe the content of this chapter is unique and relevant. Although some of the organizations discussed have evolved, the concepts of innovation in partnership and with labor unions remains a discussion point all leaders should be aware of.

ealth care in the United States is going through a period of great change, much of it driven by the multiyear rollout of the Patient Protection and Affordable Care Act (PPACA) and its mandates for who and under what structure individuals will be covered by health insurance. The authors of this chapter are perhaps uniquely situated to forecast the challenges this period of change will present to the U.S. healthcare industry and to recommend strategies for meeting those challenges; they are veterans of the trailblazing labor–management partnership between Kaiser Permanente and the Coalition of Kaiser Permanente Unions, itself a partnership composed of 27 union locals representing 105,000 employees—80% of Kaiser Permanente's unionized workforce. The partnership was born as a response to financial difficulties faced by Kaiser Permanente during the 1990s, which drove innovation in improving the quality of care while simultaneously cutting costs. As Kaiser Permanente has grown in physical facilities and lives covered, and its quality ratings have risen, it has arguably been seen as a model for the more integrated systems of healthcare delivery anticipated to be the likely adaptations that the U.S. healthcare industry will need to make to meet the PPACA's mandates on cost and quality. The partnership was at the heart of the changes in Kaiser Permanente, and it has been well studied within academia. The authors come from each side of the partnership—Kaiser Permanente management and union leadership—and have been intimately involved in its origin, growing pains, and successes.

Additionally, this chapter will review the challenges facing the healthcare industry and the labor movement, the paradoxes that must be engaged to innovate, and several of the notable innovations accomplished by the Labor/Management Partnership (LMP).

▶ Current State of the Healthcare Industry and Labor Unions

Healthcare Industry: Current Challenges and Misconceptions

On March 23, 2010, President Barack Obama signed the PPACA into law. The intended outcome of the legislation is to provide mechanisms through which uninsured individuals in the United States can secure access to healthcare insurance. It is the most significant expansion of U.S. healthcare since the advent of Medicare in the 1960s. In April 2014, the Congressional Budget Office (CBO) and the Joint Committee on Taxation (JCT) estimated that the PPACA will reduce the number of individuals without insurance by 26 million by 2024 (Congressional Budget Office, 2014). This is a dramatic change. Before the advent of the PPACA, it was estimated that more than 46 million Americans did not have basic health coverage. Because of these numbers, the law represents a significant capacity challenge to healthcare organizations across the country, potentially stressing an infrastructure that already faces issues with overcrowded emergency departments and a lack of a truly integrated healthcare delivery model. Hospitals and health systems must do their best to provide high-quality and safe patient care in an environment of declining reimbursement and rising costs. Kaufman (2011) estimated that as a result of the PPACA, most healthcare systems will be required to reduce their current cost structures by

10–15%. Specifically, Medicare payments to hospitals will be reduced under PPACA if they are unable to reduce their readmission rates for selected high-cost ailments; experience avoidable hospital conditions, such as patient falls with injury or nosocomial infections; or find themselves in the top quartile of facilities with defined avoidable hospital-acquired conditions. Such PPACA mandates regarding quality will compel hospitals to focus their attention on the most costly areas of traditional inpatient stays and identify ways to provide high-quality care at lower costs.

Although the benefits of the PPACA landmark legislation could affect millions of uninsured Americans, the responsibility for ensuring the continued viability of today's healthcare institutions rests with its leadership and diverse partnerships with nontraditional organizations such as labor unions. Even before the advent of the PPACA, Morrison (2000) suggested that the lack of effective leadership is the largest issue facing healthcare organizations in the new millennium. Effective and competent leadership and diverse partnerships are essential to overcoming the challenges presented by healthcare reform and the PPACA.

It is perhaps worth noting that, although the PPACA does contain mandates on healthcare quality, its mechanism for driving quality improvements is largely through reforms in the structure of payment for care—what gets paid for and how. For instance, if a hospital's patients suffer from pressure ulcers—a symptom of poor-quality care, because patients with pressure ulcers have in general not been well-enough attended by the staff who are charged with checking on them and moving them frequently—that hospital will not receive reimbursement from the Centers for Medicare and Medicare Services (CMS) for the care of that condition. If a patient acquires pneumonia while in the hospital, the hospital—not the patient's insurer or own finances—must pay for the resulting treatment of pneumonia. These reimbursement changes shift the financial and quality model of health care from volume and fee-for-service to a more value- and outcomes-based reimbursement model. The shift from volume to value is a significant one because it requires new ways of partnering among providers, insurers, hospitals, and communities to achieve significantly better and more affordable care outcomes. The PPACA has been structured to push more payment toward proactive and integrated care models to encourage the U.S. healthcare industry to evolve toward a focus on wellness and prevention rather than on sickness and cure. Reforms in care quality, including scientific advances, are anticipated to be a by-product of payment reform and the pressures on the system from the expected influx of newly insured people, as well as to be self-reinforcing as the law and its effects continue to roll out. Regardless of any new legislation that might overturn the specific mandates of the PPACA, the healthcare industry has begun the shift to value-based care. To meet the new pressures of affordability, quality, and population health, organizations must work together, in partnership, to innovate solutions for the industry. This affords management and labor new opportunities to develop collaborative relationships; some would argue that it requires interdependency. Without this, it will be impossible for either entity to be successful in navigating the new reality of healthcare reform.

Labor: Current Challenges and Innovation

Today's context for considerations of partnership and innovation as trade union strategies is highly dynamic and complex. The challenges are stark: unions represent just 6.7% of workers in the private sector (Henwood, 2015), down from a peak of about 35% in the mid-1950s. Throughout the 20th century, unions engaged in collective bargaining with employers to negotiate and improve wages, hours, and working conditions for their members. For decades this model proved successful, allowing unions to create good jobs and standards of living for their members. Today, with union membership at its lowest level since the Great Depression, "traditional collective bargaining has all but vanished from the economic landscape—taking raises, benefits, job security and much of the American middle class with it as it goes" (Meyerson, 2013). Although unions represent 35.7% of public sector workers, recent attacks from political opponents have rolled back public sector union rights in traditional union strongholds such as Wisconsin and Michigan. In its 2014 ruling on *Harris v. Quinn*, the Supreme Court decided that home-care workers do not have to pay any fees to the unions representing them, stripping them of rights enjoyed by other public sector workers (Greenhouse, 2014). Not just within the healthcare industry, employers (both unionized and nonunion) do not typically look to unions as drivers of innovation; in fact, they too often characterize them as obstacles to change. The economic backdrop for this set of challenges is profound income inequality and wage stagnation, characterized by a growing economy in which working people are not reaping financial rewards for the productivity gains they are helping to achieve for the organizations they work for. Couple these macroeconomic trends with the attendant loss of collective voice, security, and respect that unions help create at work, and the results resemble the broader conditions in which the kind of workplace speak-up culture required for creating innovation is suppressed. Detert and Edmondson (2007) describe how in environments in which workers are forced to focus on their own self-preservation, "we found the innate protective instinct so powerful that it also inhibited speech that clearly would have been intended to help the organization." This is one dynamic that places a divide in how organizations and workers partner to create novel solutions and can specifically affect how well healthcare organizations can adapt to the changing environment of quality and cost.

At the same time, in the context of the environment previously described, the labor movement has responded with a willingness to experiment with a broad and vibrant array of revitalization strategies. Labor is embracing innovation and adapting to current challenges through novel operating structures. Worker centers, such as the Restaurant Opportunities Center, the National Domestic Workers Alliance, and the National Guest Worker Alliance, do not yet engage in collective bargaining, but they nevertheless advocate for and give voice to workers in various industries, including winning economic judgments for workers from employers. Unions are also leading broad-based, long-term campaigns to raise standards of living for low-wage workers. The Fight for 15, which calls for a wage of $15 per hour and the right to form a union, is mobilizing workers, often through strikes, in industries including fast food, warehousing and logistics, and home care. Strikes (legally protected actions in which workers withhold their labor) were an integral part of how the labor movement grew strong in the middle of the 20th century in the face of massive, and sometimes violent, resistance from U.S. industry. Geoghegan (2014) describes a major distinction between the often open-ended, lengthy strikes that helped shape industries such as auto, steel, and mining and today's quick and broadly distributed actions targeted at the low-wage service sector. The latter "did nothing to move McDonalds. But these losses put the issue at the top of Obama's

2014 State of the Union address" (2014, p. 37). And unions have helped lead coalitions that won new $15 per hour minimum wage laws in cities including Seattle, San Francisco, and Los Angeles, which will apply not just to union workers but also to the community at large.

David Rolf, president of Service Employees International Union (SEIU) Local 775, is explicit about the imperative for organized labor to embrace innovation:

> Progressives should take a cue from business and enter an era of innovation, leveraging labor's significant institutional resources to create organizations dedicated to studying the future of organizing and work . . . By striking out into complexity instead of retreating back to what is familiar, progressives can seize this moment of crisis and win enormous victories for workers. However, labor and its allies must be willing to experiment with new models outside traditional collective bargaining, even outside the traditional idea of a union. (2014, para. 7, 13)

The labor and management relationship in health care has had some history of adversarial encounters. Nursing and other healthcare worker strikes or work stoppages have created some polarizing opinions from healthcare professionals, organizations, and patients questioning the intent and operations of organizations and the represented workforce. Traditionally, both labor and management have relied on primarily linear leadership practices that focused on singular interests, like pay, benefits, and work hours, and tried to achieve them by inaction (stalled negotiations, refusal to discuss issues, and inflexibility) or overaction (reductions in negotiated benefits, command-and-control management, work stoppages, and negative ad campaigns). Many situations do not yet possess the conditions for exceeding this traditional zero-sum, adversarial approach. Such an approach, although it may produce short-term gains for either party, may have inherent limitations in the context of the cost and efficiency pressures described by Berwick (2011) in his speech to the Institute for Healthcare Improvement:

> Our nation is at a crossroad. The care we have simply cannot be sustained. It will not work for health care to chew ever more deeply into our common purse. If it does, our schools will fail, our roads will fail, our competitiveness will fail. Wages will continue to lag, and, paradoxically, so will our health.
>
> The choice is stark: chop or improve. If we permit chopping, I assure you that the chopping block will get very full—first with cuts to the most voiceless and poorest us, but soon after to more and more of us. Fewer health insurance benefits, declining access, more out-of-pocket burdens, and growing delays. If we don't improve, the cynics win. That's what passes the buck to us. If improvement is the plan, then we own the plan. Government can't do it. Payers can't do it. Regulators can't do it. Only the people who give the care can improve the care.

Therefore, we argue that when and where the right conditions exist, innovative partnerships and more evidence-based, interest-based, and innovative leadership practices will result in a better healthcare system where workers, organizations, and patients benefit from better quality, cost, and care.

In this context of a spectrum of experimental strategies for organized labor, the labor–management partnership at Kaiser Permanente provides an intriguing model of what is achievable through collaboration focused on shared improvement and innovation goals, as well as an example of how unions and employers can, under the right conditions, exceed rather than discard traditional collective bargaining in the pursuit of common interests.

▶ Healthcare Industry: Innovation

U.S. health care and labor intersect in an unpredictable and dynamic environment, including patients, payers, providers, suppliers, and each other. These intersections provide a focused lens to examine how evidence-based innovation can occur when tension, environmental factors, and complex connections are acknowledged and leveraged for success. Given the scarcity of resources and a global economy that is far from stable, health care and labor separately and together face significant challenges driving a need to innovate. For management and labor, traditionally engaged in an adversarial relationship, coming together in partnership to tackle shared challenges could be seen as a kind of top-level, disruptive innovation from which a cascading series of innovations can follow to most effectively respond to such challenges.

To discuss diverse partnerships that drive innovation, we must have a common definition of healthcare innovation. Thakur, Hsu, and Fontenot defined healthcare innovation as the

> adoption of those best-demonstrated practices that have been proven suc-cessful and implementation of those practices while ensuring the safety and best outcomes for patients and whose adoption might also affect the performance of the organization. In other words, innovation in health care is defined as those changes that help healthcare practitioners focus on the patient while helping healthcare practitioners work smarter, faster, better, and more cost effectively. (2012, p. 564)

Healthcare innovation can take many forms, and although it is widely perceived and accepted to be a positive outcome, it carries a number of trade-offs and para-doxes. These trade-offs and paradoxes are best addressed by partnerships between groups that can coadapt to the unpredictable environment.

Innovation does not necessarily follow a logical and sequenced series of well-rationalized steps. It is important for leaders to recognize this and work to identify new approaches in the identification, adoption, and spread of innovation in health care. Dixon-Woods, Amalberti, Goodman, Bergman, and Glasziou (2011) identified three paradoxes that innovators in health care specifically are likely to encounter (**BOX 15-1**).

Paradox 1: Adoption Without Evidence

Paradox 1 addresses the phenomenon of why some new practices are quickly adopted and spread, even though there is little or no empirical evidence that the practice is effective, or even safe, while other practices from which patients could benefit are never adopted, let alone spread. There are a number of reasons why this may occur.

BOX 15-1 Paradoxes of Innovation in Health Care

Paradox 1: Uptake of the dubious, rejection of the good; adoption without evidence
Paradox 2: The wisdom and failings of democracy; stopping innovation through collaboration
Paradox 3: Health systems are never able to keep up; change as a barrier to change

Data from Dixon-Woods, M., Amalberti, R., Goodman, S., Bergman, B., & Glasziou, P. (2011). Problems and promises of innovation: Why healthcare needs to rethink its love/hate relationship with the new. *BMJ Quality & Safety, 20*, i47–i51.

The innovation may simply be the latest fad—that must-have practice or product that is so new that no evidence yet exists to support or refute it. This can often be the case with technology; new technologies experience increased hype as they enter the market, but they may not perform as expected while adoption increases. Adopters and resisters demonstrate several behaviors as new practices are introduced into the environment. Sometimes adopters defend their decision to adopt by pointing out that the innovation is better than doing nothing. Or perhaps the innovation does offer some modicum of face validity or intuitive appeal as a possible solution to the problem, so adoption provides a degree of defense against the accusation of doing nothing. The risk of action without evidence can sometimes work in opposition to the values of healthcare workers, such as do no harm.

Each of these reasons for succumbing to paradox 1 poses the risk that an organization will adopt processes or products that have yet to be fully vetted for efficiency or effectiveness. Conversely, innovation under paradox 1 could result in a failure to spread practices that have been proven effective. As a result, there is potential risk to the organization and its staff members; physicians; and, most important, the patient. At the very minimum, an innovation under this paradox could result in the disruption or displacement of other beneficial efforts. With paradox 1, innovation crowds out others fighting for a place in a landscape of limited resources, both human and capital. An unproven and hastily implemented solution can crowd out a proven or even yet-to-be proven but better solution.

Paradox 2: Stopping Innovation Through Collaboration

Paradox 2 speaks to innovation through collaboration. Dixon-Woods and colleagues (2011) assert that, although collaborating with other professionals may be an effective way of ensuring implementation and spread of an innovation, it may also be one of the most effective ways of stopping it.

The benefits of actively involving those individuals most likely to be affected by the proposed innovation and who are the most knowledgeable about the situation that the planned innovation is designed to address are apparent, including better-informed decisions and greater collective buy-in to the implementation. Actively involving subject matter experts also increases the identification of further opportunities for innovation. This social movement approach and the role of self-organizing and self-governing networks is gaining popularity in numerous settings and is gaining momentum particularly within the healthcare setting. It promotes the self-management of change, and it works well when the problems being addressed are well-known to the organization and individuals involved. In the healthcare industry, where one is attempting to change the practice of professionals, this social movement approach works well. Professionals are educated and prepared to manage their own clinical practices, which can create a negative reaction to being required to do new practices that do not originate from the individual professional. To overcome the potential resistance of dictating innovation through a hierarchy, leaders can use the social movement approach because the individuals designing and implementing the innovation are the same as those who will have to use the innovation.

Although there are many advantages to the social movement approach, it also presents its share of threats to successful innovation. Group-based, collaborative efforts like this can be and are often undermined from within the group. One of the most common innovation-stopping issues the social movement approach creates is the failure to engage stakeholders in the change process. Another threat occurs when an individual attempts to substitute his or her own agenda for the greater good of the organization and those it serves. Thus, it is critical that the innovation process be as transparent and inclusive as possible. Transparency and inclusiveness can serve to isolate and marginalize an individual who is obstructing the will of the group. Although a social movement approach to innovation in health care has been shown to be particularly successful when engaging professionals like nurses and technicians, professional boundaries and scope of practice law can be another source of contention and possible derailment.

Paradox 3: Change as a Barrier to Change

Paradox 3 is rooted in the fact that improvement requires change, and change will always create its own set of challenges. Quality improvement systems are notoriously unable to keep up with the pace of innovation. By its nature, innovation is a disruptive activity, and by the time quality improvement catches up with the innovation, things have usually changed—again. Failures in the evaluation process can only intensify this problem. The evaluation process is often too narrowly focused on a specific intervention while failing to capture the systemic effects and unintended consequences of the innovation.

The Paradoxes in Summary

In this section we examined the challenges associated with innovation in today's complex and volatile healthcare environment. Dixon-Woods and colleagues (2011) identified three paradoxes—the problems and promises—of innovation. Paradox 1 is innovation for the sake of innovating. In some cases, the innovation that is promoted and adopted is without empirical evidence that it will achieve what it seeks to accomplish. Perhaps the innovation is accepted out of pure desperation or simply to do something, which is believed to be better than doing nothing. Innovation linked to paradox 1 potentially places the entire organization, its patients, and its staff at risk by either producing direct harm or by crowding out alternative, more beneficial innovation.

Paradox 2 considers innovation though collaboration. While the authors contend that this form of innovation may result in better outcomes as the result of active involvement of subject matter experts promoting a motivation for the spread and

---

BOX 15-2 Innovation in Health Care: An Agenda for Action

- Assess innovation risk and reward for all innovation activities.
- Develop processes for assessing innovation and technology value to the organization.
- Evaluate innovation in real time, including how the innovation is affecting outcomes.
- Use social science to evaluate pilots as the innovation test of change is in progress. Focus on what resources might be needed to implement the innovation in a production environment.
- Clearly define the roles involved in innovation work and use formal leadership structures to facilitate and manage frontline workers, patients, and other stakeholders in the process.
- Identify unintended impacts of innovation by using a variety of research methods, including clinical trial methods, before spreading innovation across an organization.
- Develop innovation competencies through education, training, and experience to help overcome the barriers to change.

Adapted from Dixon-Woods, M., Amalberti, R., Goodman, S., Bergman, B., & Glasziou, P. (2011). Problems and promises of innovation: Why healthcare needs to rethink its love/hate relationship with the new. *BMJ Quality & Safety, 20,* i47–i51.

---

adoption of the innovation as the result of social mechanisms, it too has problems. Innovation under paradox 2 may result in the undermining of the innovation if the members of the collaborative fail to engage or they substitute their own agendas for the innovation, thereby effectively derailing constructive and meaningful change.

The final paradox cited by the authors considers innovation as disruptive change. Innovation and improvement *is* change. The issue, however, is that the normal quality improvement processes central to the healthcare industry are always lagging the innovation. By the time the quality improvement processes catch up to the innovation, new change has occurred, and the quality improvement cycle must start all over. **BOX 15-2** outlines the considerations for proactively addressing these issues.

▶ Evidence-Based Partnerships in Innovation: The Kaiser Permanente Example

The partnership between Kaiser Permanente and the Coalition of Kaiser Permanente Unions (the Coalition), started in 1997, has established itself as the longest-lasting and most successful labor–management partnership in the United States. This comprehensive partnership, which is defined in the national agreement between the parties as a strategy for operational collaboration at every level, has built a track record of success in performance improvement. It provides a number of different mechanisms and processes for interaction between labor and management at every level of the organization—national and regional down to the local facility levels—and each provides for extensive engagement and decisions made by consensus.

Hal Ruddick, the executive director of the Coalition, positions the partnership in the context of a trade union legacy of advocating expanded access to health care:

> Our partnership is about providing the best care and quality. In that way, it's in the tradition of the historic mission of the American labor movement, which includes ensuring quality, affordable health care for working families. We are able to do that without sacrificing good jobs with good pay and benefits. Many other affordability strategies sacrifice either quality or good jobs, or both. Our strategy is based on high-quality care, good jobs and affordability. (H. Ruddick, personal communication, June 2, 2015)

In his remarks to the Coalition's annual Union Delegates Conference in 2015, Chokri Bensaid, the Kaiser division director from the Coalition's largest local union, SEIU United Healthcare Workers West, characterized the partnership as creating tripartite benefits that go far beyond the immediate self-interest of union members:

> When we do things like bargain the best benefits in the country, we don't just do right by our members. We set the bar in our communities. We set the bar in our industry. The Kaiser contract is the contract every health-care worker aspires to have. And every time you improve that, you inject a little bit of hope in the lives of those working people who aspire to have the same contract . . . We're dealing with waste, we're dealing with improvement of workflow, we're dealing with creative ways of delivering care and being more personal to our patients, and when you cut waste out of the system, the company wins, we win, and the patients win. (Bensaid, 2015)

At the facility level, where the care meets the patient, unit-based teams (UBTs) are groups of frontline workers, managers, and physicians in a given natural work department (such as a medical–surgical unit, pharmacy, or environmental services department) who work together on improvement projects. Using the Rapid Improvement Model (RIM), UBTs identify issues in their departments, review data together, and develop goals for improvement. This process of continuously generating and evaluating data helps avoid the pitfalls of paradox 1, adoption of an innovation without evidence, because the evidence for or against a given innovation arises nearly in real time.

The UBT goals are informed by the core values of the partnership, which are working together with a focus on the patient or member to achieve the best quality and service, and to make Kaiser Permanente both the most affordable care provider and the best place to work. In the decade since UBTs were first negotiated and implemented, Kaiser Permanente has grown into an industry leader in quality and service. At the same time, the industry-best wages, benefits, and working conditions bargained for by the Coalition and enabled by this partnership serve as an example to other unions and employers as a potential standard and even a counterexample to the cuts and reductions characterizing much of the rest of the national collective bargaining environment.

The most thorough history of the first decade of this partnership is provided by Kochan, Eaton, McKersie, and Adler in *Healing Together* (2009). The authors describe the traditional collective bargaining relationship between labor and management, according to federal law through the National Labor Relations Act, as by definition adversarial, with "a clear line of demarcation" (2009, p. 22) between management's rights to run an organization and labor's rights to bargain over the impact of changes to hours, wages, and working conditions. "Such efforts are restrained by twentieth-century thinking about how work is organized, organizations are structured, and goods and services are produced and delivered" (2009, p. 23). In contrast, the partnership at Kaiser Permanente reflects more current thinking:

> Rather than dividing people into management and labor camps, contemporary models of work organization stress teamwork among people who bring different, specialized knowledge to bear at tasks at hand. That is the potential creativity that labor–management partnerships in general and the KP [Kaiser Permanente] Labor–Management Partnership in particular, seek to mobilize. (2009, p. 23)

With a foundation of approximately 3,500 UBTs covering virtually every department in Kaiser Permanente that employs members of the Coalition, this partnership has built a solid foundation based on improving established work processes. At the same time, it provides intriguing examples and opportunities for how such a collaborative strategy can be leveraged to implement more extensive innovation as well.

A review of the literature reveals both evidence of the efficacy of the labor–management partnership at Kaiser Permanente and examples of the ways that other healthcare unions and their employers have charted their own courses to collaborate to achieve shared interests. These examples show a growing critical mass of experience and proficiency in partnering around performance improvement and glimmers of what might be possible with increased focus on similar efforts to collaborate on innovation.

Adler and Heckscher (2013) situated Kaiser Permanente in the context of the challenges of organizations operating in complex environments to perform both in terms of innovation or flexibility and efficiency or control. This tension describes well the dynamics that healthcare organizations face. The authors characterize high performance in both domains as *ambidexterity*: "the ability simultaneously to exploit existing capabilities and to explore new opportunities" (2013, p. 35). Organizations dealing with complexity that are not able to develop an integrated approach to this dynamic are likely to be mired in mediocrity. According to Adler and Heckscher, ambidextrous organizations synthesize mechanistic and organic approaches through a collaborative model, a form that

> is not only a better mix, but also outperforms one-dimensional organizations at their own games. That is, an effective collaborative system is better at efficiency than a bureaucracy, because it engages members in continuous improvement and problem-solving; and it is better at innovation than a market or decentralized bureaucracy, because it coordinates knowledge more effectively across a wider scope. (2013. p. 43)

In their case study of Kaiser Permanente, Adler and Heckscher cite the labor–management partnership as one example of how the company has met its ambidexterity challenges, supporting the implementation of both management-driven initiatives and frontline improvement ideas, along with the spread of lessons and best practices (2013, p. 45). Kaiser Permanente has achieved "dramatic improvements both in exploration and exploitation dimensions" (2013, p. 47), performing at the top of the industry in core outcome measures and having developed "an impressive capacity for radical innovation" (2013, p. 47).

In a separate study, Lazes, Katz, Figueroa, and Karpur (2012) observed the labor–management partnership between Montefiore Medical Center and 1199 SEIU in the Bronx, New York, finding a similar interplay between disruptive innovation and adaptive change. Disruptive innovation "enables organizations to create new systems of care, products, or services" (2012b, p. 150), whereas adaptive change "is based on incremental changes that optimize current processes or services by improving efficiencies and eliminating waste. The use of the adaptive change approach can be instrumental in standardizing new processes and procedures that were initially created by a disruptive change approach" (2012, p. 150).

The study focuses on Montefiore as an example of an organization that, in its efforts to become a more fully and deeply integrated care delivery system, is pursuing both disruptive and adaptive change models. The strategy is based partly on increasing prevention and care management efforts to reduce costly hospitalizations—like the labor–management partnership at Kaiser Permanente, perhaps showing a way forward for the entire U.S. healthcare industry as it struggles to adapt to the mandates of the PPACA. Critical to the strategy's success at Montefiore's Contact Centers has been a "comprehensive labor–management partnership to help design and implement new work systems to provide not only a positive customer service experience for patients and providers, but an exceptional work environment for staff as well" (Lazes, Katz, Figueroa, & Karpur, 2012, p. 160).

This capacity to absorb and balance both disruptive innovation and adaptive change through the flexibility of its collaborative processes is how the LMP at Kaiser seems to have largely avoided the pitfalls of paradox 3. Labor and management collaborate at every level of the organization, from top leadership down to the unit level and back up through the hierarchy, with information flowing freely not only upward and downward, but laterally. The RIM used by the UBTs allows the most disruptive innovations to be incorporated in the most intimate ways into the basic everyday tasks involved in direct patient care. RIM and UBTs render ideas of change from abstract concepts to concrete procedures and are able to make the necessary adjustments, or adaptive changes, at that level.

Nixon's study of UBTs at Kaiser Permanente (2012) demonstrates the correlation among staff engagement, team performance, and team development. Kaiser Permanente measures staff engagement through an internal survey called People Pulse. With its database of UBTs, called UBT Tracker, which documents teams' activities and accomplishments, Kaiser Permanente can analyze both team performance on operational goals and team development as measured by an internal rubric called the Path to Performance. The study revealed the link between team development (ranked on a five-point scale ranging from foundational to high performing) and a dozen measures of staff engagement, including perceptions of how a department operates effectively as a team and staff understanding of how their jobs contribute to organizational goals. The data demonstrates the connection between staff engagement and performance on key operational metrics. For instance, staff perceptions of more efficient work procedures in their departments correlate to lower hospital mortality rates and greater patient satisfaction with the hospital experience. Similarly, higher levels of comfort among staff in raising ethical concerns to their managers link to significantly lower staff injury rates. The study makes a compelling case that investment in supporting and nurturing UBTs can drive changes in workplace culture that can lead to improved performance.

Lazes, Katz, and Figueroa (2012) looked at both Kaiser Permanente and other healthcare systems as evidence of how labor–management partnerships can produce improved clinical outcomes, better work environments, and cost savings. They concluded that "the involvement of healthcare unions, including both leaders and members, in restructuring initiatives affecting the entire delivery system yields concrete clinical improvements. Further, such improvements are directly linked to increased involvement of front-line healthcare workers in the process" (2012, p. 5). Here, too, we see evidence of improved operational performance through partnership and hints of what might be possible with an increased focus on partnering for innovation. The authors examined a number of UBTs at two Kaiser Permanente medical centers: San Rafael and San Diego. For example, in its broader efforts to improve workplace safety and reduce injury rates, the San Rafael Clinical Lab Scientist (CLS) UBT tackled lab design. The CLS UBT "has harnessed the insight of its staff members to transform a department into a safe and efficient workplace designed by its staff, for its staff" (2012, p. 16). The authors observed that the two unions at Kaiser Permanente San Rafael, through their work with UBTs, "have become more engaged in discussions around remodeling and have taken an active interest in technology issues" (2012, p. 18).

At Kaiser Permanente San Diego, the Emergency Department UBT developed and implemented a system for team communication to support adoption of a new technology: "Using a communication tree and a training tracking system to support their work, the team increased the percent of staff that had access to and were trained in iNotes from 10 percent to 94 percent from May to July 2010" (Lazes, Katz, & Figueroa, 2012, p. 28). Finally, the characterization of the labor–management partnership at Kaiser Permanente San Diego describes some of the conditions that are necessary for enabling not just joint performance improvement but collaboration to innovate as well: "UBT work has enabled employees to access and understand key financial and operations data, allowing for a more engaged and effective workforce" (2012, p. 29).

Looking again at examples outside Kaiser Permanente, Lazes, Katz, and Figueroa (2012) find value in the collaboration between Fletcher Allen Health Care and the Vermont Federation of Nurses and Health Professionals, American Federation of Teachers. This partnership is focused on Model Unit Processes (MUPs), a negotiated "innovative process whereby nurses and unit managers would meet to analyze the needs of patients and determine appropriate staffing levels by unit" (p. 33).

MUPs, which are analogous in some ways to Kaiser Permanente's UBTs, are the vehicle for nurses and their managers in given departments to "become involved not only in determining appropriate staffing levels but also in influencing the way in which units function at Fletcher Allen through the redesign of care delivery and work processes" (2012, p. 33). As an example, the parties worked together to address an overreliance on traveler nurses, a practice that both eroded union jobs and ran up hospital costs.

> In 2006, Fletcher Allen employed at least 125 travelers. The MUP teams pursued new ways of giving nurses a voice in the workplace and made specific changes to work environment and clinical practices. As a result, conditions at Fletcher Allen began to improve. At the time of publication, no travelers have been hired, open positions remain limited, and the hospital boasts a low nursing turnover rate. (2012, p. 40)

The SEIU reports on its National Hospital Quality Initiative, which was launched in 2014 to expand and strengthen its labor–management partnerships with a range of different local unions and their respective employers (Service Employees International Union, 2015). Each appears to ground its partnership in its own particular culture, experience, and strategy. For instance, SEIU Local 721 and Los Angeles County's Department of Health Services have created Care Innovation Teams (CITs) focused on reducing patient wait times and improving the patient experience in ambulatory settings. At Los Angeles County's Martin Luther King Jr. Outpatient Center, staff and managers in the hematology–oncology department were able to reduce wait times, from registration to taking vitals, from 23 minutes to 3 minutes (Service Employees International Union, 2015). In Miami, SEIU Local 1991 and Jackson Memorial Hospital have partnered to improve safe patient handling; they project $9 million to $13 million in annual savings from their project (2015). SEIU has established a National Learning Collaborative to share lessons and best practices from these various partnership experiences.

Although a partnership between labor and management is far from the industry standard, an increasing body of evidence shows that a diversity of approaches to collaboration among unions and their employers has yielded measurable improvements in targeted areas of focus, including quality, service, affordability, and staff satisfaction. As healthcare systems and unions grapple with increasingly complex competitive, clinical, and financial challenges, this model of partnership may be particularly suited to the imperative to simultaneously exploit existing capabilities and strike out into uncharted areas of innovation.

▶ Innovation in Partnership and Solidarity: The Electronic Healthcare Record Background and Implementation

Regulations and incentives within the PPACA that are meant to push the entire U.S. healthcare system toward electronic medical records (EMRs), both to cut costs and increase efficiency and effectiveness, have already gone into effect. This is another arena in which Kaiser Permanente has led innovation within the industry as the first major health system in the country to roll out a comprehensive EMR. At Kaiser, pressures to create this system came separately from the very top, at the chief executive officer (CEO) level, as well as organically from the grass roots, the bedside nurses on the front lines of patient care. The LMP can be seen as the metaphorical meeting-in-the-middle point, where the vision from above and the knowledge from below intersected in a productive manner. It provided the processes and methodology to translate overarching vision and everyday knowledge into practical design and implementation.

The account from the grass roots is carried by Kathy Sackman, RN, former president of the United Nurses Associations of California/Union of Health Care Professionals (UNAC/UHCP), who recalls a project within Kaiser Permanente in the late 1990s where paper charts were replaced with flow sheets so nurses could document patient care information faster and in fewer places. "At the time," said Sackman, "some individual Kaiser Permanente hospitals in Southern California had internal computer systems that were being used for outpatient care. As soon as we started that patient documentation project, the nurses began asking when we were going to go electronic with our charts" (Kathy Sackman, RN, personal communication May 4, 2015). Successive CEOs near the latter end of the same period had similar ideas. Dick Pettingale, Kaiser Permanente California Division president from 1999 to 2002, worked on developing such a system. Pettingale's replacement in 2002, George Halvorson, scrapped Pettingale's EMR to bring in a system he had already worked with called EPIC. This became the new basis for Kaiser Permanente's eventual in-house product, HealthConnect, which rolled out in selected California facilities in 2003.

The government mandate for all health records to go digital would not come until 2004, but Halvorson believed that a patient who visited Kaiser Permanente in any area of the country should have the same experience, with the same access to medical records, as any other. In 2002, a patient in such a situation would have had to get paper copies of all files and take them to any other Kaiser Permanente location, even in the same region, for providers to review them. In addition, inpatient care within the hospital was not connected to outpatient care that might take place in the emergency room or outlying clinics. The challenge was not just to share information internally but also across the continuum of care.

Another challenge was that some of the technology necessary to make it all possible did not yet exist. Plenty of computer and information technology (IT) professionals could write a computer program for a pop-up box to be shown on a screen or code a universal chart to be shared electronically. But there was no health IT specialty, and any technology expert had a steep learning curve when it came to understanding the healthcare side of the workflow. In addition, it was impossible to rewire many old hospitals, constructed decades before local area networks and the Internet, to share information electronically. Wireless technology, though not yet in widespread use, became the only option for sharing information within most hospitals and clinics.

Three groups of workers needed to be involved to get the EMR project off the ground: clinicians, the people who would actually use the system; business representatives, who needed to look at it from a financial perspective and determine how to change Kaiser Permanente policies to support it; and IT professionals, who needed to develop the technological infrastructure. The collaborative model from the partnership was absolutely critical to fitting all the pieces together.

HealthConnect development went through three layers of decision making. The top level was the national development validation and build delegation sessions, made up of a small group from every region, who worked to ensure that the experiences from every Kaiser Permanente region would be homogeneous. Below that was the regional development build group, modeled after the larger group structure. One representative from every emergency department in Southern California attended the regional build validation sessions, for example. Staff educators were involved, as well as local management across all regional facilities. Finally, at the local level, representatives from different units and worker groups across a single Kaiser Permanente health center participated. This allowed local staff member to give their input into how the final product would look. The meetings included employees performing a variety of jobs to be certain that all who needed to provide input would be on one of the build teams. One representative from each local facility then represented that facility at the regional build meetings. A three-level review process gave all who were affected the chance to correct problems before implementation.

Although HealthConnect carried the blessing and mandate of Kaiser Permanente's CEO and top leadership, there was significant initial resistance from those management level staff that comprised the national team working to build the system—an example of paradox 2 in action. Getting the frontline nurses involved at that level was crucial in changing this dynamic. Those nurses already involved pushed for inclusion at the highest levels so that those who would be interacting with the system the most could help build it. UNAC/UHCP president Kathy Sackman, RN, went to bat for the nurses in conversations with top leadership on the management side. Before long, nurses were sitting at the national table discussing the practicalities of how to make HealthConnect function from a worker standpoint.

"The partnership is a commitment by the employer and by the unions that the workforce will be involved," according to Sackman. "It's recognition that the employer understands that the workers know how to do the work and have ideas on how to do it better. They know how to eliminate waste in the system" (Kathy Sackman, RN, personal communication, May 4, 2015). With a project of this scale, designed to affect the workflow of every staff member who interacts with patients, engaging with the workforce from the very beginning was a necessity.

One nurse on the national build team, Troy Seagondollar, RN, ultimately became the lead for the Kaiser Permanente Southern California rollout. Even as a working RN he had an interest in health informatics. His position was a unique hybrid creation and embodiment of the LMP. He came out of the labor side, as a UNAC/UHCP-represented RN. Even during the project, his office was housed at UNAC/UHCP's headquarters, and he served as liaison for the Coalition of Kaiser Permanente Unions. Yet his salary was paid by Kaiser Permanente.

When it came time to do the rollout in the Southern California region, Seagondollar met with the nurse executives at each medical center to plan training. He explained how many people needed to be trained to do peer-to-peer support, by different job type. These workers who were trained would then explain to others with the same job type what HealthConnect was, how it worked, and how it would affect their job flow. There was training and some measure of selling the new EMR. This allowed innovators to train a wide range of people, engaging all workers in the process.

Finally, when the rollouts of HealthConnect began, there was another process implemented to help achieve success. This work would start 90 days before going live and continue for 6 weeks after the launch. Three teams would go into a medical center to do a readiness survey: IT, Kaiser Permanente HealthConnect Leads, and Deployment Support. The first team of IT workers ensured that the necessary equipment and the technical infrastructure was in place to support using the EMR. The Kaiser Permanente HealthConnect Leads worked with management to assess and mitigate the perceived impact. In addition, they would ensure congruence between local policies and procedures with expected workflow changes after the deployment of the EMR. The third team, Deployment Support, performed education and training sessions. In this phase, local staff subject matter experts would be selected to assist with the training and support of their respective peer groups; for example, nurse to nurse, lab tech to lab tech, manager to manager, provider to provider. In most instances, a team of nurses was brought together to form a nursing informatics team.

This team's charter was to continue to support their colleagues after the Deployment Teams left. The deployment of HealthConnect in each health center was just the beginning. Those who had done the peer-to-peer support during rollout were now back to their regular jobs and were embedded. When workers had problems with the system, they knew exactly who to ask for help. The clinicians were also free to keep suggesting ways to optimize HealthConnect. Those who did peer-to-peer support became change agents. They still attend regional meetings and continue working to improve HealthConnect. Their position has transitioned from the initial period of disruptive innovation into the current period of adaptive change, creating a helpful continuity from one phase to the other.

▶ Ongoing Innovation

Although paradox 3 codifies the risk that change that moves too rapidly can become a barrier to further change, well-managed innovation, conversely, opens up numerous pathways to subsequent innovation. HealthConnect has not just given different clinicians who are updating or reviewing a patient's records instantaneous access to the same information. As technology has leaped ahead, it has now allowed patients to review their own information on both the Kaiser Permanente website and a mobile app. Patients can access test results and even submit photos to aid in diagnosis, as well as exchange e-mails with their care provider or a nurse who handles patient advice.

Currently, clinicians are limited to using the EMR at desktop computers, though much of their work happens away from the desktop. A newly formed Nurse Innovation Team is working on how to make the EMR mobile, whether through tablets or other mobile devices yet to be invented. This opens up multiple questions that will need to be worked through in partnership. For example, after critical information is mobile, how can it be shared with all the care providers who need to see it? What information should be sent under given scenarios, and how can it be transmitted to a care provider quickly and with actionable data?

The final major innovation on HealthConnect has the potential to revolutionize the entire healthcare industry by creating a critical mass of data that can be mined for future evidence-based innovation. With years of data now in the system, it is possible to review and analyze it in aggregate to determine which treatments are most effective, separately and in combination, from exercise to medication. Clinicians will be better able to predict the progress of a given patient's condition using vital signs, emergency room visits during the past year, and other data already entered for similar patients in HealthConnect. Kaiser Permanente can create best practices for how to use the data to anticipate a declining condition or redirect efforts toward patients who are likely to worsen. This aggregation and use of data can be used in the future as a means of heading off paradox 1, providing solid evidence of support or refutation when it comes to further innovation within the organization.

▶ Lessons in Healthcare Innovation

The collaborative model at Kaiser Permanente also encompasses unions and unionized workers. Unions are an essential part of Kaiser Permanente's business, and they have developed a labor–management partnership that is unique in its scale and ambition (Kochan et al., 2009). The parties recognized their interdependence in a landmark partnership agreement, included in the collective bargaining contract in

1997. The collaboration enabled by this partnership has become central to the organization's efforts to meet its ever-intensifying ambidexterity challenges, providing a foundation for combining top-down initiatives by specialized technical staff (e.g., for new computerized medical records) and bottom-up input and involvement by a broad range of personnel for local improvement projects, as well as extensive lateral learning so that similar locations can share lessons learned (Adler & Heckscher, 2013).

How can the lessons from Kaiser Permanente LMP and its EMR implementation be universalized and applied in other healthcare settings, whether union or nonunion, system or facility? The first principle for innovation in a healthcare setting is also the foundational concept of the LMP: Workers know best how to do the work. Therefore, their full and free participation is not a luxury but rather an absolute necessity for innovation to weather the paradoxes that threaten all such change, survive the rough seas of disruptive innovation, and make it through to the relative calm of ongoing adaptive change.

It is perhaps ironic that, although unions and management are traditionally seen as oppositional, in the LMP setting it is the very presence of the union that serves to give employees the sense of psychological safety and security, without which true partnership and cooperation are not possible. Therefore, in a nonunion setting, it is even more important that the workers feel truly empowered to participate fully and honestly without fear of retaliation from management. Within the context of the team's focus on a given task, it must be clear to all participants that everyone is equal. Lip service to this principle will not work. If an employee contributes to the task-oriented discussion in a way that offends a manager and suffers consequences, this would be fatal to the collaborative nature of the enterprise.

Lesson: Management must make a genuine commitment to the workers involved that their full participation is encouraged without negative consequences to their standing within the organization and hold to that commitment.

Within the LMP setting, the union always chooses its own representatives for the given committee, task force, or project. Even in a nonunion, non-LMP setting, it is probably a good idea to allow this. If workers feel that their representatives are handpicked management favorites, this can undermine trust in the process and its results.

Lesson: Let workers choose their own representatives.

In the LMP process, decisions are made by consensus. Neither management nor labor can overrule a group decision. Consensus decision making can sometimes take longer than simply a vote because any one party can halt the process with a simple thumbs down. However, in a consensus decision-making setting, everyone agrees up front that all will support any decision that allows the whole group to move forward. This means that any initiative that does progress has been thoroughly vetted, and it creates greater buy-in and a more personal stake in the outcome from everyone involved. A hybrid system can also be followed, where ground rules are put in place to allow for a democratic vote under certain conditions, agreed to up front, where consensus becomes unworkable and brings the project to a dead stop.

Lesson: Consider allowing decisions to be made by consensus for thorough vetting and greater buy-in.

For the Kaiser Permanente EMR project, having a workable collaborative structure already in place was a huge advantage. The structure that had previously been set up through the LMP was modeled for the HealthConnect build. Start with a national body that oversees the project from the 37,000-foot level. Add a middle layer with regional bodies that can make the project work within a particular area. Finish with local bodies at the facility level. The key to this structure is that information should flow both ways—down from the national and regional bodies, and up from the local and regional bodies.

Even within one facility, this multilevel structure can be duplicated, with participatory groups functioning, for example, at the facility, department, and work unit levels. As with consensus decision making, this might seem to add time and complexity to the design and implementation of an innovation, but in practice it ensures that the end product receives input from multiple stakeholders at all levels of the organization and with every type of expertise that must be brought to bear so that it has depth and breadth and is robust and comprehensive.

Lesson: A multilevel structure can be useful, adaptable, and sizable to any enterprise, from a nationwide health system to a single facility.

Seagondollar, the lead on the Kaiser Permanente Southern California EMR rollout, found that one key to successful change management is understanding how individual personalities function within a group dynamic. He found that most workers fall into one of the following categories:

- Innovators: Those who are looking for change and embrace it
- Middle of the pack: Those who will buy in as long as they know what they need to do
- Late adopters: Although they really do not want to do it, they will after the initiative is tried and true
- Resisters: Will not make the change, and if it is forced on them, they may quit

One key to a successful rollout of a significant new initiative is to find and encourage the innovators in the process who want to be part of the change. These are the people who keep pushing when the project has problems, and they make it a reality. They can become the trainers, the subject matter experts, the ongoing resources for their colleagues. And they can become a means of heading off paradox 2, where individuals within a group pursuing their own agendas can derail the group initiative.

Lesson: Innovators are always present. They will often step to the fore on their own. Regardless, keep an eye out for them, find them, and encourage them to participate and even take the lead.

The UBTs at Kaiser Permanente have led to dramatic improvements in company operations (Adler & Heckscher, 2013). Based on the UBT model, HealthConnect has regional nurse domain teams that are specific to health care. For instance, case managers have their own regional nurse domain teams. Emergency nurses were their own domain. There is a domain for every specialty. These teams meet monthly to discuss anticipated changes and determine the best way to integrate those changes into HealthConnect, modify workflow, and train colleagues on the modifications. These groups talk about what is not working and suggest ways to improve. If the decision is made to do a pilot, the scope of the pilot is defined at these meetings as well.

Lesson: In addition to the multilevel decision-making bodies, it can be productive to have lateral groups based on profession or unit that meet on an ongoing basis to synthesize input into the wider process and also carry the work forward. These groups can be key to moving an innovation from disruptive to adaptive change.

▶ Leadership for Partnership and Innovation

Along the continuum from incremental performance improvement to radical innovation, a number of factors act as preconditions for effective collaboration. These include cultures and practices in which everyone, whatever their formal role, is encouraged to lead and is empowered to do so, including speaking up in an environment of psychological safety, acting and collaborating beyond the constraints of official hierarchy, and thinking with a systems mind-set. A review of recent literature highlights some of the key leadership behaviors and practices that support high performance and innovation.

Kotter (2013) speaks to the limits of hierarchy in a competitive environment characterized by an increase in both threats from a variety of directions and windows of opportunity that open and close quickly. In this context, organizations need to be structured to be reliable and efficient, and at the same time nimble and fast moving; a reliance on only the former will not allow organizations to drive the major changes that such challenges demand. People at every level of the organization need to be empowered to act and collaborate beyond the bounds of formal institutional structure. In other words, both hierarchy and network are required. Similarly, Battilana and Cascario (2013) identify the power of informal networks in driving change. In their study of change initiatives at the massive British National Health Service, they conclude, "Change agents who were central in the organization's informal network had a clear advantage, regardless of their position in the informal hierarchy" (Battilana & Cascario, 2013, p. 64).

Within the partnership between the Coalition of Kaiser Permanente Unions and Kaiser Permanente, the parties have identified a set of 37 behaviors, organized around seven core principles, to guide collaboration (Kaiser Permanente, 2003). Each of the principles calls on managers and union stewards to take shared responsibility for various dimensions of the partnership, including ensuring the success of both parties, providing patients with a superior care experience, and engaging employees in decision making. Eaton, Konistney, Litwin, and Vanderhorst (2011) conducted a study of high-performing UBTs at Kaiser Permanente. Several findings, among other structural and process factors, stand out. They identify psychological safety as key to high performance, describing "a work environment where everyone was able to speak up and had the courage to have difficult conversations. Employees stated they could say what was on their minds without fear of retaliation or retribution" (Eaton et al., 2011, p. 11). Systems thinking is also crucial: "The most successful teams we studied were interested in how their work and performance were affected by that broader system and were working collaboratively with other departments to achieve common goals" (Eaton et al., 2011, p. 10). Among the leadership dimensions identified by the authors is a shift from traditional, command-and-control management to an approach in which "managers would work to coach and motivate employees instead of micromanaging them. They trusted employees to do their jobs. Managers of the teams stated that once they were able to change how they managed employees, their job actually became easier" (Eaton et al., 2011, p. 8). This transformation is accompanied by another noteworthy aspect of leadership: "On most of the high performing teams we studied, the labor leads—who were generally selected by the unionized employees on the unit—took on such an authentic leadership role that they became essentially interchangeable with their management counterparts" (Eaton et al., 2011, p. 8).

Finally, Bevan and Fairman (2014) provide a thorough examination of how leadership needs to shift to reflect the scope and complexity of contemporary healthcare challenges. Like other authors cited here, they identify the need to marry what they term a dominant approach, characterized by top-down leadership, with an emergent model, marked by shared purpose. The mind-set is that transformational change is more likely to happen cross-organizationally than within a single organization and that hierarchical levers cannot drive change across the wider system. From this perspective, large-scale change depends on many partners (2014, p. 18). On the emergent side, they note that "the most important skill that leaders of change need to develop for the 21st century is the ability to build partnership" (2014, p. 18).

The labor–management partnership at Kaiser Permanente reflects broader organizational and industry thinking about how collaboration and distributed leadership can help spur the kind of change and innovation that contemporary circumstances demand. At the same time, this partnership has developed its own specific practices and lessons about what is required to achieve high performance. As this partnership continues to grow and evolve, we expect that it will continue to both draw from and contribute to emerging approaches to innovation leadership.

▶ Innovation Outside Health Care

Looking at the nexus of labor and innovation beyond health care, The Workers Lab is an innovation incubator and accelerator that was established as an answer to its founders who ask themselves, in the context of a shrinking labor movement and a growing low-wage economy, "why can't we take the dynamism and ingenuity fueling new products, services and institutions, and harness them to advance the interests of low-wage workers? Can we channel that creativity and rigorous experimentation to address the vexing problems facing millions of American workers?" (Maxwell, 2015, para. 3).

The Workers Lab focuses on investing in "organizing strategies, business models, and platforms that will lift wages and transform the lives of US workers" (The Workers Lab, 2015, para. 1). Backed by unions and foundations, it funds a small number of projects aimed at developing and testing new approaches to achieving economic justice for workers in low-wage industries.

Among its first round of projects in 2015, The Workers Lab funded an experiment called Top Server with the Restaurant Opportunities Center (ROC) United and the Everett Program at UC Santa Cruz, which marries workforce development to advanced technology and gamification. The mission of ROC United is to address and improve the low wages and poor working conditions suffered by restaurant workers; its Colors Hospitality Opportunities for Workers (CHOW) Institute provides free job training and development for restaurant workers to move into living wage jobs. With funding and support from The Workers Lab, ROC United will be developing an online gaming platform for the CHOW. Institute's restaurant worker members to support their efforts to develop career skills to move into higher-paying jobs in that industry.

In an article in *Fast Company*, The Workers Lab's executive director, Carmen Rojas, speaks to the benefit that can accrue to employers when they provide workers with living wages and good benefits: "When these conditions are met, corporations and revenue-generating ventures experience less employee turnover and have increased customer loyalty . . . This is great for their corporations as well as for our economy" (Dishman, 2015).

Such intentional experimentation, including the application of innovation methodologies more commonly used in for-profit endeavors, such as technology start-ups or big business, represents a significant departure from traditional organizing and collective bargaining strategies and holds the potential to provide rich lessons and insights about how to achieve sustainable and scalable victories for the labor movement in a low-wage economy marked by massive income inequality and declining rates of unionization.

References

Adler, P., & Heckscher, C. (2013, 4th Quarter). The collaborative, ambidextrous enterprise. *Universia Business Review,* 34–50.

Battilana, J., & Cascario, T. (2013, July/August). The network secrets of great change agents. *Harvard Business Review,* 62–68.

Bensaid, C. (2015, March). *How our strategy works for all workers.* Speech presented at Coalition of Kaiser Permanente Unions Delegates Conference. Anaheim, CA.

Berwick, D. (2011, December 7). The moral test. Retrieved from http://www.ahier.net/2011/12/remember-patient.html?m=1

Bevan, H., & Fairman, S. (2014). The new era of thinking and practice in change and transformation: A call to action for leaders of health and care. Retrieved from http://media.nhsiq.nhs.uk/whitepaper/index.html

Congressional Budget Office. (2014). *Updated estimates of the effects of the insurance coverage provisions of the Affordable Care Act, April 2014* (CBO Publication No. 45231). Washington, DC: Government Printing Office.

Detert, J., & Edmondson, A. C. (2007). Why employees are afraid to speak. *Harvard Business Review.* Retrieved from https://hbr.org/2007/05/why-employees-are-afraid-to-speak

Dishman, L. (2015, May 8). Meet the woman working to change low income workers' prospects. Retrieved from http://www.fastcompany.com/3046041/strong-female-lead/meet-the-woman-working-to-change-low-income-workers-prospects

Dixon-Woods, M., Amalberti, R., Goodman, S., Bergman, B., & Glasziou, P. (2011). Problems and promises of innovation: Why healthcare needs to rethink its love/hate relationship with the new. *BMJ Quality & Safety, 20,* i47–i51.

Eaton, A., Konistney, D., Litwin, A. S., & Vanderhorst, N. (2010, December). *The path to performance: A study of high-performing unit-based teams at Kaiser Permanente* [white paper]. Publication of Kaiser Permanente Labor Management Partnership.

Geoghegan, T. (2014). *Only one thing can save us: Why America needs a new kind of labor movement.* New York, NY: New Press.

Greenhouse, S. (2014, June 30). Supreme Court ruling on union fees is a limited blow to labor. *The New York Times.* Retrieved from http://www.nytimes.com/2014/07/01/business/supreme-court-ruling-on-public-workers-and-union-fees.html.

Henwood, D. (2015, January). Union membership is down again—but it still pays to be a union member. Retrieved from http://www.inthesetimes.com/working/entry/17567/union_membership_is_down_again_but_it_still_pays_to_be_a_member.

Kaiser Permanente. (2003). Labor management partnership behaviors. Retrieved from http://lmpartnership.org/sites/default/files/lmp__behaviors.pdf

Kaufman, N. S. (2011). Changing economics in an era of healthcare reform. *Journal of Healthcare Management, 56*(1), 9–13.

Kochan, T. A., Eaton, A. E., McKersie, R. B., & Adler, P. S. (2009). *Healing together: The labor-management partnership at Kaiser Permanente.* Ithaca, NY: Cornell University Press.

Kotter, J. (2013, October 18). *Accelerate* [Video file]. Retrieved from https://www.youtube.com/watch?v=o9SxvladTCg

Lazes, P., Katz, L., & Figueroa, M. (2012). *How labor–management partnerships improve patient care, cost control, and labor relations: Case studies for Fletcher Allen Health Care, Kaiser Permanente, and Montefiore Medical Center.* Ithaca, NY: Cornell University.

Lazes, P., Katz, L., Figueroa, M., & Karpur, A. (2012). Using adaptive and disruptive change strategies to create an integrated delivery system: Montefiore Medical Center's experience. In S. A. Mohrman & A. B. Shani (Eds.), *Organizing for sustainable health care* (pp. 147–168). Bringley, UK: Emerald Group.

Maxwell, M. B. (2015). Investing in the future: The Workers Lab sows the seeds of change. Retrieved from https://blog.dol.gov/2015/04/30/investing-in-the-future-the-workers-lab-sows-seeds-of-change/

Meyerson, H. (2013, September 13). Harold Meyerson: At AFL-CIO convention, labor embraces the new America. *Washington Post.*

Morrison, I. (2000). *Health care in the new millennium: Vision, values, and leadership.* San Francisco, CA: Jossey-Bass.

Nixon, J. P. (2012, January). *Culture matters: An investigation into UBTs, workplace culture and performance.* Presented at the Executive Committee of the Labor Management Partnership Strategy Group, Oakland, CA.

Rolf, D. (2014, June 18). What if we treated labor like a startup? *The Nation.* Retrieved from http://www.thenation.com/article/180316/omcibator-labor#

Service Employees International Union. (2015). *Improving care, lowering costs: How front-line hospital workers are transforming healthcare.* Washington, DC: Author.

Thakur, R., Hsu, S. H., & Fontenot, G. (2012). Innovation in healthcare: Issues and future trends. *Journal of Business Research, 65*(4), 562–569.

The Workers Lab. (2015). Innovating for worker justice. Retrieved from http://theworkerslab.com/program/

CHAPTER 16

Disrupting the Undisruptable— Innovation and Healthcare Education

Sandra Davidson

▶ Introduction

This chapter is a compilation of questions, issues, evidence, innovations, and a vision for the future and how care providers could be educated to create the preferred future of health care. It builds on many of the themes presented throughout this text and that are interpreted here within an educational context. There is a Buddhist saying that is helpful in framing the discussion in this chapter: If you want to know your past, look into your present conditions. If you want to know your future, look into your present actions.

The chapter will start with an overview of the current contextual challenges and opportunities in health sciences education. Then it will turn its attention to the future. What do emerging trends, evidence, innovation, and contemporary learning theory tell us about how we might act to disrupt and transform the education of health disciplines?

▶ Disrupting the Undisruptable: The *Titanic* That Never Sank

It is very apropos to use the *Titanic* analogy here. When the *Titanic* sank in April 1912, it was state of the art and represented the highest achievement in engineering and design at the time. In many ways, our education system is like the *Titanic*: It was state of the art at the beginning of the 20th century! However, the education system did not meet with an icy adversary as the *Titanic* did. Instead, it has been lovingly cared for, maintained, and kept in working order for more than 100 years. Perhaps every decade or so, it has received a new coat of paint or its fixtures have been up-dated based on the latest fashion. Educators have reconfigured an assessment here or a learning strategy there. But, under all the embellishments, it is still a large boat with a steam-powered engine (linear, content-laden, behaviorist education). When you think of formal health-sciences educational programs, I would venture to guess that *innovative* and *future-focused* are not the first words that come to your mind. How is it that our formal educational programs have resisted change for so long? There are a myriad of factors—organizational, political, financial, and philosophical—that have made all higher education (not just healthcare faculties) largely recalcitrant and *undisruptable* for the majority of the 20th century. In recent years, there has been an increasingly loud narrative exclaiming that "higher education is broken!" I would argue that it is not broken—it functions very well. The problem is that the system of higher education was constructed in the shadow of the industrial revolution, and it is a system that is obsolete. Just like the well-maintained vintage ocean liner, it may be functional and get the job done, but it is no match for the state-of-the-art energy-efficient super liners that can traverse the world's oceans in a fraction of the time and with greater amenities and energy efficiency. Malcom Oliver's blog (https://malcolmoliver.wordpress.com/titanic-vs-oasis-of-the-seas/) provides a won-derful comparison between the *Titanic* and modern-day Oasis class ocean liners. The parallels to higher education are striking, as you can see in **TABLE 16-1**.

There is growing acknowledgment in health professions education that we can no longer simply rearrange the deck chairs on the *Titanic*. We need to create new patterns of interaction and meaning, new ways of being, and new language that res-onates with the current and emerging realities of 21st-century health care. It is time to adopt a new mode of travel that is more representative of where we want to go.

The Futurist publishes its annual outlook list in December each year. The list is a compilation of forecasts collected by the World Future Society. It is not intended to predict the future but rather to provoke thought and inspire action for building a better future starting today. The 2015 outlook list included this statement: "teleportation is getting closer, photon by photon" (Scott, 2014). Scott elaborated further:

TABLE 16-1 Comparison of 20th-Century to Modern Systems

	Titanic	Modern Ocean Liner	Traditional Higher Education	Future of Higher Education
Size/Scale	46,000 gt	225,000 gt	One size fits all	Learner-centric; individualized learning
Amenities	Cabins were cramped, did not have private baths or toilets; only two baths for the 700 third-class passengers (one for men and one for women)	2,700 passenger cabins, with air-conditioning, TV, en suite sink, toilet, and a shower in every cabin	Standard programming, large lecture sections, variation or deviation discouraged; volume-driven model	Individualized learning and accommodation of needs; transportability of learning (e.g., micro-credentialing, digital badges); focus on student experience
Classes	Three-class ship	One-class ship	Quality based on ability to pay (e.g., Ivy League, state universities, technical colleges)	Democratization of learning; standardization of excellence
Technology	Morse code via radio was new technology	Satellite GPS, telephones, and wireless Internet	Space-bound (classroom driven); seat-time models of learning (credit hours)	Ubiquitous, customizable, flexible learning; mastery/competency based

Moving physical matter from one place to another has long been the impossible dream of science fiction, but physicist Juan Yin of the University of Science and Technology of China claims to have teleported entangled photons over a distance of about 60 miles. While vacationers should make more-traditional travel arrangements for the foreseeable future, teleportation technologies will advance over the next several decades. (2014)

Imagine what we might accomplish in healthcare education if we were to adopt this metaphor to guide our way forward.

In this section I will present some ideas, issues, and opportunities for how the evidence-innovation dynamic can beam healthcare education into the future. To start, let us revisit the relationship between evidence and innovation from a complex relational perspective. **FIGURE 16-1** is presented here as a reminder of the socially constructed meaning-making space that exists within our systems: the hurly-burly of organizational life. In the knowledge era, we have access to a wide range of sources of evidence (both formal and informal). In the knowledge era, evidence acts as the foundation upon which educational practices, policies, processes, and programs should be based. Just as in practice environments, there is always the danger of slipping back into habitual and unexamined practices on the grounds that we have always done it this way. It is in the conversational spaces of the organization (in this case, universities, colleges, programs, and classrooms) that meaning about and from evidence is made. The relational dynamics may result in adoption, adaptation, or even avoidance of evidence-based practices, depending on the ebb and flow of enabling and constraining patterns of meaning. Adaptation of evidence often occurs in several ways that can lead to innovation.

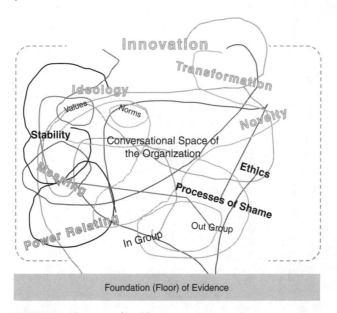

FIGURE 16-1 The mess of healthcare innovation.

First, the foundational evidence may be partial or incomplete, or gaps may exist. For example, there may be compelling and high-quality evidence that suggests gamification is an effective learning strategy, but the population used in the research may not be second-year pharmacy students. Educators would then need to interpret and extrapolate what the utility of these research findings might be for their population of learners. Through conversations, educators might consider and deliberate about learner preferences and characteristics and local best practices, or they may engage experts to provide consultation. Suppose that the educators in this example decided to adapt the gamification learning strategy in ways they believe could best meet the needs of their students. In so doing, an educational innovation occurs. As the educators monitor the impact on student learning, satisfaction, and feasibility (cost, ease of use, etc.), local evidence is generated. From here, further cycles of innovation may occur to further tailor and fine-tune the educational intervention, or if the initial innovation was deemed successful, the educators may decide to publish an article sharing the intervention and associated outcomes. Thus, what was an innovation becomes evidence.

A second scenario for innovation may arise out of a void in the evidence. Perhaps the conversational space of the organization is filled with dissatisfaction with a current practice. For example, perhaps a traditional learning activity (such as lecture) is being used by educators who are charged with teaching pharmacotherapeutics to a class of 100 students. The educators have noted that students' achievement of learning outcomes (and probably satisfaction) is wanting. Perhaps the educators explore the literature and find that there is no strong evidence to suggest that the lecture is an effective learning strategy. But what could they do with a large class that would be more effective? For this example, let us say that they are unable to find evidence that provides guidance for effectively teaching pharmacotherapeutics to large classes of undergraduate nursing students. In other words, there is a void in the available evidence.

Instead of continuing to teach using a practice that is not evidence based (lecture), the group of instructors who team-teach this course might explore literature about adult learning and student-centered learning principles (theory). From this basis, they may use their innovation skills (such as design thinking, experience mapping, and prototyping) to develop an innovative teaching strategy that is founded on sound theory and student preferences and values. This might be a combination of using technology (social media) and student learning collectives, for example. Perhaps it takes several iterations of this teaching approach before improved outcomes are noticed. This is the ongoing process of tinkering (another innovation strategy). Eventually this teaching strategy may become a local best practice for teaching large classes in the nursing program and shared among instructors in the community of practice.

These two examples are just two of the infinite possibilities of how the evidence-innovation dynamic might be actualized from a complex relational perspective in education. **FIGURE 16-2** is an adaptation of Melnyk and Fineout-Overholt's (2005) well-known evidence-based practice framework. I have adapted it to illustrate how these same considerations and contextual awareness can be applied in healthcare education. This is a useful graphic organizer for educators seeking to engage in evidence-based education.

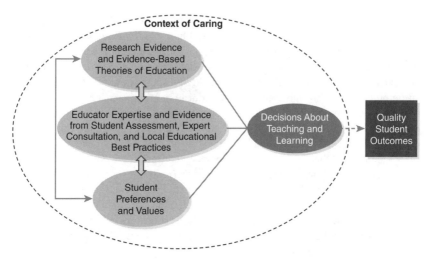

FIGURE 16-2 The merging of science and art: Evidence-based practice within an educational context.

Modified from Melnyk, B. and Fineout-Overholt, E. (2005). *Evidence-based practice in nursing and healthcare*, p. 15. Philadelphia, PA: Lippincott, Williams & Wilkins.

▶ Reflections on What Is and Why We Need Disruption

As I reflect on what is, I am reminded of the words of former Czech president Václav Havel from a speech he gave in 1994: "It is as if something were crumbling, decaying, and exhausting itself—while something else, still indistinct, were rising from the rubble" (Havel, as cited in Scharmer, 2007, p. 1). Scharmer elaborates further: "The crisis of our time reveals the dying of an old social structure and way of thinking, an old way of institutionalizing and enacting collective social forms. Frontline practitioners—managers, teachers, nurses, [and] physicians . . . share a sense of the current reality. They can feel the heat of an ever-increasing workload and pressure to do even more" (2007, p. 2).

I believe this characterizes the vibe in healthcare education today. Health professions instructors (as both practitioners and teachers) are doubly aware of the pressures to do more with less and the ultimate futility of continuing to educate and practice as we have in the past. In this section I will highlight some of the contextual challenges, debates, and pain points that permeate the current reality of healthcare education. The pressure to do even more, I believe, comes from the friction created when old ways of being and doing rub up against the new. Instructors may feel conflicted and bewildered as they try to make sense out of the ambiguity of what has been versus what is becoming. In an effort to cover all the bases (often out of fear and uncertainty), instructors end up doing double work—maintaining the practices of the past while attempting to engage with new educational innovations, ideas, and practices. As a result of spreading our time, attention, and energies too broadly, we often feel that nothing gets done particularly well. How do we make decisions about what educational practices to let go of, what to keep, and what is worth developing? We will return to this question later.

And what of students? What is the experience of our students who have arrived in our classrooms (both physical and virtual) full of purpose and excitement? Health professions students often arrive with an idealized view of the profession they seek to join. As students progress through their programs of study, they become increasingly aware of the frenetic nature of both healthcare education and practice. They see instructors trying to cover all the content and find themselves cramming for tests. In their learning experiences in clinical settings, they see care providers who are trying to do more with less. Rarely do they see their clinical mentors step off the treadmill long enough to catch their breath. Students' idealized visions of their profession are quickly replaced with cynicism and trepidation as they are immersed in the brine of toxic healthcare workplaces and as they absorb their mentors' professional malaise.

Of course, education does not occur in a vacuum. Health professions instructors and students teach and learn within complex contextual structures, namely, the educational system and the practice environment. Each of these structures is constituted of unique processes, policies, and personalities that make up the overall environment. Our current organizational realities are dominated by hierarchy and mechanistic structures in both practice and education. A common metaphor used to describe the structures and hardened divisions in these organizations today is that of the silo. In these columnar and encapsulated structures, there is little communication or diffusion between practice and educational contexts. Is it any wonder that the literature and research in healthcare education is replete with references to the education–practice gap?

Even within each silo, there are layers and levels of division. At each level, we find ourselves separated by the siloed distinctions: surgery unit or medical unit, inpatient or outpatient services, clinical course or theory course. We are habituated to organizing and constructing our world around what makes us different. It is not surprising, then, that we struggle to find common ground, to collaborate, or to seek synergies. **FIGURE 16-3** depicts the contextual silos and the intersilo distinctions that perpetuate this divisive mind-set. Although there is some communication and movement among the grand silos (for example, students who graduate from the educational system move to the practice context), there is a disconnect

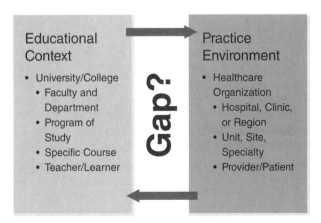

FIGURE 16-3 Education and practice silos.

(gap) between the silos because they function as closed systems. This model is representative of current mainstream health care and healthcare education, and it is emblematic of our mechanistic and Newtonian legacy. To use an industrial analogy, our machines are obsolete. They still function quite well, but their purpose and form are suited to a bygone era. Before exploring the social, organizational, and learning technologies that are state of the art, let us delve a little deeper into our current predicament.

In 2008, the Association of Academic Health Centers (AAHC) published a report on the state of the health workforce (2008). The report is aptly titled *Out of Order, Out of Time*. It provides an excellent overview of the contextual challenges in health professions education. I will use some of the key findings of the AAHC report to frame the discussion that follows here.

▶ The Canary in the Mine Shaft: Dissatisfaction in Health Care

The healthcare industry has experienced waning workforce satisfaction for several decades. Healthy workplace environments and overall work–life satisfaction are crucial for both the recruitment of future health professionals and for the retention of existing providers (Association of Academic Health Centers, 2008). However, numerous surveys across all disciplines point to growing dissatisfaction. In an international study conducted among hospital-based nurses, almost one in three nurses younger than the age of 30 reported that they were planning to leave their jobs within the year (Aiken Clarke, Sloane, Sochalski, & Busse, 2001). Likewise, Unruh, Zhang, and Chisolm (2016) reported that between 30% and 50% of newly licensed RNs leave their job or the nursing profession entirely within 3 years of graduating. In a 2014 survey, 66% of pharmacists rated their workload level as high or excessively high. Further, 45% of pharmacists reported that their current workload had negative or very negative effects on mental/emotional health (Midwest Pharmacy Workforce Research Consortium, 2015).

Overall, six workplace characteristics have been identified as the most prevalent barriers to the recruitment and retention of healthcare providers (AAHC, 2008):

- The healthcare system is too hierarchical, with too much rigidity or little room for growth or innovation.
- The work is too traditional; new graduates, particularly, find practice environments to be antiquated and stifling.
- The work is too physically demanding.
- The 24/7 nature of many healthcare settings results in undesirable schedules for some health professions. There is still a negative stigma about shift work.
- Financial remuneration may be low or has plateaued.
- The pace of work is demanding and stressful.

The healthcare system, as it is currently experienced by many providers, feels untenable, yet there is no distinct resolution or relief in sight. From a health professions education perspective, the challenges are many. How do educators recruit prospective students into health professions yet still present an appealing (and realistic) vision of what their future professional practice will be like? How do educators manage the tensions among textbook idealism, preparing the practitioners of the future, and the often grim reality of current practice environments? What is the quality and effectiveness of clinical experiences for students, given the widespread dissatisfaction and role strain of practicing healthcare providers? These are just a few of the countless questions that keep many educators up at night.

LEARNING ACTIVITY

In small groups, spend 15 to 20 minutes addressing the following three questions:

How do educators recruit prospective students into health professions yet still present an appealing (and realistic) vision of what their future professional practice will be like?

How do educators manage the tensions among textbook idealism, preparing the practitioners of the future, and the often-grim reality of current practice environments?

What is the quality and effectiveness of clinical experiences for students, given the widespread dissatisfaction and role strain of practicing healthcare providers?

Please share your own experiences (as students, providers, leaders) in relation to these issues. Are there best practices you could suggest?

▶ Quality and Consistency of Education Amid Faculty Shortages

Faculty shortages are present and intensifying across all health disciplines. The shortages are driven by a number of factors. Prominent among them are the aging of the existing faculty workforce, coupled with the declining pipeline of future faculty members to replace them upon retirement.

In nursing, the age of faculty members has been increasing steadily. Based on a 2015–2016 survey, the average ages of doctoral nurse faculty members holding the ranks of professor, associate professor, and assistant professor were 62.2, 57.6, and 51.1 years, respectively (American Association of Colleges of Nursing, 2017). As a result, large numbers of nursing faculty are retiring. The Canadian Association of Schools of Nursing (CASN) 2016–2017 survey reported similar trends: 58.0% of nursing faculty members with permanent positions (e.g., tenure track) were 50 years of age or older; 41.1% were 55 years or older and 21.0% were 60 years or over (Canadian Association of Schools of Nursing, 2018). Similar trends are present in dentistry; pharmacy; and allied health professions such as nutrition, respiratory therapy, dental hygiene, and radiography (Association of Academic Health Centers, 2008).

These mass retirements across all health disciplines necessitate a focus on the recruitment and development of new faculty. However, retiring faculty members are not being replaced at a rate sufficient to even maintain current enrollment numbers, not to speak of future growth of educational programs (Association of

Academic Health Centers, 2008). The reasons for the paucity of qualified new faculty are many. Salary inequities are prime among them. Across all disciplines, clinical salaries are higher than academic salaries. Given that most health disciplines require faculty members to have at least a master's degree and ideally a doctorate, the added time and expense of earning this advanced education (e.g., lost wages due to prolonged study, along with tuition and student loans) tends to diminish the financial appeal of academic work even further.

There also seems to be a general lack of enthusiasm for academic healthcare positions. Just as in the clinical realm, low job satisfaction has been reported among health professions faculty members. "Stress, unrealistic job expectations, and difficulties managing academic life and personal life contribute to this problem. There is evidence that many junior faculty members have difficulty securing the research grants that are necessary for promotion and tenure" (Association of Academic Health Centers, 2008, p. 46). Unfortunately, and mostly unconsciously, healthcare instructors tend to role model the less desirable aspects of academic life for students. If students perceive the work of academics to be characterized by burdensome teaching schedules, nonexistent work–life balance, the constant scrambling for scarce research funds, and impossible publication expectations, there is little mystery as to why so few students are interested in academic healthcare positions.

With respect to the quality and continuity of health professions education, the combination of aging and retiring seasoned instructors and the lack of qualified new instructors to replace them constitutes a crisis not only of numbers but also of quality. In an article in *The Chronicle of Higher Education*, Dr. Pascarella, a professor at the University of Iowa, was quoted as saying, "It took me a while to become a decent teacher. I just hate to think of the students I've screwed up" (Berrett, 2013). Many instructors in the health disciplines today would echo Dr. Pascarella's sentiments.

Becoming a good teacher requires a substantial investment of time and effort to develop one's abilities. Particularly in health sciences, there exists another challenge toward achieving good teaching. The majority of health professions instructors are not formally educated to be educators. That is, our primary discipline is not education; we are physical therapists, physicians, nurses, social workers, and pharmacists who have figured out how to teach, largely through informal learning, such as trial and error, self-study, and student feedback. New instructors who are fortunate enough to have good mentors may have had a somewhat less tumultuous introduction to teaching. However, with the impending retirements of many seasoned instructors, health professions are also losing those who can most wisely mentor and support new educators. Dr. Valiga, in her address to the NLN's National Advisory Council on Nurse Education and Practice in April 2002, summed up the situation:

> Without preparation in the faculty role . . . without role models and mentors to help them manage the unique issues one faces in that role . . . without strong commitment to a role where teaching is primary and one's own clinical practice is secondary . . . and without a science to undermine their practice, individuals whose preparation was as a nurse practitioner or clinical nurse specialist struggle to implement the faculty role. (Valiga, 2002, p. 4)

EXEMPLAR: THE FACULTY NAVIGATOR PROGRAM (FNP)

In response to the challenges outlined by Valiga in her 2002 statement, a group of nurse educators in Alberta, Canada, developed a unique and effective program to support the transition of clinical nurses into teaching nursing—most often as clinical instructors. The Faculty Navigator Program (FNP) arose out of the need to support and retain clinical instructors in the nursing program at Red Deer College.

Transition from Practice to Education

The challenges of the transition from practice to education are significant and may include an identity struggle and a sense of loss and grief (Cranford, 2013). Ramage (2004) described a process of "disassembling" the nursing identity and then "rediscovering" and "realizing" the new "self" as educator. Many clinical nurses who venture into academia have not had courses in classroom instruction or education on how to be an effective clinical instructor (Hessler & Ritchie, 2006). This lack of training may contribute to role strain and conflict and cause valuable instructors to retreat to their clinical roles that seem less complicated (Esper, 1995). Schoening (2009, 2013) described novice educators as being on a journey down a new career path with no guide to help them navigate in the new world of education to reach their destination in the transition to formation of an identity as a nurse educator. Significantly, the sense of feeling like an educator changed the teaching practice. The emphasis became the process of learning, rather than simply the product. The focus shifted from their behavior as a teacher to the students' experience as a learner. In other words, there was a shift from being a clinician to being an educator.

Davidson (2011) described teacher formation as a personal and professional transformation that results in the formation of a nurse educator—"not a nurse who teaches or a teacher who happens to be a nurse and not a nurse/educator, but a nurse educator" (p. 166). Davidson believed that understanding the process of formation is significant in the quest to transform the discipline of nursing and nursing education.

The FNP: Supporting Teacher Formation

Building on the concept of self-efficacy (Bandura, 1977; Nugent, Bradshaw, & Kito, 1999) and Benner's (1984) exploration of the novice-to-expert process for nurses, the FNP initially focused on increasing competence and confidence in the role of nurse educator and on developing processes and strategies to support retention of faculty. Nurse educators may have personal efficacy based on their clinical expertise but less teacher efficacy (Nugent, Bradshaw, & Kito, 1999). For nurse educators to be effective, both personal and teaching self-efficacy are required.

The FNP began as a pilot project in 2012 and was initially developed as a strategy to support new and novice faculty in the transition from clinician to nurse educator to enhance retention. The goal was to increase teacher self-efficacy. Over time, the program has had an increased focus on supporting faculty in the development of an educator identity, the outcome of which is to enhance the student learning experience.

A navigator is defined as one who is able to "find and follow a path through a difficult place to deal effectively with a complicated situation" (macmillandictionary.com) or is an informal guide (oxforddictionaries.com). In this program the faculty navigator assists faculty to navigate the complexity of the teaching and learning process by helping to find resources, encouraging supportive relationship building, exploring the transition from clinical practice to education practice, and supporting the development of the educator role identity (e.g., teacher formation).

(continues)

EXEMPLAR: THE FACULTY NAVIGATOR PROGRAM (FNP)   *(continued)*

The two-year pilot project focused on a group of new and novice (less than five years of teaching experience) nursing educators. Positive program evaluation data of the pilot resulted in formal adoption and ongoing support/funding of the program, and currently the FNP is available to any nursing instructor in any of the nursing programs (BSN and PN) at Red Deer College.

Structure of the FNP

The program consists of two components: individual consultations and a community of practice. In terms of individual consultations, the faculty navigator is available to attend a lab or classroom teaching session, a clinical learning experience, or any teaching/learning situation. As well, the faculty navigator is available for in-the-moment consultations via phone, text, e-mail, or office drop-in. The purpose of these individual interactions is to engage in a dialogue about the experience of being an educator, discuss strategies currently used to support student learning and the effectiveness of the strategies, discuss options, and address specific issues and concerns.

The second component of the FNP involves facilitation of a community of practice. Wenger (2006) described three key elements: (1) members share an interest and a body of knowledge, (2) members help each other and build relationships that allow them to learn from each other, and (3) members of a community of practice share a variety of resources and experiences. The community of practice sessions were held every 4–6 weeks. Integration of an appreciative inquiry approach to the conversations was important in the ongoing engagement of the nurse educators with the community of practice sessions. Appreciative inquiry (Cooperrider & Whitney, 1999) attempts to highlight the best of what is currently occurring and build on this to enhance practice.

Topics for discussion were initially proposed by the faculty navigator and focused on topics related to teaching strategies. An article from nursing education literature was sent out with the meeting request to support the outcome of engaging in evidence-based practice in nursing education. After the initial sessions (4–5 months), the focus of the FNP shifted to a greater emphasis on supporting faculty members in the development of their identity as nurse educators. The shift in focus stems from a variety of contextual factors, including an increased emphasis on learner-centered approaches to teaching (Weimer, 2013), increased understanding of the learning process from neuropsychology, a changing student population, increased use of technology in the teaching and learning process, and current discussions about the purpose and direction of nursing education.

Fast-Forward to 2019

Since the initial pilot project at Red Deer College in 2012, refinement of this program has taken place. Red Deer College is now on its second generation of faculty navigators (the original two having retired in 2015 and 2016) and the program is still going strong. Program evaluation data has informed the refinement of the FNP and participant outcomes are positive: Regrettable clinical instructor turnover is almost nil, and instructors and students alike report improved quality of teaching and better student learning outcomes.

Diffusion of this innovative program has also happened. Presentations about the FNP at local and regional nursing education conferences led to the adoption of the program at two additional nursing schools in Alberta. In 2016, the faculty navigators and administrators from these schools developed a two-day Faculty Navigator Training Workshop. Over 40 nurse educators and administrators from across Western Canada attended the workshop, and many returned to their institutions and created their own versions of the FNP. A second Faculty Navigator Workshop was held again in 2018 where participants from the 2016 workshop were invited to share progress and best practices, while at the same time inviting new participants to learn FNP basics. In essence, faculty navigators have now created their own community of practice, and the FNP movement continues to grow.

Additional acknowledgements for this section are Elizabeth Hagell, and Sheila McKay, both faculty emeriti (and the first Faculty Navigators) at Red Deer College.

▶ Interprofessional Education and Practice: The Key to Meeting Future Needs

A wide variety of national and international groups have highlighted the need for and promise of interprofessional education and practice over the past 25 years (Association of Academic Health Centers, 2008, 2013; Institute of Medicine, 2001, 2011; Interprofessional Education Collaborative Expert Panel, 2011; Tresolini & Pew-Fetzer Task Force, 1994; World Health Organization, 2010). As evidenced by this broad array of reports, it is evident that dialogues have been occurring for several decades around interprofessional education and practice. In light of these long-running interests in interprofessional activities, one might wonder why we are not further ahead.

Interprofessional or multiple disciplinary education, more generally, tends to occur in isolated pockets, and initiatives seem to be short term. It is often the case that an interprofessional education initiative flourishes for several years under the auspices of a grant or research project, but institutional interest and resources wane after the project period ends (Association of Academic Health Centers, 2008; Interprofessional Education Collaborative Expert Panel, 2011). Again, many of the identified barriers to true collaborative practice and interprofessional education programs can be traced back to our siloed and hierarchy-heavy organizations and professions. The following is a summary of the major barriers to interprofessional education (Interprofessional Education Collaborative Expert Panel, 2011; World Health Organization, 2010):

- Institutional-level challenges: Leadership support, buy-in, and resource allocation
- Practical concerns: Scheduling, space, synchronizing multiple curricula
- Faculty development: Teaching interprofessional process is different than traditional discipline-specific didactic methods
- Lack of collaborators: One discipline may want to participate, others may not; single-discipline schools may not be able to provide interprofessional education opportunities
- Regulatory challenges: Discipline-specific regulators may not view interprofessional competencies as essential for practice
- Assessment: What exactly is being assessed (knowledge, skills, and behaviors), and how do we assess interprofessional learning?

Our organizational structures, mind-sets, policies, and long-held assumptions about the nature of health care and education are the biggest impediments to change. In other words, we are getting in the way of our own success.

However, there is reason for optimism. Slowly but surely, there is progress. There are individuals, teams, and even organizations that are leading the way in overcoming these traditional barriers to interprofessional education and collaborative practice. In relation to the themes and focus of this text, healthcare innovation is just one type of collaborative practice. There is great synergy between interprofessional education and educating the future leaders of healthcare innovation. Innovation is a team sport, so to speak. It follows, then, that the basic knowledge, skills, and attitudes that enable teams to be innovative are also the foundation of high-functioning collaborative care teams. Innovation theory and practice may well be the vehicle that propels us from teaching through the past toward preparing the next generation of healthcare providers who are fully capable of transforming health care. Clinical reasoning, creativity, multiple disciplinary collaboration, evidence-based practice, and leadership amid complex systems are but a few of the competencies deemed essential in 21st-century healthcare practice. These new competencies and realities for practitioners require that we transform the ways in which individuals are educated for and enter into health professions in the knowledge era and beyond.

▶ **Where Do We Go from Here?**

Benner, Sutphen, Leonard, and Day (2010) published the most significant work on the transformation of nursing education since Bevis and Watson's work in the 1980s. Through their research, Benner and colleagues crafted a compelling, and at times scathing, exposé of the current realities and inadequacies of nursing education in light of the state of the U.S. healthcare system and the clinical settings in which nurses practice. The following are the four transformational "shifts for integration" (2010, p. 82) that arose in their study:

- "Shift from a focus on covering decontextualized knowledge to an emphasis on teaching for a sense of salience, situated cognition, and action in particular situations" (2010, p. 82).
- "Shift from sharp separation of clinical and classroom teaching to integration of classroom and clinical teaching" (2010, p. 83).
- "Shift from an emphasis on critical thinking to an emphasis on clinical reasoning and multiple ways of thinking that include critical thinking" (2010, p. 84).
- "Shift from an emphasis on socialization and role taking to an emphasis on formation" (2010, p. 86).

This list is yet another reminder of the pathologies of either/or, mechanistic, and siloed thinking that has led to the current situation in healthcare education. In the view of Benner and colleagues, "to become a good nurse, one must develop not only technical expertise but also the ability to form relationships and engage in practical ethical and clinical reasoning" (2010, p. 86). These findings point to the need for more relational ways of being and learning. More and more, the work of nurses and all healthcare providers is relational in nature, so the value of creating a learning environment that allows students to learn and practice in relational ways seems self-evident. However, to accomplish this means that we must (in many instances) reinvent our relationships in health professions education and health care. That encompasses relationships with students, academic peers, clinical colleagues, leaders, patients, communities, and regulators.

▶ Revisiting the Organization as Conversation

Organization as conversation is a useful way to reframe our thinking about what happens in our day-to-day interactions in the places where we work and learn. This perspective is theoretically grounded in complexity science (complex responsive processes, to be specific) and social constructionism. From this relational complexity perspective, reimagining our constellation of relationships starts with new language. New language is a powerful tool for creating the potential for novelty and change. If we want to transform healthcare education into something beyond the mechanistic, siloed, either/or, and boundaried reality, a change of language may be useful in generating new ways of being.

Language is a conduit for shared meaning making. That is, the ways that people talk together and the language they use can dramatically shape how they perceive their circumstances. Perception then comes to bear on the actions we choose and the attitudes we adopt in response to our perceived circumstances. Language is the foundation of the stories (narratives) we tell and the metaphors we use to make sense of the world around us; reciprocally, our experience in the world is shaped by the stories and metaphors we choose. Take, for example, the language used earlier to describe the existing dynamic between education and health care: the education–practice *gap*. As we perpetuate this narrative of disconnection and division, the gap becomes more real as we continue to behave accordingly. What would happen if we spoke about the education–practice *connection*? Imagine if we began to act within that connection rather than widening the gap? Another example of how language serves to reinforce our experiences of the world is the analogy of the discipline, unit, or specialty as a silo.

Palmer suggested that we must endeavor to "debunk the myth that institutions are external to and constrain us, as if they possessed powers that render us helpless—an assumption that is largely unconscious and wholly untrue" (2007, p. 3). This raises another facet of the power of language. Narratives and myths can serve to either enable or constrain our actions. Have you ever heard a peer or colleague say, "I should have done X, but the system would not let me," or perhaps, "I was only following policy." In other words, we may use policies, processes, or other organizational constraints to abdicate our personal responsibility for unprofessional behavior. Rather than continuing to tell victim stories about how we have been done wrong by the system, we can choose to view ourselves as the organization (education or practice or both) that we are a part of. Said differently, the system is not some faceless overlord or mythical force that keeps us under a spell. Instead, from a complex relational perspective, the organization is made up of people (you and me) working together toward a common purpose or goal. In this sense, we are the system; the system is us. This vantage point places the power to change the system in our hands. The language we use, the relationships we foster, and the day-to-day choices we make can act as vectors that help us move toward the preferred future of health professions education.

LEARNING ACTIVITY

1. Individually reflect on the idea of analogies and metaphors as a way to describe our experiences. What metaphors or analogies have you heard, or used yourself, to describe the following?
   - Clinical practice (unit culture, interprofessional practice, hospital administrators, etc.)
   - Educational experiences (e.g., teaching, learning, assessment, labs)
   Take a few minutes to write down the analogies and metaphors that came to mind.
2. Share your analogies and metaphors with a peer or in a small group. Were your metaphors similar? Can you discern an overall theme across them?
3. Take some time to discuss what you think this collection of analogies and metaphors tells us about health care and education.
4. With a peer or in a small group, share your personal visions of what you want the future of health care and healthcare education to be like.
5. Try to generate metaphors or analogies that would capture what that preferred future would look and feel like. You may want to share and compare your future-focused analogies and metaphors in a large group discussion.

In the sections that follow, I will discuss various facets of healthcare education in hopes of discerning a way forward. The relational complexity perspective described in the previous section brings a new layer of meaning to the Buddhist saying shared at the beginning of this chapter: ". . . If you want to know your future, look into your present actions." We have a choice in each and every moment. We can choose to perpetuate the past, in which case the future will yield more of the same, or we can choose different ideas, relationships, theories, and narratives that will bring about something new. The concepts, theories, practices, and research highlighted in the rest of this chapter are meant to provide incitement for readers to engage further with new or different ideas and perspectives. I urge you to talk about, try, question, tinker with, and add to them from whatever your particular vantage point in health care happens to be (student, teacher, practitioner, leader, or patient).

▶ The Nature and Aims of Healthcare Education Revisited

Given the contextual aspects of the current state of health professions education outlined earlier, it seems reasonable to start by reexamining the goals of healthcare education. Slattery suggested that "the demoralization of educators, disenfranchisement of students, and the dissatisfaction of stakeholders [in healthcare education and practice] are all indications that something is terribly wrong" (2013, p. 285). It is clear that we cannot keep doing what we have always done. Returning to the idea that we seem to be always trying to do more and more, and the question of how we decide what to let go of, let us first explore the function of content in health professions education.

The premise of teaching in the past has been driven by covering content. Like many other practices of the previous century, the assumption that teachers cover content is ingrained and indeed part of the professional identity of many educators (Weimer, 2013). Covering the content is another metaphor that shapes our perceptions. "Thinking that content is there to be 'covered' does not cause us to use the content in ways that promote learning or develop important learning skills" (Weimer, 2013, p. 117). Tied in with covering content are long-held assumptions about content, such as that more is better or that course quality is determined by how content rich it is. We have ample educational research from the past 30 years which states that what is transmitted to students through covering (lecturing) is not retained beyond a few days or weeks (Finkel, 2000). Instructors are often reticent to give up favorite topics or content. The irony is that in merely covering the content, we have already been giving them up (Weimer, 2013).

As an alternate metaphor, Weimer asked, "What if our introductions to our fields were characterized by the features of a good introduction of one person to another? A good introduction offers a few details about the new person that makes her sound interesting—someone you'd like to meet and possibly get to know" (2013, pp. 117–118). This analogy is doubly appealing because it frames content relationally. We want our students to develop relationships with the content of our beloved disciplines. Although we as educators may be responsible for the initial introduction to the discipline, we hope that students develop their own friendships and connections with the content of health care.

What is the function of content, then, if not to be covered? First, content is (and always has been) essential to develop a knowledge base around a specific topic or discipline. Surgeons could not practice surgery without the requisite knowledge base. However, we must assist our students to engage in the content in a deeper way to develop an enduring knowledge base. Concept-based, problem-based, and context-based learning strategies are a few examples of deeper ways to engage students in the content. Second, content acts as a medium for learning how to learn and also for helping students understand the work of a discipline. Content is necessary for students to engage in cognitive apprenticeship (learning to think like a pharmacist, doctor, or social worker). Learning to learn is especially noteworthy and tied to another important aspect of the nature of content in healthcare education. That is the exponential growth and short life span of content (knowledge) in the 21st century.

▶ Teaching in the Knowledge Era: Learning in a Wired World

Since the 1990s we have been living in the knowledge era. All health disciplines have experienced an unprecedented explosion in the generation and availability of research and information in general. More and more practitioners see themselves as knowledge workers rather than task-driven care providers. The exponential growth of knowledge and the ubiquitous access to it has been enabled by amazing advancements in technology. Access to an ocean of information is literally at our fingertips. Clinical apps for our phones (such as drug guides; clinical practice guidelines; and, yes, even Google), vast research databases, and access to experts and networks of peers are as close as our pocket. The knowledge era has presented us with a new dynamic between information and learning, and we must overcome long-held assumptions about how we think about information, knowledge, and learning.

The life span of relevant knowledge has greatly diminished. For instance, the amount of new technical information produced doubles roughly every 2 years. This means that, for students who are in a 4-year degree program, half of what they learn in their first year of study may be outdated by their third year (Tucker, 2008). The shortening half-life of information further suggests that focusing on covering content is less useful than using content to learn how to learn. This also means that healthcare education programs must prepare students to engage in lifelong learning and ongoing professional development to remain competent.

Knowledge is no longer a commodity, but it has become an application to be accessed and used as needed and purged when no longer useful (Brown, 2005). Brown used the term *navigationism* as a way to frame how we might educate students to thrive in the knowledge economy. He described information navigation as a new type of literacy for the 21st century: "I believe that the real literacy of tomorrow will have more to do with being able to be your own private, personal reference librarian, one that knows how to navigate through the incredible, confusing complex information spaces and feel comfortable and located in doing that" (Brown, 2006, p. 112).

Brown suggested that the learning paradigm is shifting beyond constructivism (knowledge production) to knowledge navigation. **TABLE 16-2** compares the landscape of learning as seen from different paradigms.

Siemens (2005) suggested an additional learning theory that aligns with and builds upon navigationism. Siemens integrated principles from chaos, network, complexity, and self-organizing theories and applied these to learning in the knowledge era.

From this integrated complexity perspective, Siemens described learning as actionable knowledge that is focused on connecting specialized information sets, "and the connections that enable us to learn more are more important than our current state of knowing" (Siemens, 2005, p. 5). The principles of connectivism (Siemens, 2005; Brown, 2006) are described as follows:

- Learning is a process of connecting specialized nodes or sources of information.
- The capacity to know more is more critical than what is currently known.
- Nurturing and maintaining connections is needed to facilitate continual learning.
- The ability to see connections among fields, ideas, and concepts is a core skill.
- Currency (accurate, up-to-date knowledge) is the intent of all connectivist learning activities.
- Decision making is a learning process. Choosing what to learn and the meaning of incoming information is seen through the lens of a shifting reality. Although there is a right answer today, it may be wrong tomorrow because of changes in the information climate that affects decision making.

It is also important to highlight our shifting understanding of valid sources of knowledge (evidence) in light of emerging learning paradigms, technology, and the knowledge era. In the past, it was easier to discern reputable sources of knowledge, mostly because there were fewer of them. Knowledge production was much slower, and the means for knowledge production and dissemination were available only to experts (e.g., elite academics and researchers). There was a time in the not-so-distant past that information presented in a textbook could be assumed to be expert and up to date. Recall that in the first half of the 20th century, knowledge doubled every 30

TABLE 16-2 Characteristics of Knowledge and Learning From Three Perspectives

Paradigms	Past (Knowledge Adoption)	Present (Knowledge Production)	Future (Knowledge Navigation)
Learning	Memorizing, studying. Aim is a change in behavior of the learner.	Inquiry and research, active learning. Aim is the construction of new personal knowledge and meaning.	Exploring, connecting, evaluating, manipulating, integrating, and navigating knowledge.
Nature of knowledge	Knowledge creation was for elite experts. Knowledge was already there and ready to be learned.	Previous (existing) knowledge is built upon. Active learning enables the creation of new meaning or knowledge.	Sources of knowledge are everywhere. The focus is on navigating the vast amounts of information and making sense of it.
Learner	Focused on gaining knowledge.	Constructs new meaning by actively engaging with knowledge.	Solves contextual real-life problems via active engagement, networking, communication, and collaboration.
Teacher	Sage on stage. Subject expert; primary source of knowledge.	Guide on side. Not the only source of knowledge; guides both what and how to learn.	Coach in touch. Coaches and mentors in skills of sense making, information facilitation, knowledge configuration.

Modified from Brown, T. H. (2006). Beyond constructivism: Navigationism in the knowledge era. *On the Horizon, 14*(3), 108–120.

years. The concern of textbooks being obsolete almost as soon as they are printed would have seemed ludicrous to publishers in the 1920s.

However, today that is a reality. In response to the exponential growth of knowledge, many of our more traditional sources of knowledge and evidence have adapted by moving to online publishing processes that are faster and more nimble. Many peer-reviewed professional journals have leveraged technology to accelerate the peer review process and shorten the time between submission of a paper and its publication. Most journals today have electronic versions and use online and early release features to expedite the dissemination of new research.

The traditional sources of evidence and knowledge (books and journals) are now one of many sources. The rise of Web 2.0 technologies has democratized the access to knowledge production. Almost everyone with an Internet connection has the ability to self-publish a book, create a website or blog, participate in social media conversations, and generally contribute to the ongoing production of knowledge. This means that the critical appraisal of the electronic sources of evidence (and knowledge sources in general) becomes an important skill, not just for healthcare professionals but for everyone.

The term *digital literacy* has been used to describe and enumerate the skills, attitudes, and knowledge needed to be an active and informed participant in the digital world. Digital literacy is "the ability to use information and communication technologies to find, evaluate, create, and communicate information, requiring both cognitive and technical skills" (Visser, 2012, para. 2). Specific to healthcare education and practice, the ability to "use diverse technologies appropriately and effectively to retrieve information, interpret results, and judge the quality of that information" (Visser, 2012, para. 4) is critically important in the current learning paradigm and also the future paradigm (navigationism and connectivism). Coaching and mentoring students to develop their digital literacy is a role that health professions instructors must be ready to take on. This means that instructors must develop and practice digital literacy.

DISCUSSION

Digital literacy is described as a set of skills that are both *technical* and *cognitive*. This includes the actual mechanics of using technology to access information and thinking about it in sophisticated ways (e.g., clinical reasoning and critical, creative, and ethical thinking).

- What barriers have you experienced to developing and using digital literacy skills?
- Were they mostly technical or cognitive?
- How did you overcome them?
- How might you partner with others in your organization to create an environment that supports the ongoing development of digital literacy?

Another aspect of digital literacy that is of particular importance in health care is e-health literacy, that is, the ability to find, understand, and appraise health information from electronic sources and apply the knowledge gained to address health problems (Norman & Skinner, 2006). Not only do future healthcare providers need to be e-health literate, but they must also have the skills to coach and mentor others (patients, peers, communities) in this endeavor. Active learning opportunities that help students to develop their e-health literacy and digital literacy skills are critical and should be integrated into health professions education.

In this chapter we have discussed the need to rethink the function of content in healthcare education programs. Keeping in mind the aspects of navigationism and e-health literacy, consider the following:

1. How might you develop a learning activity that would use content as a vehicle to help students solve a real-world problem? For example, have a student collaborate with a newly diagnosed type I diabetic patient who is experiencing low blood glucose levels in the morning (content). The patient and her family do not understand why this is happening, and they have asked about a suggestion they read in an online patient chat room for new diabetics (real-world problem).

2. Have the student and patient work together to find, understand, and appraise health information from electronic sources (digital literacy) and apply the knowledge gained to address health problems (e-health literacy).

▶ Teaching into the Future: Relationship-Centered Care and Interprofessional Practice

It has been suggested that interprofessional practice and relationship-centered care may hold the potential to be transformational forces in health care. For this potential to be tested and hopefully realized, future healthcare providers need to be educated in ways that are resonant with these practices. This section presents emerging learning theories, and teaching and learning practices that create the context for students and educators to develop relational competence.

Relational Education

Relationship-centered health care has been described by Tresolini and the Pew-Fetzer Task Force (1994) in terms of three pivotal relationships in health care: the patient–provider relationship, the provider–provider relationship, and the provider–community relationship. Each type of relationship requires the provider to apply specific knowledge, skills, and attitudes for positive relationships to be formed and maintained. Gergen (2009) likewise asserted that there are relationships (or circles) that enable relational education:

Circle 1: Teacher and student

Circle 2: Relationships among students

Circle 3: Classrooms and community

Circle 4: Classrooms and the world

Indeed, as Gergen (2009) added, there are actually unceasing circles or relationships that may be envisioned in relational education (e.g., teacher to teacher, administrator to teacher, regulators to administrators, administrators to students, etc.).

The point of describing and highlighting certain relationships is simply to illustrate the idea that when we focus on relationships (as opposed to individuals) as the organizing feature of health care or healthcare education, we can envision new possibilities and potential.

Social construction theory posits that knowledge and reason can be viewed as relational achievements rather than entities held in the minds of individuals. From this standpoint, the "primary aim of education is to enhance the potentials for participating in relational processes—from the local to the global" (Gergen, 2009, p. 243). Most of our educational systems are built upon the individualist, siloed mentality and traditional hierarchies that place knowledge in the minds of individuals. From this view, learning is something that can be managed, measured, and precisely orchestrated using tools such as a curriculum, course syllabus, and meticulous lesson plans. In this traditional (behaviorist) view of learning we draw a clear distinction between the "knowing teacher and the ignorant pupil . . . and we presume that a knowing mind is good preparation for a successful future" (Gergen, 2009, p. 241). From a complex relational point of view, learning is a relational process of communicative interaction. It is participative action rather than mere reproduction of memorized steps (mimicry). Knowledge arises in the participative communicative interactions that take place among people in moment-to-moment interactions (Stacey, 2001).

A helpful analogy for this socially constructed and complex relational view of learning is education as a rhizome (Cormier, 2008). Cormier suggested that in collaborative learning, "knowledge becomes negotiation" (2008, p. 1) in that the learning process itself is ongoing negotiation. A rhizome is a plant that has no center, no boundaries; rather, it is constrained only by the limits of its environment (habitat). Rhizomes are comprised of a number of semi-independent nodes that are each capable of growing and spreading on their own (Cormier, 2008). When this analogy is applied to education, knowledge can only be negotiated. The contextual and collaborative learning experience is a social and personal process of knowledge creation "with mutable goals and constantly negotiated premises" (2008, p. 1).

In the rhizomatic model of learning, the curriculum is not driven by predefined inputs from experts; it is constructed and negotiated in real time by the contributions of those engaged in the learning process. This community acts as the curriculum, spontaneously shaping, constructing, and reconstructing itself and the subject of its learning in the same way that the rhizome responds to changing environmental conditions (Cormier, 2008).

For all health professions to engage in the healthcare transformation that is called for, educators will need to take up new ways of teaching and participating in educational processes. Tresolini and the Pew-Fetzer Task Force (1994) highlighted that the educational environments we construct serve to reinforce the underlying assumptions about both learning and care. As such, relationship-centered care is reflected in learner-centered education. "The caring relationship between practitioner and patient is modeled by the nurturing environment that students, faculty, and practitioners themselves create through the quality of their relationships" (1994, p. 42). Similarly, learning goals that are mutually established by a community of teachers and learners can be used to teach the parallel process of collaborative goal setting in provider–patient relationships (Tresolini & Pew-Fetzer Task Force, 1994).

From a collaborative practice and interprofessional perspective, the same logic applies. Collaborative practice is reflected in collaborative learning experiences.

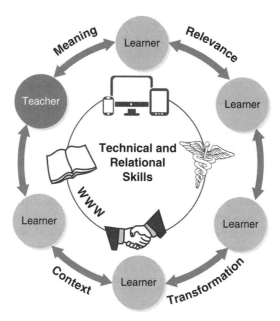

FIGURE 16-4 Learning in the knowledge era.

A wide array of collaborative learning processes exist (communities of practice, learning collectives, self-organized learning environments, etc.). Any type of collaborative learning configuration leverages the power of co-constructed knowledge and social meaning making. Collective learning also provides an opportunity to develop relational competence (for example, emotional intelligence, self-regulation, deep listening, improvisation, and authentic presence).

FIGURE 16-4 visually represents how the various ideas and perspectives on teaching and learning discussed in this chapter might come together. A brief description of the elements in the figure is as follows:

- Learning is not solely content driven, but content provides a context for learning both technical skills and relational skills. It is about learning to learn while learning how to be (in the profession).
- There are multiple sources of evidence and information (some are technology enabled, others are relational), for example, electronic databases, clinical applications, and texts that could be technology enabled. Peers, practitioners, patients, and teachers are also sources of knowledge (relational).
- Digital learning resources and technology are integrated into learning in a way that helps students understand how practitioners can (and do) use technology to solve real-world problems. Digital literacy and e-health literacy are integral to learning in the knowledge era.
- Student and peer knowledge contribute to learning. Peers learn from each other and cocreate new meaning together. The teacher's knowledge is not privileged as the only source. The teacher is a co-learner and participates in the meaning-making process.

- Student-centered learning environments are context rich. Learning is situated in ways that make it relevant to the learner and to his or her future practice.
- Learning is collaborative and inherently relational. Meaning and knowledge are socially constructed. Participation in learning creates new patterns of meaning and patterns of relating that have the potential to transform both the individual and the system (we are the system).

Safe Learning Environments Celebrate Failure

Failure is an essential element of learning. However, students, educators, and practitioners typically view failure as negative and something to be avoided. We know that deep (enduring) learning occurs when we are active and engaged in doing learning. In passive education, there is no skin in the game, so to speak. There is less risk of failure, and there is also less learning. When we are engaged in trying, tinkering, and testing new ideas, of course, there will be mistakes. Those mistakes are the source of learning! Through ongoing engaged involvement in the learning process, we begin to develop mastery. Chapter 8 focuses on failure as an essential component for innovation.

Mastery develops more quickly in an environment where active engagement is high, mistakes are recognized as part of the process of learning, and students receive just-in-time formative feedback about their learning. This feedback can come from multiple sources (especially in the knowledge era). For instance, a student's own self-reflection and self-awareness are powerful sources of feedback. Peer feedback is also critical and is readily available, especially in collaborative learning environments. Patients, preceptors, mentors, and teachers are also sources of feedback. One of the largest barriers to students tapping into the many sources of feedback and thus improving their learning is a mental construct that is often perpetuated from outdated learning paradigms. That is, the teacher (expert) is the only valid source of feedback. As previously noted, in the knowledge era this is simply not the case. However, many of us have been habituated to pay attention to the teacher (expert) and the hierarchical mind-set that students are subservient to the all-knowing expert. This mind-set causes us to tune out other useful and important sources of feedback that are literally everywhere.

Grades and assessment practices have also contributed to the prevalent fear of mistakes. In most grading structures, mistakes are punished with lower grades. In traditional educational models, the proxy measure for learning has been grades (based most often on summative, formal evaluations, such as exams). Summative measures alone do not provide feedback about performance until after the fact. Exams, high-stakes testing, and other forms of summative evaluation provide no opportunity to learn from mistakes or develop mastery. Summative evaluation provides only a snapshot of the current state of performance, knowledge, and mastery. These assessments are useful and necessary in certain instances (such as determining if a medical or nursing student has accumulated the requisite knowledge and skills to enter the profession). However, an overreliance and use of summative evaluation has contributed to a prevailing sense of fear and trepidation about both assessment processes and mistakes. This is manifested in a variety of different ways that all function to shut down learning and diminish performance. A classic example is test anxiety.

Emerging theories of cognition are revealing that the process of learning is not a logical and progressive sequence. Rather, learning consists of processes that are nonlinear, intuitive, and emotional. The brain does not separate emotion from cognition structurally or perceptually (Caine & Caine, 1991). In essence, the emotion of fear that is often related to evaluation processes and mistakes impedes our ability to access our higher-order thinking (reasoning, critical thinking, problem solving). The prevailing belief in education for many years has been that we were capable of getting over our emotions and bracketing them out of the learning equation. Brain and learning research is now showing that emotions are integrally important in learning. Just as negative emotions can have a detrimental impact on our learning, positive emotions associated with learning experiences can have a powerful positive influence.

Educators can integrate this new evidence about emotion and learning to create more conducive learning environments. Creating a sense of emotional safety in a learning environment can enhance a student's ability to access higher-order thinking and more fully engage in the act of learning. From a relational point of view, safe and welcoming environments also support the development of relationships and improve collaboration. Safe learning environments can replace the fear of making mistakes with curiosity and excitement about failures. As such, students remain engaged in the learning process and open to feedback that will move them toward mastery.

I have not failed. I've just found 10,000 ways that won't work.

—**Thomas Edison**

▶ Strengthening the Practice–Education Connection

Leaders who work with complex systems in today's world must develop a set of competencies to effect the changes they aspire to make. These competencies are: understanding the evidence–innovation–leadership dynamic, self-leadership, innovation capacity, communication and connection, and building momentum for change.

The development of such competencies is essential for leaders to strengthen the practice–education connection. Existing leaders in health care may undertake additional formal education (e.g., a master's or doctoral program) to develop these competencies. In doing so, they become enmeshed again in the education setting and can cross-pollinate their clinical perspectives and realities that will inform the development and refinement of formalized education programs that are more attuned to practice needs and realities. Leaders in education systems need to develop these competencies as well. Education leaders who develop these competencies will be more attuned to the changing needs of the healthcare system and can also build their capacity to begin to change the stagnant ivory tower thinking that is still prevalent in many institutions of higher education. Ideally, with a concerted focus on these competencies, we will create a relationship that no longer resembles two individual silos but a relational structure that represents the practice education dynamic (**FIGURE 16-5**). In essence, there is integration, not separation. From a complex relational perspective, the individual and the social (larger organization) are one and the same. Similarly, education and practice are aspects of the same phenomenon: health care.

It is not just leaders who need to support and live in the education–practice dynamic. Each of us, from whatever our vantage point in health care, needs to take

FIGURE 16-5 The education–practice dynamic in health care.
© Chuhail/iStockphoto

up more integrative and connected ways of talking and relating. A critical opportunity to strengthen the practice–education dynamic can be found in changing how we relate to the next generation of healthcare educators. Currently, there is reason for much concern; there is a faculty shortage across many health disciplines, and academic careers seem less appealing in the eyes of potential new educators. How can we change this? Focusing on strengthening the practice–education dynamic may be the place to start. In short, if we view our organizations from this dynamic rather than a siloed perspective, it is a whole new game. Continuing to socialize incoming faculty into an outdated and overmatched academic culture serves only to put healthcare programs further behind. Even the most thorough, well-crafted new faculty orientation program and mentorship by the most seasoned faculty become counterproductive if they are based on our traditional, mechanistic ways of being. In this new era healthcare education, we are all novices in some way. Our greatest hope for transformation within health care may lie with those we now call novices. New instructors who have current knowledge of clinical realities and existing relationships with practitioners could offer a wealth of insight and potential for the integration of healthcare practice and education (**TABLE 16-3**). We have much to learn from each other (students, peers, leaders, patients, and colleagues). We need only to take the time to connect, listen, and talk with each other. Transformation may only be a conversation away.

New language can open up the experiential space and create opportunities for disrupting our day-to-day habitual ways of being in healthcare education. Bolman and Deal provided a poignant example of the power of disrupting our habitual ways of being: "A mess can be defined as both a troublesome situation and a group of people who eat together" (2003, p. 40). It is my greatest hope that through ongoing disruptive conversations and cultivation of relational practices, healthcare education will look and feel more like the latter.

TABLE 16-3 Summary of the Current Shifts in Healthcare Education

From	Toward
Teacher centered	Learner centered
Knowledge as a commodity	Knowledge as an application
Lone learning	Collaborative learning, team-based learning
Decontextualized facts	Context-based application, solving real-life problems
Technical skills	Technical and relational skills
Silos	Rhizomes
Practice–education gap	Practice–education dynamic
Covering content	Learning to learn, navigationism, connectivism, concept-based learning

References

Aiken, L. H., Clarke, S. P., Sloane, D. M., Sochalski J. A., Busse, R., Clarke, H. . . . Shamian, J. (2001). Nurses' reports on hospital care in five countries. *Health Affairs, 20*(3), 43–53. https://doi.org/10.1377/hlthaff.20.3.43

American Association of Colleges of Nursing. (2017, April). *Nursing faculty shortage fact sheet.* Washington, DC: Author. Retrieved from https://www.aacnnursing.org/News-Information/Fact-Sheets/Nursing-Faculty-Shortage

Association of Academic Health Centers. (2008). *Out of order, out of time: The state of the nation's health workforce.* Washington, DC: Author.

Association of Academic Health Centers. (2013). *A call to action. Out of order, out of time: The state of the nation's health workforce 2013.* Washington, DC: Author.

Bandura, A. (1977). Self-efficacy: Toward a unifying theory of behavioral change. *Psychological Review, 84*(2), 191–215. https://doi.org/10.1037/0033-295X.84.2.191

Benner, P. E. (1984). *From novice to expert: Excellence and power in clinical nursing practice.* Menlo Park, CA: Addison-Wesley.

Benner, P., Sutphen, M., Leonard, V., & Day, L. (2010). *Educating nurses: A call for radical transformation.* Stanford, CA: Jossey-Bass.

Berrett, D. (2013, November 22). Teaching clearly can be a deceptively simple way to improve learning. *The Chronicle of Higher Education,* 1–4. Retrieved from http://chronicle.com/article/Teaching-Clearly-a/143209

Bevis, E. O., & Watson, J. (1989). *Toward a caring curriculum: A new pedagogy for nursing.* New York, NY: National League for Nursing.

Bolman, L. G., & Deal, T. E. (2003). *Reframing organizations: Artistry, choice and leadership.* San Francisco, CA: Jossey-Bass.

Brown, T. H. (2005). Beyond constructivism: Exploring future learning paradigms. *Education Today, 2,* 1–11.

Brown, T. H. (2006). Beyond constructivism: Navigationism in the knowledge era. *On the Horizon, 14*(3), 108–120.

Caine, R. N., & Caine, G. (1991). *Making connections: Teaching and the human brain*. Alexandria, VA: ASCD Press.

Canadian Association of Schools of Nursing. (2018, November). *Registered nurses education in Canada statistics 2016–2017*. Ottawa, ON: Author. Retrieved from: https://www.casn.ca/2018/12/registered-nurses-education-in-canada-statistics-2016-2017/

Cooperrider, D. L., & Whitney, D. K. (1999). *Appreciative inquiry: A positive revolution in change*. Oakland, CA: Berrett-Koehler.

Cormier, D. (2008). Rhizomatic education: Community as curriculum. *Innovate, 4*(5). Retrieved from http://nsuworks.nova.edu/cgi/viewcontent.cgi?article=1045&context=innovate

Cranford, J. S. (2013). Bridging the gap: Clinical practice nursing and the effect of role strain on successful role transition and intent to stay in academia. *International Journal of Nursing Education Scholarship, 10*(1). https://doi.org/10.1515/ijnes-2012-0018

Davidson, S. (2011). *The experiences of novice nursing faculty: A complexity perspective* (Order No. 3504674). Available from ProQuest Dissertations & Theses Global. (992876092). Retrieved from http://ezproxy.lib.ucalgary.ca/login?url=https://search-proquest-com.ezproxy.lib.ucalgary.ca/docview/992876092?accountid=9838

Esper, P. S. (1995). Facing transition—nurse clinician to nurse educator. *Journal of Nursing Education, 34*(2), 89–91. https://doi.org/10.3928/0148-4834-19950201-12

Finkel, D. L. (2000). *Teach with your mouth shut*. Portsmouth, NH: Boyton/Cook.

Gergen, K. J. (2009). *Relational being: Beyond self and community*. New York, NY: Oxford Press.

Hessler, K., & Ritchie, H. (2006). Recruitment and retention of novice faculty. *Journal of Nursing Education, 45*(5), 150–154.

Institute of Medicine. (2001). *Crossing the quality chasm: A new health system for the 21st century*. Washington, DC: National Academies Press.

Institute of Medicine. (2011). *The future of nursing: Leading change, advancing health*. Washington, DC: National Academies Press.

Interprofessional Education Collaborative Expert Panel. (2011). *Core competencies for interprofessional collaborative practice: Report of an expert panel*. Washington, DC: Author.

Melnyk, B., & Fineout-Overholt, E. (2005). *Evidence-based practice in nursing and healthcare*. Philadelphia, PA: Lippincott, Williams & Wilkins.

Midwest Pharmacy Workforce Research Consortium. (2015, April 8). *Final report of the 2014 national sample survey of the pharmacist workforce to determine contemporary demographic and practice characteristics and quality of work-life*. Minneapolis, MN: Author. Retrieved from http://www.aacp.org/resources/research/pharmacyworkforcecenter/Documents/FinalReportOfTheNationalPharmacistWorkforceStudy2014.pdf

Norman, C. D., & Skinner, H. A. (2006). E-health literacy: Essential skills for consumer health in a networked world. *Journal of Medical Internet Research, 8*(2), e9.

Nugent, K. E., Bradshaw, M. J., & Kito, N. (1999). Teacher self-efficacy in new nurse educators. *Journal of Professional Nursing, 15*(4), 229–237. https://doi.org/10.1016/S8755-7223(99)80009-X

Oliver, M. (n.d.). Malcolm Olivers' water world [Blog post]. Retrieved from: https://malcolmoliver.wordpress.com/titanic-vs-oasis-of-the-seas/

Palmer, P. J. (1998). *The courage to teach*. San Francisco, CA: Jossey-Bass.

Palmer, P. J. (2007, November/December). A new professional: The aims of education revisited. *Change: The Magazine of Higher Learning*. Retrieved from http://www.changemag.org/archives/back%20issues/november-december%202007/full-new-professional.html

Ramage, C. (2004). Negotiating multiple roles: Link teachers in clinical nursing practice. *Journal of Advanced Nursing, 45*(3), 287–296. https://doi.org/10.1046/j.1365-2648.2003.02889.x

Scharmer, C. O. (2007). *Theory U: Leading from the future as it emerges*. Cambridge, MA: Society for Organizational Learning.

Schoening, A. (2009). The journey from bedside to classroom: Making the transition from nurse to nurse educator. *Educational Administration: Theses, Dissertations, and Student Research*. Paper 7. Retrieved from http://digitalcommons.unl.edu/cehsedaddiss/7

Schoening, A. M. (2013). From bedside to classroom: The nurse educator transition model. *Nursing Education Perspectives, 34*(3), 167–172. https://doi.org/10.5480/1536-5026-34.3.167

Scott, G. (2014). Outlook 2015. *The Futurist, 48*(6). Retrieved from http://www.wfs.org/futurist /2014-issues-futurist/november-december-2014-vol-48-no-6/outlook-2015

Siemens, G. (2005). Connectivism: A learning theory of the digital age. *International Journal of Instructional Technology and Distance Learning, 2*(1). Retrieved from http://www.itdl.org /Journal/Jan_05/article01.htm

Slattery, P. (2013). *Curriculum development in the postmodern era: Teaching and learning in the age of accountability.* New York, NY: Routledge.

Stacey, R. D. (2001). *Complex responsive processes in organizations: Learning and knowledge creation.* London, UK: Routledge.

Tresolini, C. P., & Pew-Fetzer Task Force. (1994). *Health professions education and relationship-centered care.* San Francisco, CA: Pew Health Professions Commission. Retrieved from http:// www.rccswmi.org/ uploads/PewFetzerRCCreport.pdf

Tucker, P. (2008, December). Forecast #6: Professional knowledge will become obsolete almost as quickly as it's acquired. *The Futurist.* Retrieved from http://blogs.britannica.com/2008/12 /forecast-6-professional-knowledge-increasingly-obsolete

Unruh, L., Zhang, N., & Chisolm, L. (2016). Job and professional leaving among newly licensed RNs: A structural equation model. *Western Journal of Nursing Research, 38*(1), 5–26. https://doi .org/10.1177/0193945914559290

Valiga, T. M. (2002, April 11). *The nursing faculty shortage: National League for Nursing perspective.* Retrieved from http://www.nln.org/research/facultyshortage.html

Visser, M. (2012). Digital literacy definition. Retrieved from http://connect.ala.org/node/181197

Weimer, M. (2013). *Learner-centered teaching: Five key changes to practice* (2nd ed.). San Francisco, CA: Jossey Bass.

Wenger, E. (2006). *Communities of practice: A brief introduction.* Retrieved from https://www.ohr .wisc.edu/cop/articles/communities_practice_intro_wenger.pdf

World Health Organization. (2010). *Framework for action on interprofessional education & collaborative practice.* Geneva, Switzerland: Author. Retrieved from http://www.who.int/hrh /resources/framework_action/en/

Index

G

H

Q